A Special Issue of
The Quarterly Journal of Experimental Psychology
Section A
Human Experimental Psychology

Hearing and Speech

Edited by

Quentin Summerfield

MRC Institute of Hearing Research
University of Nottingham

LAWRENCE ERLBAUM ASSOCIATES, PUBLISHERS
Hove and London (UK) Hillsdale (USA)

Lawrence Erlbaum Associates Ltd., Publishers
27 Palmeira Mansions
Church Road
Hove
East Sussex, BN3 2FA
U.K.

British Library Cataloguing in Publication Data

Summerfield, Quentin
Hearing and speech.
I. Title II. Quarterly Journal of Experimental Psychology
150.724

ISBN 0-86377-178-5 (Hbk)

Printed and bound by BPCC Wheatons, Exeter

Contents

---

* *This special issue was originally compiled for the third issue of volume 43 of The Quarterly Journal of Experimental Psychology, so page numbering starts on page 321.*

THE QUARTERLY JOURNAL OF EXPERIMENTAL PSYCHOLOGY, 1991, *43A* (3) 321–325

Introduction

Quentin Summerfield

Many scientists carry out research on psychological issues in hearing and speech, yet only rarely is their work reported in the *Quarterly Journal.* This special issue seeks to redress the imbalance. It contains papers contributed by scientists working in Britain, the U.S.A., and the Netherlands. The papers were among those submitted in response to a call for papers. The criteria for inclusion were that papers should report new results and that they should pass the *Journal*'s usual process of anonymous peer review. In addition, they should be written in a style that would make their contents accessible to a readership with a broad spectrum of interests in experimental psychology. Thus, the aim is not to provide a comprehensive overview, nor to highlight a few emerging topics, but instead to illustrate the diversity of current research on hearing and speech and to encourage further submissions in this area. This editorial serves to introduce the nineteen papers.

Several of the papers take as their starting point the idea that the peripheral auditory system can be modelled as a bank of linear, overlapping, bandpass filters each tuned to a different centre frequency. When listeners are required to detect a signal, they would, optimally, attend to the output of the single filter giving the best signal-to-noise ratio. Although this model can explain performance in many situations, recently it has been shown to fail in others. The papers by Brian Moore and his colleagues and by Joe Hall and John Grose illustrate two such conditions. Moore and his colleagues show that it is harder to detect a change in the depth of modulation of a sinusoidal signal if a second sinusoid, remote in frequency from the first, is given a similar modulation. Hall and Grose describe the inverse situation. In the phenomenon of "comodulation masking release", a tone must be detected in a noise-band whose amplitude is modulated; applying the same pattern of modulation to a second band of noise, remote in frequency from the first, makes the signal easier to detect. In both cases, therefore, spectro-temporal patterning remote from the signal frequency affects the ability of listeners to detect the signal, and the assumption that listeners attend to the output of a single filter breaks down.

Sid Bacon and Michael Smith describe experiments on the phenomenon of "overshoot", the increased difficulty of detecting an increment in energy near the start of a sound compared to later points in its duration. They too conclude that across-channel effects are operating, in that the overshoot involves peripheral adaptation extending over a range of frequencies around the signal frequency.

Denis McKeown and Chris Darwin are also concerned with interactions between the outputs of auditory filters, but in the perception of speech sounds. They demonstrate that it is possible to produce systematic changes in the identity of a vowel by altering the phase relationship between adjacent harmonics close to the first formant. The effect occurs despite the fact that the harmonics excite different auditory filters. The authors consider the possibility that the results are due to changes in the amount of lateral suppression between resolved harmonics.

The paper by Peter Assmann addresses a different issue in the perception of vowels. Some authors have argued that closely-spaced formants are treated in speech perception as a single spectral peak at the frequency of their "centre of gravity", even though they would be represented as distinct peaks at an earlier stage of auditory analysis. Assmann argues against this conclusion. He shows that changes to the amplitude of one of two closely spaced formants do not produce the changes in vowel identity expected if the two formants were represented by a single peak.

For several years, David Green has studied the ability of listeners to detect changes in the spectral-amplitude profile of a set of tones. The ability of listeners to detect a change in the level of one tone is helped by the presence of tones at remote frequencies. The paper by David Green and Bruce Berg maps out differences in performance as a function of the position of the critical tone in the complex. The related paper by Niek Versfeld and Adrianus Houtsma studies performance as a function of the number of components, their spacing, and their slope.

Virginia Richards and her colleagues describe experiments on the detection of a tone in a narrow band of noise. Here, only within-channel cues are present and no across-channel reference is available, yet performance is hardly affected by randomly varying the overall level of tone and noise between observation intervals. Listeners cannot, therefore, be detecting the tone purely from the increase in energy in the output of the filter centred on the tone. They are likely in addition to be using cues for detection conveyed by the temporal patterning of the waveform in the output of the filter. Richard's paper describes experiments designed to determine whether energy-based cues can play *any* role in the detection process.

Sensitivity to the temporal patterning of filtered waveforms is an important element of binaural localization, at least at low frequencies. The paper by

Trevor Shackleton and his colleagues describes experiments in which listeners judged the location and "width" of images produced by pairs of brief tones presented one to each ear. One interesting result is the demonstration that tones separated by extreme inter-aural time differences are perceived as separate (suggesting that the process of binaural fusion has broken down) but nonetheless influence each other's perceived location (suggesting an interaction between the input to each ear).

Michael Beauvois and Ray Meddis describe a computational model of the formation of auditory streams. When listeners are presented with a rapidly alternating sequence of high and low tones, they may hear two separate sequences, one of high tones and one of low tones, occurring concurrently. Their model starts with a bank of bandpass filters. It aims to account for the phenomenon of streaming in terms of physiological mechanisms that might plausibly be found in the peripheral auditory system, without recourse to central processes of pattern analysis.

From these papers, the concept of the auditory filter emerges with a central place in hearing research. The bank of auditory filters performs an initial frequency analysis prior to cross-channel analyses responsible for computing the spectra of sounds, for grouping energy from the same source in different frequency regions, and thus for separating signals from other sounds. Listeners with hearing impairments of cochlear origin often have difficulty with these tasks. Over the last decade there has been debate about the extent to which their poorer than normal performance is a consequence of elevated detection thresholds or of supra-threshold distortions such as impaired frequency selectivity; that is, auditory filters with broader than normal bandwidths. The paper by Judy Dubno and Amy Schaefer contributes to this debate. It shows that at the high stimulus levels at which impaired listeners must be tested, frequency selectivity in normal-hearing listeners is poorer than at lower presentation levels, though generally better than that of the impaired listeners. Nonetheless, the authors argue, some previous comparisons where normal and impaired listeners were tested at different levels may have exaggerated the consequences of impaired selectivity in the impaired listeners.

Fan-Gang Zeng and Christopher Turner also report experiments with hearing-impaired listeners. Their aim is to understand the processes by which listeners can discriminate the loudness of sounds over a range of 120dB when the dynamic range of the majority of peripheral auditory nerve fibres is only 30–40dB. They study listeners with unilateral hearing impairments. In their impaired ear, the listeners can detect sounds over a restricted range of frequencies, yet their loudness judgements are unaffected. The authors conclude that the spread of excitation along the cochlear partition is not the primary cue for loudness. As an alternative, they present a model in which use is made of a population of neurons with a range of different thresholds to distinguish loudness over a wide dynamic range.

Michael Dorman and his colleagues describe experiments on use of speech cues by profoundly deaf patients whose inner ears are stimulated directly with electrical signals through a cochlear implant. Their experiments confirm that such patients achieve only an impoverished representation of the speech spectrum in the mid- to high-frequency range. One consequence is that they rely more heavily than normal on gross features such as the overall shape of the spectrum and the abruptness of onsets in judging the place of articulation of stop consonants. In contrast, their use of spectro-temporal cues conveyed at lower frequencies is more nearly normal.

Margaret Walsh and Randy Diehl are concerned with the interpretation of speech cues by listeners with normal hearing. There is disagreement about the relative importance of the duration of the formant transitions and the abruptness of the amplitude rise in cueing the distinction between stop consonants (e.g./b/) and semi-vowels (e.g./w/). Walsh and Diehl show that transition duration is the major cue with rise-time playing a secondary role. They find an analogous pattern when the speech stimuli are replaced by single tones tracing out the path of the first formant and listeners judge the abruptness of the onset. The authors conclude that there may be an auditory basis to listeners' categorization of the speech stimuli.

Ken Grant and his colleagues are concerned to identify signals of low dimensionality that can be extracted from a speech signal and used to supplement the ability to "speechread" (i.e. lipread). They explore the effects of extracting the variations in amplitude in different frequency bands in the speech signal and using them to modulate the amplitude of a single tone that is presented to the subject along with a video of the talker. These signals provide significant benefit to lipreading by conveying aspects of the speech signal that have no correlates in the pattern of visible articulatory movements. The experiments show that benefit is greatest when the tone is centred on the frequency band from which the amplitude envelope was derived.

Louis Braida's paper describes two models of audio-visual integration in the perception of consonants. He asks whether integration occurs before or after the information in each modality is categorized phonetically. He demonstrates that several different sets of data are best explained by a model of pre-categorical integration.

The last three papers address issues in the psychology of speech and language. Arthur Samuel uses his development of the "phonemic restoration" paradigm to study the levels of analysis to which attention can be directed in speech perception. Surprisingly, despite thousands of trials of training, listeners cannot attend at a phonemic level and cannot, therefore, prevent phonemic restoration from occurring. As the author concludes, "people are fundamentally suited to deriving lexical representations". James

Flege outlines some of the problems encountered in establishing the forms of phonetic knowledge acquired by learners of a second language and describes experiments that seek to establish at what stage in second-language learning, if ever, the phonetic categories of the new language are established. Finally, Peter Howell and Keith Young describe experiments in which they seek to identify the prosodic cues that talkers use to signal that they have made an error in speaking. They show that pauses are used to signal the start of a correction and that stress is used to mark the corrected item. A perceptual experiment demonstrates that listeners are more likely to deduce the correct form when these cues are present.

Every paper went through at least one stage of peer review, some through more than one. I am grateful to all those who commented on papers and helped to clarify and strengthen them. Their names will appear in a future issue of the *Quarterly Journal.*

Taken together, the papers illustrate how the multidisciplinary basis of research on hearing and speech extends from auditory physiology and psychoacoustics through speech perception and phonetics to linguistics. I hope that the appearance of this Special Issue will encourage authors to submit further papers on psychological issues in hearing and speech to the *Quarterly Journal* in the future.

THE QUARTERLY JOURNAL OF EXPERIMENTAL PSYCHOLOGY, 1991, *43A* (3) 327–347

Across-channel Masking of Changes in Modulation Depth for Amplitude- and Frequency-modulated Signals

Brian C.J. Moore, Brian R. Glasberg, Tracey Gaunt, and Tim Child

University of Cambridge, Cambridge, U.K.

This study examines a form of masking that can take place when the signal and masker are widely separated in frequency and cannot be explained in terms of the traditional concept of the auditory filter or critical band. We refer to this as across-channel masking. The task of the subject was to detect an increment in modulation depth of a 1000-Hz sinusoidal carrier. The carrier could either be sinusoidally amplitude modulated or sinusoidally frequency modulated at a 10-Hz rate. Modulation increment thresholds of this "target" signal were measured for the target alone, and in the presence of two interfering sounds with carrier frequencies of 230 and 3300 Hz. When the interfering sounds were unmodulated, they had no effect on modulation increment thresholds. When the interfering sounds were either amplitude or frequency modulated, thresholds increased. Amplitude modulation (AM) increment thresholds were affected by both amplitude-modulated and frequency-modulated interference. Similarly, frequency modulation (FM) increment thresholds were affected by both amplitude-modulated and frequency-modulated interference. For both types of signal, the interference was tuned for modulation rate; across-channel masking was greatest when the interfering sounds were modulated at rates close to 10 Hz, and declined for higher or lower rates. However, the tuning was rather broad. When the target and interfering sounds were modulated at the same rate, there was no effect of the relative phase of the modulators. Two possible explanations for the results are discussed. One is based on the idea that carriers that are modulated in a similar way tend to be perceptually "grouped". The other is based on the idea that there are "channels" in the auditory system tuned for AM and FM rate. Neither explanation appears completely satisfactory.

Requests for reprints should be sent to Brian C.J. Moore, Department of Experimental Psychology, University of Cambridge, Downing Street, Cambridge CB2 3EB, U.K.

This work was supported by the Medical Research Council (U.K.). We thank Sid Bacon, Tom Baer, Ervin Hafter, Joe Hall, David Wessel, and Bill Yost for helpful comments on an earlier version of this paper.

It is widely held that the auditory system behaves as though it contains an array of overlapping bandpass filters. The characteristics of these filters have been estimated using a number of different psychophysical methods (Patterson & Moore, 1986), and they are often referred to as auditory filters. A traditional model of auditory masking for narrowband signals assumes that the observer monitors the output of a single auditory filter centred at or close to the signal frequency, and that threshold corresponds to a constant signal-to-masker ratio at the output of that filter (Fletcher, 1940; Patterson & Moore, 1986). According to this model, the outputs of auditory filters tuned well away from the signal frequency should neither enhance nor degrade signal detection.

In the last few years, several authors have described situations where the assumptions of this model clearly fail. In some cases, the outputs of auditory filters tuned away from the signal frequency can be used to *enhance* signal detection, as in profile analysis (for a review see Green, 1988) or comodulation masking release (CMR) (Hall, Haggard, & Fernandes, 1984; for a review see Moore, 1990). In other cases, the outputs of auditory filters tuned away from the signal frequency *degrade* signal detection. This degradation seems to happen mainly when the masker is modulated in some way (Yost & Sheft, 1989; Moore, Glasberg, & Schooneveldt, 1990). This paper is especially concerned with masking produced by the modulation of masker components distant in frequency from the signal frequency.

Yost and Sheft (1989) showed that the threshold for detecting sinusoidal amplitude modulation (AM) of a sinusoidal carrier was increased in the presence of another carrier, amplitude modulated at the same rate, even when the second carrier was remote in frequency from the first. They called this modulation detection interference. They showed that modulation detection interference did not occur if the second carrier was unmodulated. They suggested that this interference might be a consequence of perceptual grouping; the common AM of target and interfering sounds might make them fuse perceptually (McAdams, 1984; Bregman, Levitan, & Liao, 1990), making it difficult to "hear out" the modulation of the target sound. Wilson, Hall, & Grose (1990) have demonstrated a similar phenomenon for the detection of frequency modulation (FM). They showed that the threshold for detecting sinusoidal FM of a given carrier frequency could be elevated in the presence of a second carrier that was also frequency modulated. The effect showed some tuning for carrier frequency, being greater when the carrier frequencies of the target and interfering sounds were close, but it persisted even when the carriers were widely separated in frequency (by more than one octave). The effect also showed tuning for modulation rate, being greatest when the modulation rates of the target and interfering sounds were close.

Moore et al. (1990) carried out a series of experiments measuring the threshold of a brief 700-Hz signal as a function of its temporal position relative to the modulation cycle of a 700-Hz masker 100% amplitude modulated at a 10-Hz rate. When extra components, also 100% amplitude modulated at 10-Hz, were added to the masker, signal detection was often impaired, even when all of the added components were remote in frequency from 700-Hz. The effect was usually greater when the added components were modulated in phase with the 700-Hz component than when they were modulated with a different phase. Moore et al. called this effect across-channel masking, as it did not seem to be explicable in terms of the output of the single auditory filter centred at the signal frequency.

It seems likely that the across-channel masking found by Moore et al. (1990) is related to the modulation detection interference described by Yost and Sheft (1989). For the signal and maskers used by Moore et al., the main cue for signal detection was probably the change in the pattern of envelope modulation produced by adding the signal to the masker. The flanking modulated components appear to interfere with the ability to detect the change in modulation pattern (an effect opposite to CMR). Henceforth, we will use the term across-channel masking as a general descriptor of situations where the presence of components remote from the target frequency impairs the ability to detect changes at the target frequency.

In the present paper we determine how thresholds for detecting an *increase* in modulation depth (sinusoidal AM or FM) of a given carrier frequency are affected by modulation of carriers with frequencies well away from that of the target carrier. The target sound was modulated in both observation intervals of a trial, and the task was to identify the interval in which the modulation depth was greater. The following questions were addressed:

1. When the target and interfering sounds are modulated at the same rate, is the threshold affected by the relative phase of their modulation? Sounds that are modulated in phase often appear to fuse more strongly than sounds that are modulated out of phase or incoherently (McAdams, 1984; Bregman, Abramson, Doehring, & Darwin, 1985; Moore et al., 1990). If across-channel masking depends on perceptual grouping processes, we might expect that it would be strong for carriers modulated in phase, and less strong for carriers modulated out of phase. Yost and Sheft (1989) found little effect of (AM) modulator phase in their experiments, but Wilson et al. (1990) did find an effect of (FM) modulator phase, the threshold for detecting FM decreasing progressively with increasing phase disparity between the modulation of the target and the modulation of the interfering sound.

2. How does the magnitude of across-channel masking vary with changes in the modulation rate of the interfering sounds relative to that of the target? This is relevant to the issue of whether there are "channels" in the auditory system tuned for modulation rate, as has been suggested on the basis of both

neurophysiological evidence (Moller, 1976; Kay, 1982; Rees & Moller, 1983; Schreiner & Urbas, 1986) and psychophysical adaptation experiments (Kay & Mathews, 1972; Tansley & Suffield, 1983; see, however, Wakefield & Viemeister, 1984). Yost, Sheft, and Opie (1989) found that thresholds for detecting AM were elevated most by interfering sounds amplitude modulated at similar rates to the target. Similarly, Wilson et al. (1990) found that thresholds for detecting FM were elevated most by interfering sounds frequency modulated at similar rates to the target. In both studies, however, the tuning was rather broad. We thought that by modulating the target in both observation intervals we might more fully engage the hypothetical channels (see below), thereby increasing the amount of across-channel masking and giving an effect with sharper tuning in the modulation domain.

3. Can frequency-modulated carriers at remote centre frequencies interfere with the detection of changes in AM depth, and vice versa? This is relevant to the issue of whether there are separate channels for AM and FM (Kay & Mathews, 1972; Tansley & Regan, 1979; Gardner & Wilson, 1979). If there are separate channels, we might expect that the detection of changes in AM depth would be affected by amplitude-modulated interfering sounds but not by frequency-modulated interfering sounds. Similarly, FM depth discrimination would be affected by frequency-modulated interfering sounds but not by amplitude-modulated interfering sounds.

PILOT EXPERIMENTS

In order to decide on appropriate experimental conditions, a number of pilot experiments were conducted. Initially, we set up some conditions very similar to those used by Yost and Sheft (1989) and Yost et al. (1989). In a two-alternative forced-choice (2AFC) task, the subjects were required to discriminate an unmodulated 1-kHz sinusoidal carrier from a carrier that was sinusoidally amplitude modulated at a 10-Hz rate. The duration of each stimulus was 1000 msec, with a 300 msec interstimulus interval. The threshold for detecting the AM was measured in the presence of a second carrier, which was either 100% or 50% amplitude modulated at a 10-Hz rate and was centred either at 230 or 3300 Hz. We chose centre frequencies for the interfering sounds that were non-harmonically related to the carrier of the target, and that were sufficiently remote from the target for interactions in the peripheral auditory system to be minimal. Like Yost and his colleagues, we found across-channel masking, but the effect was somewhat smaller than reported by them (possibly because they used 500-msec stimuli and we used 1000-msec stimuli) and therefore required many trials per subject to be clearly demonstrated. As we anticipated that the amount of across-channel masking would decrease if the target and interfering sounds were modulated at different rates (or with different modulator types, AM or FM), we wanted to establish a larger initial effect, to give some "headroom" for measuring decreases.

Our impression when listening to the stimuli was that the target sound fused with the interfering sound during the interval when the target was modulated, but did not fuse (or fused less strongly) when it was unmodulated. This is consistent with the perceptual grouping hypothesis of Yost and Sheft (1989). Hence, the task became one of detecting which interval contained an unmodulated sound. It occurred to us that across-channel masking might increase if the target was modulated in *both* intervals, and the task was to detect an increase in modulation depth. We will refer to this task as modulation increment detection. In this task, the target would be expected to fuse with the interfering sound in both intervals, making the task more difficult. Our pilot results confirmed this expectation. Therefore we decided to use such a task for the main experiments.

Even with the modulation increment detection task, the amount of across-channel masking was still not very large. To try to increase it further, we investigated the effect of using two interfering sounds, one centred at 230 Hz and one at 3300 Hz. We found that this did produce an increase in across-channel masking. Indeed, the across-channel masking produced by two interfering carriers was greater than might have been expected from a simple summation of their individual effects. However, we did not explore this fully. In our main experiments, the interfering sound, when present, always consisted of two carriers, one centred at 230 Hz and one at 3300 Hz.

Finally, we conducted a pilot experiment in which the reference modulation depth of the target and the modulation depth of the interfering sounds were varied. We found that the across-channel masking tended to be greatest when the interfering sounds had a greater modulation depth than the reference modulation depth of the target. A ratio of about two in modulation depth always gave substantial across-channel masking. Hence we decided to use such a ratio in our main experiment.

MAIN EXPERIMENTS

In the main experiments, we measured thresholds for detecting an increase in modulation depth for two types of target signal (AM and FM) in the presence of two types of interfering sound (AM and FM). Each combination of signal type and interference type was measured in a separate experiment, giving four experiments altogether: amplitude-modulated target, amplitude-modulated interference; frequency-modulated target, frequency-modulated interference; amplitude-modulated target, frequency-modulated interference; and frequency-modulated target, amplitude-modulated interference.

Method

Stimuli and Conditions. The expression defining an amplitude-modulated sound is:

$$[1+m\sin(2\pi f_m t+\varphi)]\sin(2\pi f_c t+\theta)$$

where t is time, f_c is the carrier frequency, f_m is the modulator frequency, m is the modulation index, and φ and θ are terms determining the starting phases of the modulator and carrier, respectively; in these experiments, φ and θ had random values. In generating the electrical signal, a DC voltage, corresponding to the "1" in the equation, is added to the modulator before multiplication with the carrier.

The expression defining a frequency-modulated sound is:

$$\sin[2\pi f_c t+\theta+\beta\sin(2\pi f_m t+\varphi)]$$

where t, f_c, and f_m have the same meaning as above, β is the modulation index (equal to the peak deviation in frequency from f_c divided by the modulation rate), and θ and φ are terms representing initial phases, which again had random values in these experiments.

The target signal was always an increase in modulation depth of 1000-Hz carrier sinusoidally modulated at a 10-Hz rate. For AM, the reference modulation index, m, was 0.25, that is, relative to the unmodulated carrier the envelope amplitude varied between 0.75 and 1.25. For FM, the modulation index, β, was 2.0, that is, the frequency varied between 980 and 1020 Hz. These reference modulation depths were chosen as satisfying two constraints: (1) The modulation in the reference condition was clearly audible, having a magnitude several times the threshold for detecting the respective modulation type. (2) It was possible to have a large increase in modulation depth without reaching 100% modulation (in the case of AM) or without components spreading significantly outside the critical bandwidth around the target frequency (in the case of FM).

The interfering sound consisted of two carriers, one centred at 230 Hz and one centred at 3300 Hz. When they were amplitude modulated, each had a modulation index of 0.5, twice the reference modulation index of the (AM) target. When they were frequency modulated, the 230-Hz carrier had a peak deviation of ± 11.2 Hz, and the 3300-Hz carrier had a peak deviation of ± 112 Hz. These modulation depths were chosen so that, as a proportion of the carrier frequencies, they were roughly twice the reference modulation depth of the (FM) target. The relative modulation depth was made slightly greater at the lower carrier frequency to allow for the fact that the detection of FM, expressed as a proportion of carrier frequency, worsens somewhat at low frequencies (Shower & Biddulph, 1931; Moore & Glasberg, 1989). The two carriers comprising the interfering sound were always modulated in phase.

All carriers were presented at a level of 60 dB SPL. An amplitude-modulated carrier has a slightly higher intensity than the corresponding unmodulated carrier. To prevent changes in intensity providing a cue for discrimination of modulation depth, carriers that were amplitude modulated were "intensity compensated" to eliminate changes in overall intensity with changes in modulation depth (Viemeister, 1979); for a carrier modulated with modulation index m, the intensity was decreased by the factor $(1+m^2/2)$.

In each experiment there were two sets of conditions. In the first, the interfering sounds were either absent, unmodulated, or had a fixed modulation rate of 10 Hz (the same as that of the target). The following conditions were included in this first set:

1. Reference condition: no interfering sounds present.
2. The interfering sounds were present but unmodulated.
3. The interfering sounds were modulated in phase with the target.
4. The modulation of the interference was advanced by 90° relative to the modulation of the target.
5. The modulation of the interference was delayed by 90° relative to the modulation of the target.
6. The interference was modulated 180° out of phase with the modulation of the target.

In the second set of conditions, the interference was modulated at a different rate from that of the target, and the phase of the modulators was random. Modulation rates for the interfering sounds were 2, 5, 8, 10.05, 12, 15, 20, 30, and 50 Hz. The rate of 10.05 Hz was chosen so that the relative modulator phase of the target and interference would drift markedly across trials, effectively randomizing the relative modulator phase. This was done to make the results comparable across the different modulation rates.

On each trial, two stimuli were presented, separated by a silent interval of 300 msec. Each stimulus had a 1000-msec steady-state portion and 20-msec raised-cosine rise/fall ramps. In one stimulus the 1-kHz carrier was modulated at the reference modulation depth. In the other, the modulation depth was greater. The order of the two stimuli was random. The phase of the modulators relative to the gating waveform was random.

Modulation and carrier frequencies were generated using three Farnell DSG1 signal generators, a Levell TG66 oscillator and a Hameg oscillator. AM was achieved using analog multipliers (Analog Devices AD 534L). For AM, the DC component of the modulator was derived from a 16-bit digital-to-analog converter (DAC). The output of the signal generator producing the modulator was split into two parts. One was amplified by 10 dB and then passed through a programmable attenuator (Charybdis, model D) and a relay before being recombined with the other part (which determined the reference modulation depth of the target) and with the DC component of the modulator, using an active adder (AD 507); the setting in the attenuator determined the increase in modulation depth in the signal interval. The relay determined the interval in which the signal would be presented. The overall level of the target was controlled by a second Charybdis model D programmable attenuator; this attenuator was used to hold the level constant (within ±0.125 dB) as the modulation depth was altered. The modulation depth of the interfering sound was controlled by passing the sinusoidal component of the modulator through a manual attenuator (Hatfield model 2125).

To produce the frequency-modulated target, the output of the signal generator producing the modulator was split into two parts. One part was amplified by 10 dB and then passed through a Charybdis model D programmable attenuator and a relay before being recombined with the other part. The combined modulator was then passed through a Hatfield 2125 manual attenuator and applied to the voltage-controlled input of a Farnell DSG1 oscillator. The setting in the manual attenuator determined the reference modulation index, and the setting in the programmable attenuator determined the increase in modulation index during the signal interval. The relay determined which interval would contain the signal. The modulation index of the interfering sounds was determined in a similar way using Hatfield 2125 manual attenuators.

Stimuli were gated using analog multipliers (AD 543L). Two multipliers were used in series giving an on-off ratio exceeding 100 dB. The gating voltage was derived from a 12-bit DAC under control of a Texas Instruments 990/4 computer, which also operated the relay determining the signal interval.

Subjects were tested individually in a double-walled sound attenuating chamber. Stimuli were delivered via one earpiece of a Sennheiser HD414 headset.

Procedure. An adaptive 2AFC procedure was used to estimate the 79.4% correct point on the psychometric function. A run always started with a large increment in modulation depth in the signal interval. After 3 successive correct responses the setting in the programmable attenuator was increased (which decreased the increment in modulation depth in the signal interval); after each incorrect response it was decreased. The initial step size was 5 dB. After 4 reversals, the step size was decreased to 2 dB, and 8 further reversals were obtained. The mean attenuator setting at the last 8 reversals was used to estimate the change in modulation index (delta m or delta β) corresponding to threshold. At least three estimates were obtained for each condition, and the threshold was calculated as the geometric mean of the three. When the standard deviation of the log values exceeded 0.2, at least one further estimate was obtained, and all estimates were averaged. The standard error of the log values was typically less than 0.1.

Subjects. Three young subjects with normal hearing at all audiometric frequencies were used. Two were inexperienced in psychoacoustic tasks and performed the experiment as part of an undergraduate research project. The other subject had extensive experience in psychoacoustic tasks and was paid for his services. During initial training, performance in the reference condition stabilized quite rapidly, but thresholds continued to decrease for some time in the conditions with interfering sounds. All subjects were given at least 20 hours' practice prior to collection of the data reported here. After this time performance appeared to be stable; no systematic improvements were noted during the course of the experiment.

Results

As individual differences were apparent, the results are shown separately for each subject in Figures 1–3. Thresholds are expressed as the change in modulation index at threshold divided by the modulation index of the standard [i.e. as (delta m)/m or (delta β)/β]. This is not necessarily the best way to express the results, but it does give a reasonable way of comparing the AM and FM increment thresholds.

Consider first the results for AM increment detection without any interfering sound (squares in the left panels above 0 on the abscissa). Thresholds were between 0.15 and 0.21. These values are slightly lower (i.e. our subjects were more sensitive) than those reported by Ozimek and Sek (1988) for a 1000-Hz sinusoidal carrier, but they used a different experimental method (method of adjustment). Our thresholds are very slightly larger than those reported by Grantham and Bacon (1988) and by Wakefield and Viemeister (1990) for AM increment detection with a broadband noise carrier; they used a forced-choice procedure similar to ours, but tracking 71% correct instead of 79% correct. Overall, our thresholds in the absence of interfering sounds are consistent with those in the literature.

AM increment thresholds in the presence of interfering sounds that were unmodulated (right-pointing triangles in the left panels) were almost the same as when no interfering sounds were present. This is what would be expected from the wide frequency separation of the target and interfering sounds, which would have led to minimal interaction in the peripheral auditory system.

Consider now the results for FM increment detection in the absence of any interfering sound (squares in right panels). Relative thresholds were between 0.1 and 0.15. In other words, subjects could detect an increase in FM depth

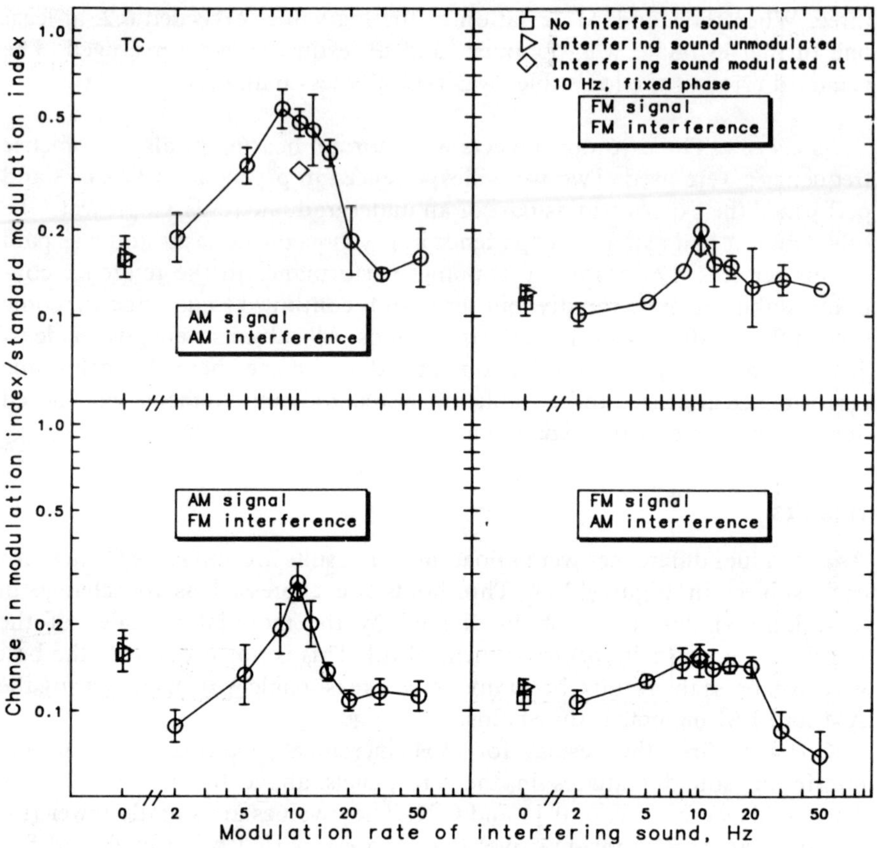

FIG. 1. Results for subject TC. Thresholds, expressed as the change in modulation index at threshold divided by the standard modulation index, are plotted on a logarithmic scale as a function of the modulation rate of the interfering sound (log scale). The box in each panel indicates the signal type and interference type. Squares show thresholds in the absence of any interfering sound, and triangles show thresholds with the interfering sound unmodulated. Diamonds show thresholds for interference modulated at a 10-Hz rate, the same as the target, averaged across the four values of modulator phase. Error bars show ± 1 SE.

from ± 20 Hz to about ± 22.4 Hz. We know of no comparable results in the literature. Unmodulated interfering sounds had a negligible effect on the FM increment thresholds.

When the interfering sound was modulated at the same 10-Hz rate as the target, there were substantial increases in threshold for both AM and FM increment detection. For each signal type, this occurred for both amplitude-modulated and frequency-modulated interfering sounds. However, there was

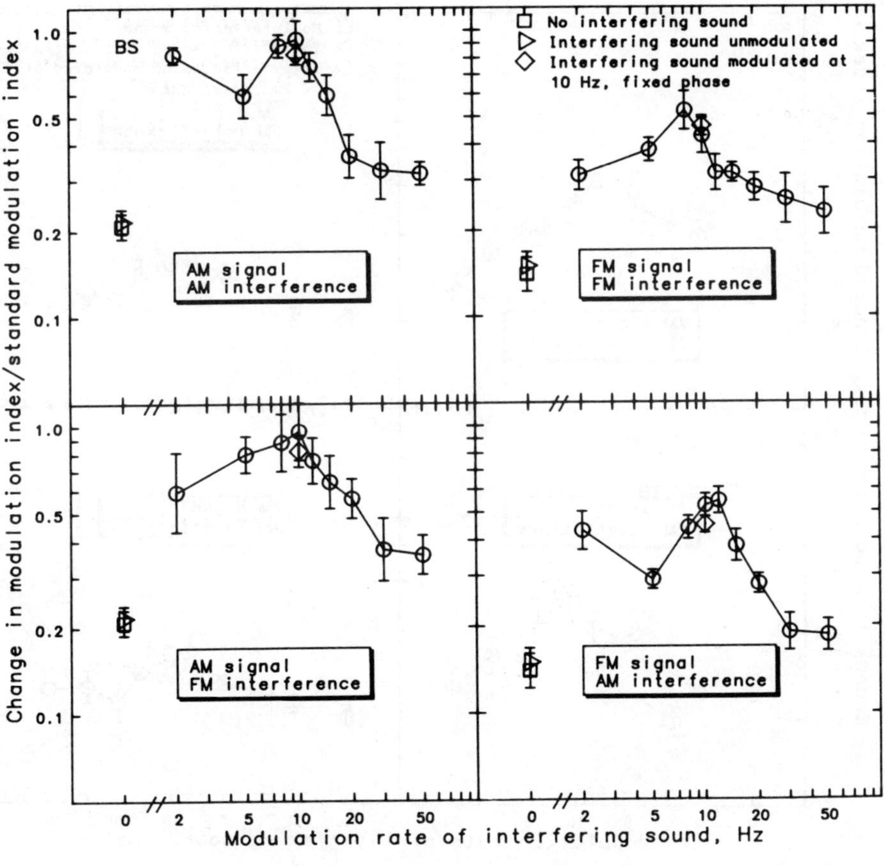

FIG. 2. As Figure 1, showing results for subject BS.

no clear effect of modulator phase. Table 1 gives the results for each subject and each modulator phase.

An analysis of variance was conducted with four factors: subjects, type of signal (AM or FM), type of interference (AM or FM), and phase of the modulator (0°, 180°, −90°, or 90°). The effect of signal type was tested against the Signal × Subjects term and was found to be significant, $F(1, 2) = 838, p < 0.001$. The effects of interference type and of phase were not significant.

The lack of a phase effect is difficult to reconcile with an explanation of across-channel masking in terms of perceptual grouping. Carriers that are amplitude modulated or frequency modulated in phase tend to be perceived as more strongly fused than carriers that are modulated with different phases

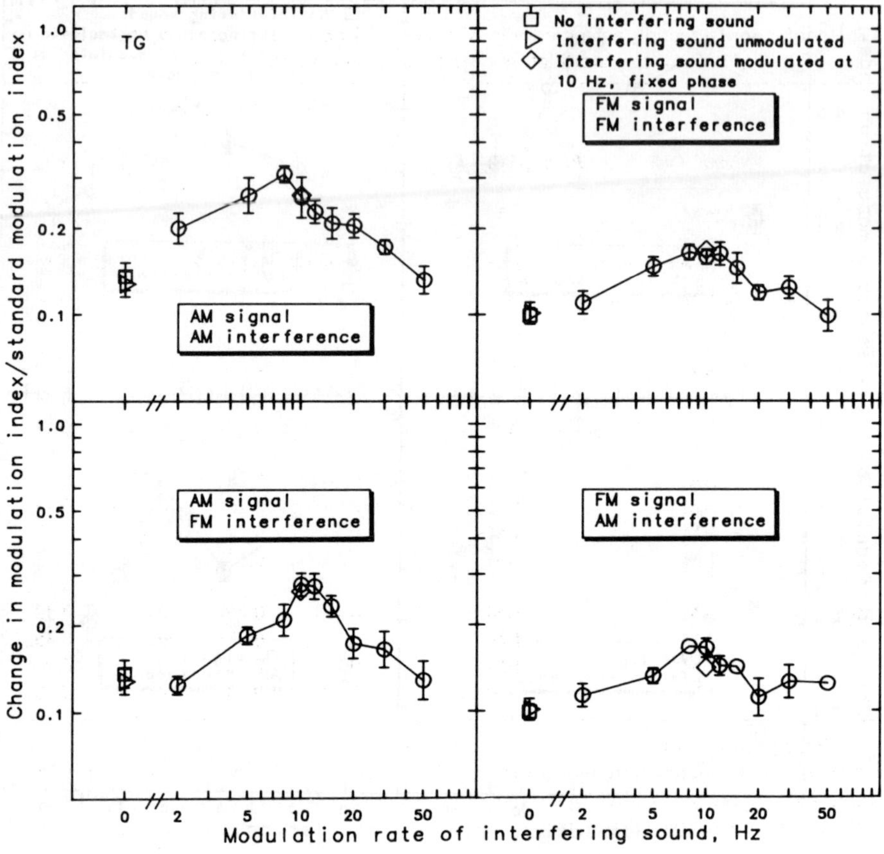

FIG. 3. As Figure 1, showing results for subject TG.

(McAdams, 1984; Bregman et al., 1985; Moore et al., 1990). Thus, if perceptual grouping were responsible for the masking, more masking would have been expected for in-phase modulators than for out-of-phase modulators. As there was no effect of modulator phase, results have been averaged for all phase conditions and are shown by the diamonds in Figures 1–3.

Consider now the influence on AM increment thresholds of amplitude-modulated interfering sounds modulated at rates other than 10 Hz (circles in top-left-hand panels). There were substantial increases in AM increment threshold for all subjects, with BS showing the largest effects and TG the smallest. The effect showed tuning for modulation rate; for all subjects, the masking was greatest when the interfering sound was modulated at rates close to 10 Hz and decreased for higher or lower rates. However, the tuning was not very sharp; all subjects showed significant threshold elevations for

TABLE 1
Thresholds for Detecting an Increase in Modulation Depth[a] as a Function of the Relative Phase of the Modulators of the Target and Interfering Sounds

Subject	*Signal Type*	*Interference Type*	*Modulator Phase* 0°	180°	−90°	90°
TC	AM	AM	0.36	0.36	0.32	0.26
	AM	FM	0.24	0.33	0.25	0.24
	FM	FM	0.18	0.21	0.18	0.19
	FM	AM	0.18	0.15	0.14	0.15
BS	AM	AM	0.86	0.62	0.98	0.88
	AM	FM	0.80	0.82	0.88	0.80
	FM	FM	0.44	0.48	0.43	0.44
	FM	AM	0.42	0.55	0.44	0.43
TG	AM	AM	0.26	0.28	0.26	0.24
	AM	FM	0.29	0.26	0.26	0.25
	FM	FM	0.18	0.18	0.15	0.17
	FM	AM	0.14	0.15	0.14	0.13
Mean	AM	AM	0.43	0.40	0.43	0.38
	AM	FM	0.38	0.41	0.39	0.36
	FM	FM	0.24	0.26	0.20	0.24
	FM	AM	0.22	0.23	0.21	0.20

[a] Either AM or FM.

Note: Both sounds were modulated at a 10-Hz rate. The change in modulation index at threshold is expressed relative to the modulation index of the standard and is given for three subjects and for the (geometric) mean.

rates between 5 and 15 Hz. For TC, the masking was negligible for the lowest interference modulation rate (2 Hz) and the three highest rates (20–50 Hz). For TG, the masking occurred for all rates except the highest rate used. For BS, significant masking occurred for all modulation rates. Again, it is difficult to reconcile these results with an explanation based on perceptual grouping. There is no obvious reason why carriers modulated at markedly different rates should fuse perceptually.

The results are consistent with the idea that there are channels in the auditory system tuned for modulation rate. It is possible that, at some stage in the auditory system, these channels combine the information from different centre frequencies (Yost et al., 1989). The amount of across-channel masking would then depend on the selectivity of the channels in the modulation domain. That such selectivity exists has been demonstrated in recent experiments by Houtgast (1989) and Bacon and Grantham (1989).

Consider now the results for AM increment detection in the presence of frequency-modulated interfering sounds (bottom left panels). The results show very clearly that frequency-modulated interfering sounds can impair AM increment detection. The pattern of results obtained as a function of the modulation rate of the interfering sounds was similar to that found for amplitude-modulated interference; the across-channel masking was tuned for modulation rate, but the tuning was rather broad. For subject BS, the amount of masking was similar for the amplitude-modulated and frequency-modulated interfering sounds. For TG and TC, the amount of masking was somewhat less for frequency-modulated than for amplitude-modulated interfering sounds.

Consider now the thresholds for FM increment detection in the presence of interfering sounds (right panels). The pattern of results resembles that found for AM increment detection, except that overall the effects are smaller. FM increment detection was affected both by frequency-modulated and amplitude-modulated interfering sounds, and the effect was tuned for modulation rate. For BS, the threshold elevations were substantial for both types of interference, and the effects extended over the whole range of modulation rates used (2–50 Hz). For TC and TG, the effects were smaller and occurred mainly for modulation rates between 5 and 15 Hz. For all three subjects, the effects were similar for frequency-modulated and amplitude-modulated interference.

These results seem to be inconsistent with the idea that the across-channel masking effects are mediated by channels tuned for modulation rate, with separate channels for AM and FM. If that were the case, then frequency-modulated sounds should not have interfered with AM detection and vice versa. We will return to this point later.

To assess the statistical significance of the results obtained using interfering sounds modulated at rates other than 10 Hz, an analysis of variance was conducted with the following factors: subject, signal type (AM or FM), interference type (AM or FM), and modulation rate. The significance of the main effects of signal type, interference type and modulation rate was assessed by testing against the corresponding interaction term with the subjects factor. For example, the effect of signal type was tested against the Subjects × Signal interaction term. There were significant main effects of signal type, $F(1, 2) = 72.2$, $p < 0.025$, and of modulation rate, $F(8, 16) = 13.72$, $p < 0.01$. The effect of interference type was not significant.

GENERAL DISCUSSION

Implications for the Perceptual-Grouping Hypothesis

The results reported above appear to be inconsistent with an explanation of across-channel masking in terms of perceptual grouping. Contrary to what would be predicted for this hypothesis, there was no effect of the relative phase of the modulation of the target and interfering sounds, and the interference persisted when the modulation rates of the target and interfering sounds were substantially different. Similar results have been reported for AM detection with amplitude-modulated interference by Yost and Sheft (1989) and Yost et al. (1989). However, Wilson et al. (1990) did find an effect of modulator phase for FM detection with frequency-modulated interference. The reason for this discrepancy is not clear.

However, it may be premature to reject the perceptual-grouping hypothesis at this stage. The evidence that the phase of the modulators plays a critical role in perceptual grouping is not very strong, particularly in the case of frequency-modulated sounds. For example, McAdams (1989) investigated the relative perceptual prominence of individual "target" vowels in a mixture of three vowels, He found that the target vowel was more prominent when all components of that vowel were coherently frequency modulated. However, the prominence of the target vowel did not depend significantly on whether the "background" vowels were unmodulated, modulated in-phase with the target, or modulated independently of the target. In other words, a difference in modulator phase between the target and background sounds did not increase the prominence of the target relative to the case where the target and background were modulated in phase. Carlyon (1991) has presented evidence that listeners cannot discriminate two carrier frequencies that are frequency modulated in phase from two carriers that are frequency modulated out of phase when the carrier frequencies are not harmonically related (as was the case for our stimuli). If subjects cannot detect differences in modulator phase, then modulator phase is unlikely to be an important factor in perceptual grouping.

There is direct evidence that listeners can detect differences in AM phase for carriers that are widely separated in frequency (Strickland, Viemeister, Fantini, & Garrison, 1989; Green, Richards, & Onsan, 1990). Furthermore, Bregman et al. (1985) have presented evidence that modulator phase can be important for the perceptual grouping of amplitude-modulated signals. However, Bregman et al. used modulation rates much higher than those used here. Thus, it remains unclear whether perceptual grouping depends on modulator phase at low modulation rates. Until this is known, it is difficult to evaluate the significance of our finding that across-channel masking of AM and FM increment detection is not affected by the relative phase of modulation of the target and interfering sounds.

The broad tuning of the interference effect does create clear difficulties for an explanation based on perceptual grouping. Bregman et al. (1990) have studied the effects of differences in AM rate on the perceptual fusion of two sinusoidal carriers. They found that fusion was strongest when the carriers were amplitude modulated at the same rate (114 Hz or 125 Hz) and fell off sharply when the carriers were modulated at rates differing by 7% (smaller differences were not tested). Thus the tuning in the modulation domain found by them appears to be much sharper than that found by us. Of course, the overall difference in modulation rate makes their results and ours difficult to compare. Nevertheless, their results lend support to the argument that the across-channel masking found by us is too broadly tuned in the modulation domain to be explained in terms of perceptual grouping mechanisms. If perceptual grouping mechanisms were responsible, then components that did *not* arise from the same sound source would frequently be grouped together. This would lead to many errors in perceptual grouping.

One might argue that for many everyday sounds, such as more than one person talking at the same time, the AM of the different sources would be complex rather than sinusoidal, and the AM spectra would show considerable overlap across sources. Thus fine selectivity in the modulation domain might not be particularly helpful in producing accurate perceptual grouping. It may be that the pattern of modulation, rather than its rate, is the critical factor. However, even a small difference in modulation rate is *sufficient* to produce a difference in pattern of modulation. Evidently, such a difference in pattern was not sufficient to eliminate across-channel masking in our experiments. Again, this suggests that perpetual grouping does not provide a satisfactory explanation of our results.

The Evidence for Channels Tuned to AM or FM

Our results do not support the idea that across-channel masking occurs in channels that are tuned for the detection of either amplitude-modulated or frequency-modulated sounds; frequency-modulated interference affected AM increment detection, and vice versa. However, it should be remembered that FM is translated in the auditory system into AM within individual auditory filters. For example, a frequency-modulated carrier whose frequency falls on the upper skirt of a given auditor filter will produce AM at the output of that filter (Zwicker, 1956). This translation of FM to AM is often explained using the concept of the excitation pattern. The latter is a representation of the distribution of activity evoked by a sound in the peripheral auditory system as a function of characteristic frequency. The excitation pattern can be defined as the amount of output of the auditory filters as a function of their centre frequency (Moore & Glasberg, 1983; Patterson & Moore, 1986). When a sinusoidal carrier is shifted in frequency, the whole excitation pattern is shifted along the frequency axis. For example, an upward shift in frequency results in an increase of excitation level on the high-frequency side of the pattern and a decrease on the low-frequency side (Zwicker, 1956).

Channels that were truly selective for AM or FM could distinguish the two types of modulation by comparing changes in excitation level on the two sides of the excitation pattern. For AM, the changes are in phase on the two sides of the excitation pattern, whereas for FM they are in opposite phase

(Zwicker, 1956; Moore & Glasberg, 1989). It is possible, however, that the hypothetical channels do not actually compare the phase of modulation at different parts of the excitation pattern. For example, the AM channels might be activated by AM at the output of *any* auditory filter. In this case, a frequency-modulated sound would activate AM channels. The effect of frequency-modulated interfering sounds on AM increment detection might result from such activitation.

To evaluate this idea, we used the excitation pattern model described by Glasberg and Moore (1990). We calculated that the FM of the 3300-Hz carrier would have resulted in a modulation of excitation level of about 12 dB (between maximum and minimum excitation levels) on the low-frequency side of the excitation pattern. This is actually slightly greater than the peak-to-valley ratio of our amplitude-modulated interfering sounds, which was about 9.5 dB. The modulation of excitation level produced by the 3300-Hz frequency-modulated carrier would be smaller on the high-frequency side of the pattern. Also, the AM produced by the 230-Hz frequency-modulated carrier would have been smaller as the auditory filters have larger relative bandwidths at low centre frequencies (Glasberg & Moore, 1990). Nevertheless, these calculations indicate that the masking of AM increment detection by frequency-modulated interfering sounds might be explained by the translation of FM to AM in the auditory system.

Consider now the changes in FM increment detection produced by amplitude-modulated interfering sounds. It is possible that there are not channels selective to FM per se. Rather, FM may be detected and discriminated using the changes in excitation level evoked by FM in the auditory system (Zwicker, 1956; Moore & Glasberg, 1989). In other words, FM is translated into AM, and discrimination is based on the AM. Amplitude-modulated interference might then affect FM increment detection by the same mechanism that amplitude-modulated interference affects AM increment detection.

To evaluate this idea further, we calculated the amounts of AM that would have been evoked by the frequency-modulated standard ($\beta = 2$) and by the signal-plus-standard at threshold (in the absence of interfering sounds). Again, this was done using the excitation pattern model described by Glasberg and Moore (1990). The change in excitation level was always greatest on the low-frequency side of the excitation pattern—that is, for auditory filters centred below the carrier frequency (1000 Hz). We present results only for a filter centred at 850 Hz; results would be similar in form for other centre frequencies below 1000 Hz. The calculated changes were compared to the AM increment thresholds in the absence of interfering sounds. The results are summarized in Table 2.

The peak-to-valley ratio of the amplitude-modulated standard ($m = 0.25$) was 4.4 dB. The increase in peak-to-valley ratio at threshold was between 0.63 and 0.98 dB, depending on the subject. The peak-to-valley ratio evoked

TABLE 2
Comparison of the Thresholds for Detecting Increments in Modulation Depth for Amplitude- and Frequency-Modulated Signals in the Absence of Interfering Sounds

	AM		*FM*	
Subject	*P/V*	*delta P/V*	*P/V*	*delta P/V*
TC	5.17	0.73	5.62	0.56
BS	5.42	0.98	5.76	0.70
TG	5.07	0.63	5.56	0.50

Note: For the frequency-modulated signals, the table gives the calculated amounts of AM at the output of an auditory filter centred at 850 Hz, i.e., below the signal frequency. The peak-to-valley ratio of the amplitude-modulated standard was 4.44 dB. The calculated peak-to-valley ratio evoked by the frequency-modulated standard was 5.06 dB. Thresholds are given both as the peak-to-valley ratio (P/V) of the standard-plus-signal (dB) and as the change in peak-to-valley ratio (delta P/V) at threshold.

by the frequency-modulated standard was calculated to be 5.06 dB. The increase in peak-to-valley ratio at threshold was between 0.50 and 0.70 dB, depending on the subject. Thus, there is a reasonable correspondence between the two sets of results. The changes in peak-to-valley ratio at threshold are consistently slightly smaller for FM than for AM increment detection, but the discrepancy is small and could easily be accounted for by individual differences in frequency selectivity. Overall, the results are consistent with the idea that increments in amount of FM are detected by virtue of the increments in depth of AM they produce in the auditory system. If this is the case, then it is not surprising that amplitude-modulated sounds can interfere with FM increment detection.

Although the overall pattern of our results is consistent with an explanation based on the translation of FM to AM in the auditory system, other research suggests that FM-induced AM is not equivalent to true AM. For example, the data reviewed earlier on perceptual grouping suggests that coherence of AM across frequency bands plays a role in perceptual grouping, whereas coherence of FM probably does not.

Interactions between AM Channels?

Yost et al. (1989) have suggested that across-channel masking might occur in the following way. The stimulus is first processed by an array of auditory filters, which separates widely spaced frequencies. Then the envelope at the output of each filter is extracted. When modulation is present, AM channels are excited, which are tuned for modulation rate. All filters responding with the same modulation rate excite the same AM channel, regardless of the filter centre frequency. Thus across-channel masking would occur within these AM channels.

Yost et al. suggested that AM channels receiving inputs from auditory filters tuned to widely different centre frequencies could be involved in perceptual grouping; each AM channel output would represent an "auditory object". However, there seem to be significant problems with a model of this kind. Firstly, if the modulation were preserved at the inputs to the AM channels, then we would expect an effect of the relative phase of the target and interfering sounds. No such effect was found. This implies either that the channels do not exist, or that the modulation (and its rate) at the output of each auditory filter is detected and extracted *before* the AM channels; the information about modulation rate fed to the AM channels would not then specify modulator phase.

A second problem with this model is connected with the broad tuning for modulation rate found in these experiments, and those of Yost et al. (1989); we have already argued that this broad tuning is inconsistent with an explanation based on perceptual grouping. If the channels are not used for perceptual grouping, it is hard to imagine what their purpose might be. As argued above, they do not appear to be involved in modulation detection per se, as there is no effect of relative modulator phase.

Concluding Remarks

Our results clearly show that modulation increment detection can be impaired by modulated carriers widely separated in frequency from the target. This represents a failure of traditional models of masking based on the concept of listening through a single auditory filter. The results do not support the idea that there are independent channels for detecting AM and FM; FM interfered with AM increment detection, and vice versa. This aspect of the results may be explained using the idea that FM is transformed into AM in the auditory system. The lack of an effect of relative modulator phase and the broad tuning of the interference effect in the modulation domain are difficult to explain in terms of perceptual grouping, or in terms of channels tuned for modulation rate.

REFERENCES

Bacon, S.P. & Grantham, D.W. (1989). Modulation masking: Effects of modulation frequency, depth and phase. *Journal of the Acoustical Society of America*, *85*, 2575–2580.

Bregman, A.S., Abramson, J., Doehring, P., & Darwin, C.J. (1985). Spectral integration based on common amplitude modulation. *Perception and Psychophysics*, *37*, 483–493.

Bregman, A.S., Levitan, R., & Liao, C. (1990). Fusion of auditory components: Effects of the frequency of amplitude modulao. *Perception and Psychophysics*, *47*, 68–73.

Carlyon, R.P. (1991). Discriminating between coherent and incoherent frequency modulation of complex tones. *Journal of the Acoustical Society of America, 89*, 329–340.

Fletcher, H. (1940). Auditory patterns. *Reviews of Modern Physics, 12*, 47–65.

Gardner, R.B. & Wilson, J.P. (1979). Evidence for direction-specific channels in the processing of frequency modulation. *Journal of the Acoustical Society of America, 66*, 704–709.

Glasberg, B.R. & Moore, B.C.J. (1990). Derivation of auditory filter shapes from notched-noise data. *Hearing Research, 47*, 103–138.

Grantham, D.W. & Bacon, S.P. (1988). Detection of increments and decrements in modulation depth of SAM noise. *Journal of the Acoustical Society of America, 84*, S140.

Green, D.M. (1988). *Profile analysis.* Oxford: Oxford University Press.

Green, D.M., Richards, V.M., & Onsan, Z.A. (1990). Sensitivity to envelope coherence. *Journal of the Acoustical Society of America, 87*, 323–329.

Hall, J.W., Haggard, M.P., & Fernandes, M.A. (1984). Detection in noise by spectro-temporal pattern analysis. *Journal of the Acoustical Society of America, 76*, 50–56.

Houtgast, T. (1989). Frequency selectivity in amplitude-modulation detection. *Journal of the Acoustical Society of America, 85*, 1676–1680.

Kay, R.H. (1982). Hearing of modulation in sounds. *Physiological Reviews, 62*, 894–975.

Kay, R.H. & Mathews, D.R. (1972). On the existence in human auditory pathways of channels selectively tuned to the modulation present in frequency modulated tones. *Journal of Physiology, 225*, 657–667.

McAdams, S. (1984). *Spectral fusion, spectral parsing, and the formation of auditory images.* Doctoral dissertation, Stanford University, Stanford, CA.

McAdams, S. (1989). Segregation of concurrent sounds. I. Effects of frequency modulation coherence. *Journal of the Acoustical Society of America, 86*, 2148–2159.

Moller, A.R. (1976). Dynamic properties of the responses of single neurones in the cochlear nucleus of the rat to AM and FM tones. *Hearing Research, 10*, 301–330.

Moore, B.C.J. (1990). Comodulation masking release: Spectro-temporal pattern analysis in hearing. *British Journal of Audiology, 24*, 131–137.

Moore, B.C.J. & Glasberg, B.R. (1983). Suggested formulae for calculating auditory filter shapes and excitation patterns. *Journal of the Acoustical Society of America, 74*, 750–753.

Moore, B.C.J. & Glasberg, B.R. (1989). Mechanisms underlying the frequency discrimination of pulsed tones and the detection of frequency modulation. *Journal of the Acoustical Society of America, 86*, 1722–1732.

Moore, B.C.J., Glasberg, B.R., & Schooneveldt, G.P. (1990). Across-channel masking and comodulation masking release. *Journal of the Acoustical Society of America, 87*, 1683–1694.

Ozimek, E. & Sek, A. (1988). AM difference limens for noise bands. *Acustica, 66*, 153–160.

Patterson, R.D. & Moore, B.C.J. (1986). Auditory filters and excitation patterns as representations of frequency resolution. In B.C.J. Moore (Ed.), *Frequency selectivity in hearing* (pp. 123–177). London: Academic Press.

Rees, A. & Moller, A.R. (1983). Responses of neurons in the inferior colliculus of the rat to AM and FM tones. *Hearing Research, 10*, 301–310.

Schreiner, C.E. & Urbas, J.V. (1986). Representation of amplitude modulation in the auditory cortex of the cat. I. The anterior auditory field (AAF). *Hearing Research, 21*, 227–241.

Shower, E.G. & Biddulph, R. (1931). Differential pitch sensitivity of the ear. *Journal of the Acoustical Society of America, 2*, 275–287.

Strickland, E.A., Viemeister, N.F., Fantini, D.A., & Garrison, M.A. (1989). Within- versus cross-channel mechanisms in detection of envelope phase disparity. *Journal of the Acoustical Society of America, 86*, 2160–2166.

Tansley, B.W. & Regan, D. (1979). Separate auditory channels for unidirectional frequency modulation and unidirectional amplitude modulation. *Sensory Processes, 3*, 132–140.

Tansley, B.W. & Suffield, J.B. (1983). Time course of adaptation and recovery of channels selectively sensitive to frequency and amplitude modulation. *Journal of the Acoustical Society of America, 74*, 765–775.

Viemeister, N.F. (1979). Temporal modulation transfer functions based upon modulation thresholds. *Journal of the Acoustical Society of America, 66*, 1364–1384.

Wakefield, G.H. & Viemeister, N.F. (1984). Selective adaptation to linear frequency-modulated sweeps: Evidence for direction-specific channels? *Journal of the Acoustical Society of America, 75*, 1588–1592.

Wakefield, G.H. & Viemeister, N.F. (1990). Discrimination of modulation depth of SAM noise. *Journal of the Acoustical Society of America, 88*, 1367–1373.

Wilson, A.S., Hall, J.W., & Grose, J.H. (1990). Detection of frequency modulation (FM) in the presence of a second FM tone. *Journal of the Acoustical Society of America, 88*, 1333–1338.

Yost, W.A. & Sheft, S. (1989). Across-critical-band processing of amplitude-modulated tones. *Journal of the Acoustical Society of America, 85*, 848–857.

Yost, W.A., Sheft, S., & Opie, J. (1989). Modulation interference in detection and discrimination of amplitude modulation. *Journal of the Acoustical Society of America, 86*, 2138–2147.

Zwicker, E. (1956). Die elementaren Grundlagen zur Bestimmung der Informationskapazität des Gehörs. *Acustica, 6*, 365–381.

Revised manuscript received 6 July 1990

THE QUARTERLY JOURNAL OF EXPERIMENTAL PSYCHOLOGY, 1991, *43A* (3) 349–372

Relative Contributions of Envelope Maxima and Minima to Comodulation Masking Release

Joseph W. Hall III and John H. Grose
University of North Carolina Medical School, Chapel Hill, North Carolina, U.S.A.

Comodulation masking release (CMR) is a phenomenon that demonstrates the sensitivity of the auditory system to across-frequency differences in the temporal modulation pattern of a complex waveform. In this paper, we review briefly some of the data on the physical parameters that affect CMR and describe models that have been proposed to account for CMR—namely, models based upon envelope equalization/cancellation, across-frequency envelope correlation, and "dip listening". The present literature is ambiguous with regard to the relative importance of energy in the peak and dip regions of the waveform envelope. We therefore performed a series of experiments to investigate this issue. In the first experiment, we examined CMR for signals that resulted either in a uniform increment or in uniform decrement in the masking noise centred on the signal frequency. This was accomplished by using a 20-Hz-wide noise band centred on 700 Hz as both the masker and as the signal, adjusting the phase angle between the signal and masker to either 0° (increment) or 180° (decrement). Conditions were examined where either zero, one, two, four, or six comodulated flanking bands were present. Results indicated positive CMRs for all conditions in which a comodulated flanking band was present. CMR increased as the number of flanking bands increased for intensity increments, but not for intensity decrements. The remaining experiments examined conditions where signals were present only in masker peaks, or only in masker dips. The results of these experiments indicated relatively large CMRs when the signal occurred in dip regions, but no CMR when the signal occurred in peak regions. Whereas some of the results of the above experiments would be difficult to account for in terms of the dip listening hypothesis of CMR, the present findings did indicate that the stimulus cues that give rise to CMR appear to be derived primarily from the dip regions of the masking noise.

Requests for reprints should be sent to Joseph W. Hall III, The Division of Otolaryngology/ Head & Neck Surgery, University of North Carolina Medical School, Chapel Hill, NC 27599, U.S.A.

This work was supported by grants from the U.S. Air Force and the National Institutes of Health. We thank Greg Schooneveldt, Søren Buus, and Quentin Summerfield for helpful comments on a previous version of this manuscript.

Several different auditory masking procedures using tonal or random noise maskers have been used to measure the frequency selectivity of the ear (Fletcher, 1940; Green, McKey, & Licklider, 1959; Margolis & Small, 1975; Patterson, 1976; Wegel & Lane, 1924; Zwicker, 1974). Results from these masking procedures indicate that the auditory system behaves in some situations like a bank of bandpass filters. When trying to hear, for example, a pure-tone signal masked by broadband noise, we appear to base detection upon the auditory filter providing the best signal-to-noise (S/N) ratio. This is usually the filter centred at or near the frequency of the signal (Moore & Glasberg, 1983; Patterson & Nimmo-Smith, 1980; Scharf, 1970). This concept assumes that only the masking energy passed by the auditory filter centred on the signal frequency influences the detection of the signal. However, this assumption does not appear to hold when the masking noise is not random, but has a modulation pattern that is coherent across frequency—that is, when noise components in one spectral region fluctuate synchronously with noise components in other spectral regions. Under this circumstance, noise components outside the auditory filter centred on the signal frequency can actually facilitate signal detection and produce a release from masking. The improvement in detection that occurs in comodulated noise is referred to as Comodulation Masking Release, or CMR (Hall, Haggard, & Fernandes, 1984a). Detection in comodulated noise appears to be based not only upon the activity within the critical band centred on the signal, but also upon the pattern of activity across a range of critical bands, an interpretation pertaining also to Profile Analysis (Green, 1988; Green, Kidd, & Picardi, 1983; Green, Mason, & Kidd, 1984; Spiegel & Green, 1981). CMR demonstrates the existence of across-channel, or across-frequency, processing of waveform envelope in auditory signal detection.

Two brief examples will illustrate the CMR effect. In one example (Hall et al., 1984a), the threshold of a 1000-Hz signal is determined as a function of the bandwidth of a modulated masking noise. In this example, comodulated noise is created by multiplying a broadband noise by a lowpass noise (0–50 Hz). As the bandwidth of the modulated noise is increased from 100 Hz to about 800 Hz, threshold improves by about 9 dB. In the second example, the threshold of a 1000-Hz signal is determined in a narrow noise band centred on 1000 Hz (on-signal band). Adding a second narrowband noise that has an envelope identical to that of the first band improves threshold by 3 to 7 dB (Cohen & Schubert, 1987; Hall, Grose, & Haggard, 1990; Hall et al., 1984a; McFadden, 1986; Moore, Hall, Grose, & Schooneveldt, 1990; Schooneveldt & Moore, 1987). CMR also occurs when the comodulated flanking energy is presented to the ear contralateral to the ear of signal presentation (Cohen & Schubert, 1987; Hall et al., 1990; Hall, Haggard, & Harvey, 1984b; Schooneveldt & Moore, 1989b).

A number of parametric studies on CMR in the normal auditory system have been reported, and some of the main findings are summarized below:

1. *Number of Flanking Bands and Total Bandwidth.* Generally, CMR increases as the total masking bandwidth or number of individual comodulated flanking bands increases (Carlyon, Buus, & Florentine, 1989; Haggard, Hall, & Grose, 1990; Hall et al., 1990; Hall et al., 1984a; Schooneveldt & Moore, 1989b), although one study did not show an effect of band number (McFadden, 1986). Hall et al. (1990) found that the greatest increase in CMR occurs when increasing the number of flanking bands from one to two (approximately 4 dB increase); for further increases in flanking band number CMR increases approximately proportionately to the square root of the number of bands. The results of Haggard et al. (1990) indicate that the important variable is not the total bandwidth of the noise, but, rather, the number of critical bands contributing information.

2. *Spectral Separation between On-signal and Flanking Bands.* Several experiments have indicated that CMR decreases as the spectral separation between the on-signal and flanking bands increases (Hall et al., 1990; Hall et al., 1984a; Schooneveldt & Moore, 1987). There are probably two contributions to this effect. One contribution is apparently related to a within-channel effect (Schooneveldt & Moore, 1987). Schooneveldt and Moore suggested that when the on-signal and flanking bands are close together, their representation in the auditory system is characterized by a regular beating pattern; the presence of the signal may then be cued by the disturbance in the beating pattern caused by the signal. However, Hall et al. (1990) have provided evidence that there is a proximity effect even for the across-channel contribution to CMR. This is based upon two considerations: (1) that the proximity effect occurs not only for a single flanking band, but also for conditions where two flanking bands are presented symmetrically around the on-signal band—Schooneveldt and Moore (1989b) have shown that within-channel beating cues are negligible for such stimuli; (2) that proximity effects also occur when flanking bands are presented to the contralateral ear (Hall et al., 1990), negating the possibility of peripheral within-channel interactions.

3. *Frequency of Modulation.* For masking noises composed of a narrow on-signal band and one or more comodulated flanking bands, CMR increases as the bandwidths of the individual noise bands decrease (Hall, Cokely, & Grose, 1988; Schooneveldt & Moore, 1987). This effect was interpreted as being due to the decrease in average rate of envelope fluctuation as noise bandwidth decreases. For masking noises generated by modulating a wideband noise by a relatively low-frequency modulator, some studies have indicated that CMR magnitude decreases monotonically as the

frequency of modulation increases (Hall & Grose, 1989; Hall & Haggard, 1983; Schooneveldt & Moore, 1989a). These results are consistent with an interpretation that CMR increases as a function of decreasing rate of masker fluctuation. However, Carlyon et al. (1989) have suggested that a within-channel cue contributes to this effect in modulated noise, and that CMR (derived exclusively from across-channel cues) is relatively independent of modulation rate (at least for a signal frequency of 4000 Hz, and modulation rates at and below 100 Hz). Data of Hall and Grose (1989) suggest that the effect of modulation rate is relatively large at a signal frequency of 500 Hz, but considerably smaller at a signal frequency of 2000 Hz. Further research exploring the issue of modulation rate would be of interest, particularly as there are important methodological/stimulus differences between studies that have examined this effect.

4. *Across-Frequency Differences in Masker Spectrum Level.* Early studies on across-frequency variation in noise level indicated that CMR effects remained when the spectrum levels of the on-signal and flanking bands differed by from 10 to 30 dB (Hall, 1986; McFadden, 1986; Schooneveldt and Moore, 1987). Hall (1987) found that CMR was affected less by across-frequency level differences when frequency spacings between the on-signal and flanking bands were relatively wide. It was hypothesized that with relatively narrow frequency spacing, spread of excitation from the more intense band may significantly alter the response to the less intense band, thereby reducing the correlation of the envelopes. Recent studies using multiple flanking bands (Moore & Shailer, in press) or very widely spaced noise bands (Cohen, 1989) indicate that CMR persists even for level disparities of from 40 to 60 dB.

5. *Across-Frequency Delay in Masker Envelope.* CMR occurs when the envelopes of the on-signal band and the flanking band are comodulated. A basic question concerns whether CMR still occurs when the on-signal and flanking bands are comodulated, but some amount of time delay exists between the envelopes. Haggard, Harvey, and Carlyon (1985) investigated conditions where the envelope delay was 0, 90, 180, or 270°. The results of this study indicated that CMR was reduced substantially for the delay conditions. McFadden (1986) and Moore and Schooneveldt (1990) also found that CMR fell off relatively steeply for across-frequency delays in envelope. These studies indicate a very limited ability of the central auditory system to compensate for across-frequency time-shifts in masker envelope.

CMR and Auditory Grouping

CMR appears to be related to what has been termed auditory grouping, auditory object formation, or auditory scene analysis (Bregman, 1978; Bregman, Abramson, Doehring, & Darwin, 1985; Bregman & Campbell,

1971; Dannenbring & Bregman, 1978; McAdams, 1984). Studies in these areas often investigate physical attributes of sound that result in the assignment of different spectral components to a common acoustic source. One such acoustic feature is common amplitude envelope trajectory (Dannenbring & Bregman, 1978; Darwin, 1983). Although early investigations of CMR proposed a link between CMR and auditory scene analysis, there have been few investigations that have addressed this area. A recent study exploring such a relation was reported by Hall and Grose (1990). In this study it was shown that the CMR resulting from a set of seven comodulated narrow bands of noise (the on-signal band and six flanking bands) could be reduced by the interjection of two additional flanking bands (termed codeviant bands), which were comodulated with respect to each other, but not with respect to the on-signal band and its comodulated flanking bands. It was hypothesized that this reduction in CMR was due to a failure of the auditory system to parse the on-signal band from the co-deviant bands. In support of this hypothesis, CMR recovered appreciably when factors that should theoretically aid the separation of the on-signal band and its comodulated flanking bands from the codeviant bands were brought to bear. For example, when further codeviant bands were added, the codeviant bands became perceptually segregated from the comodulated bands, and CMR increased. This is similar to the "capture" phenomenon, which has been described previously in the auditory grouping literature. As another example, CMR increased when the comodulated and codeviant bands received independent temporal gating patterns. This is similar to auditory segregation effects that arise from onset asynchrony. The results of Hall and Grose (1990) indicated that some processes contributing to CMR occur after, or receive feedback from, stages of processing that affect auditory grouping.

Models of CMR

At this point there is no single, comprehensive model that accounts for the across-frequency processes that presumably underlie CMR. Hall et al. (1984a) hypothesized that detection of a signal in comodulated noise is based upon an across-frequency difference in modulation pattern. One model (Buus, 1985; Hall, 1986) accounting for extraction of such an across-frequency difference in envelope is similar to Durlach's (1963) equalization/cancellation (EC) model of the masking-level difference. This CMR model proposes that the envelopes at different frequency regions are extracted, and that the envelope at the signal frequency is then subtracted from the envelope at flanking frequencies: a relatively large result from this subtraction would indicate the presence of a signal. Another general model, proposed by Richards (1987), assumes that the auditory system first extracts the various constituent envelopes and then correlates the envelope at the signal frequency with the envelope at the flanking frequency. Here, the presence of a signal would be indicated by a relatively low correlation value. The above models assume that CMR depends upon the extraction of an across-frequency difference cue. Buus (1985) also proposed a "dip listening" model incorporating envelope extraction, but not specifically requiring the identification of an across-frequency envelope difference. According to this model, the comodulated flanking band is used by the auditory system to identify low-energy or dip regions in the waveform of the on-signal masker. The dip regions of the on-signal band, which provide the best S/N ratio, are given a relatively high weighting in the detection decision, and the peak regions are given low weighting. This detection strategy would effectively increase the S/N ratio.

Although many of the CMR results presently available indicate that an across-channel process contributes to detection of signals in comodulated noise, few of the data actually help to test the relative merits of the various models that have been proposed to account for CMR. Richards (1987) noted that the envelope decorrelation caused by the signal at threshold in CMR experiments was very similar to that which she obtained in determining the ability of listeners to detect across-frequency decorrelation in waveform envelope. This would provide general support for an envelope correlation hypothesis. Moore and Emmerich (1990), however, have argued that CMR and envelope correlation discrimination are probably based upon different mechanisms, noting that a decrease in noise bandwidth causes CMR to increase, but envelope correlation discrimination to become more difficult. The results of a study that investigated CMR for multi-component signals (Hall, Grose, & Haggard, 1988) indicated that the EC model did better than either the correlation model or dip listening model in accounting for the CMR for pure tone signals presented in narrow bands of comodulated noise. The results of several investigations (Hall & Grose, 1988; Moore, 1990; Moore & Schooneveldt, 1990) suggested that the auditory system may use several different stimulus variables to detect signals in comodulated noise, and that models incorporating a single variable (e.g. envelope correlation) may be insufficient to account for all CMR results. An example supporting this contention is apparent in the data of Grose and Hall (1989), where data from some listeners favoured an EC mechanism, but the data of other listeners favoured a dip listening mechanism. In this study, using AM maskers, the depth of modulation in the on-signal band was fixed at 63%, and the depth of modulation in the flanking bands was either 63% or 100%. By the dip listening hypothesis, CMR should have been greater for the case where the flanking bands had 100% AM; by the EC hypothesis, on the other hand, CMR should have been greater for the case where the flanking bands had 63% AM. The results were ambiguous, in that the data of some subjects favoured the dip listening hypothesis, whereas the data of others favoured the EC hypothesis.

The Role of Energy in Envelope Peaks and Dips

One further set of results is pertinent to the question of the importance of energy in the dip regions of the masker envelope. The study by Grose and Hall (1989) investigated CMR for a set of nine comodulated AM tones (10-Hz sinusoidal modulation). In one set of conditions, CMR was examined for a signal composed of three short (50-msec) tone bursts that were added in phase to only the peaks of the on-signal AM tone, or only to the dips of the on-signal AM tone. Interestingly, a CMR was observed for signals added during envelope dips, but not for signals added during envelope peaks. This result was replicated in a study by Moore, Glasberg, and Schooneveldt (1990). These investigators showed further that no CMR was obtained even when the signal presented in the peak was inverted with respect to the carrier (even though such signal presentation resulted in a significant across-frequency decorrelation of envelope in the peak region of the waveform). Moore et al. also found that although a signal that increased the level in the dip region of the envelope resulted in a CMR, a signal that *decreased* the level in the dip region did not.

The result that no CMR occurs for signals presented only in the peak region of the envelope is somewhat surprising when considered in the light of a previous study by Hall and Grose (1988). In this study the signal was exactly the same narrowband noise as the on-signal masker, added in phase with the masker. Thus the signal resulted in an increase in amplitude that was uniform over the entire duration of the signal. As we have pointed out previously (Hall & Grose, 1988), CMR conditions where a noise band is added to itself are somewhat of a special case and are particularly similar to Profile Analysis experiments (where a pure tone is added to itself). One way of accounting for a CMR for such a stimulus is in terms of envelope subtraction *without* prior equalization, where the envelope at a flanking frequency is subtracted from the envelope at the signal frequency; when a signal is present, the subtraction results in a remainder, which could cue detection.[1] With regard to the dip listening hypothesis, it is important to note that the level increase due to the signal in such conditions is no greater in the dip regions than in the peak regions of the masker envelope. Therefore, no cue is present for a dip listening CMR mechanism, as the S/N ratio is constant across both peak and dip regions of the masker envelope. Even so, CMRs were observed which were similar in magnitude to those obtained for the more typical pure-tone signal, where the S/N ratio is substantially better in the masker dip regions. At first glance, it is difficult to reconcile this result

---

[1] Masking Level Differences (MLDs) are also found in the case where a narrow noise band is added to itself (Hall & Fernandes, 1983; McFadden, Jeffress, & Ermey, 1971). Under this circumstance, the EC model of the MLD (Durlach, 1963) would also have to assume subtraction (of stimulus fine structure) without prior equalization.

with the results of studies that show that CMR occurs only when signal energy is present in the masker dips. One possible interpretation is that in the case of a noise added to itself, only the increment occurring in the masker dip region actually contributes to the CMR, even though the energy in the masker peak region should theoretically carry information of equal value. Although it is consistent with the data, this interpretation has the drawback that it assumes that the auditory systems fails to utilize available information. The experiments reported below were intended to provide a better understanding of the relative contributions of information in dip and peak regions of the waveform envelope.

EXPERIMENT 1

CMR for a Noise Signal Added In-phase or Out-of-phase to an Identical Masker

Whereas the experiments of Grose and Hall (1989) and Moore et al. (1990) indicated that signal information in masker dip regions is of particular importance, the results of Hall and Grose (1988) showed that substantial CMRs could occur even when the S/N ratio was no better in the dip regions than in the peak regions. As a first step in investigating this apparent inconsistency, we thought it important first to bring under control an obvious methodological difference between the studies of Hall and Grose (1988), on the one hand, and the studies of Grose and Hall (1989) and Moore et al. (1990a), on the other. In the previous studies investigating signals presented only in peak regions, several flanking bands were present (Grose & Hall, 1989; Moore et al., 1990); in the study where the signal caused a uniform increment over peak and dip regions (Hall & Grose, 1988), however, only one flanking band was present. In the present experiment, we again investigated CMR for signals resulting in a constant level change over all portions of the masking stimulus, but now we varied the number of flanking bands present, in order to make a more valid comparison to the studies in which the S/N ratio was much better in masker dip regions (e.g. Grose & Hall, 1989; Moore et al., 1990). The experiment also investigated the effect of adding a signal that would *decrease* the amplitude of the on-signal band with respect to the amplitudes of its comodulated flanking bands. This was intended to ascertain the generality of the finding of Moore et al. (1990) that decreases in the amplitude of the on-signal band do not result in CMR.

Methods

Subjects. Three subjects, who were experienced in CMR tasks and had normal audiograms, participated.

Stimuli. The signal was a 400-msec 20-Hz-wide noise band centred on 700 Hz. The signal had a cosine-squared rise/fall time of 50 msec. In the baseline condition, the masker was a single 20-Hz-wide noise band centred on 700 Hz and had a waveform that was identical to that of the signal. The signal was added either in phase or out of phase (180° phase shift derived via an operational amplifier) to the masker (resulting in either an amplitude increment or decrement in the masker level). There were four conditions in which a single flanking band was added (at 500, 600, 800, or 900 Hz). There were two conditions in which a pair of flanking bands were added (either at 600 and 800 Hz, or at 500 and 900 Hz). There were two conditions in which four flanking bands were added (either at 500, 600, 800, and 900 Hz, or at 400, 500, 900, and 1000 Hz). Finally, there were two conditions in which six flanking bands were added (either at 400, 500, 600, 800, 900, and 1000 Hz, or at 300, 400, 500, 900, 1000, and 1100 Hz). Pilot data were also collected for cases where the flanking bands were not comodulated with the on-signal band. These thresholds were very similar to those obtained for the condition where only the on-signal band was present. Therefore, thresholds were not obtained for non-comodulated flanking bands in the actual experiment.

Noise bands were created using a multiplication/filtering method. First, a multiband noise stimulus having bands centred on 300, 400, 500, 600, 800, 900, 1000, and 1100 Hz was created by multiplying (Analog Devices AD534LH) a digitally-synthesized complex tone composed of 3300, 3400, 3500, 3600, 3800, 3900, 4000, and 4100 Hz by a bandpass noise from 2990 to 3010 Hz. The bandpass noise was derived by digitally filtering wideband noise (IHR noise generator), using an IHR Universal Digital Filter (Trinder, 1983). Following multiplication, the upper sidebands were filtered out, leaving 20-Hz wide bands centred on the frequencies mentioned above. These bands were recorded digitally on tape (using a Sony VCR in conjunction with a digital PCM unit). In order to create the comodulated band centred on the signal frequency (700 Hz), a 3700-Hz pure tone was multiplied by the same bandpass noise (2990–3010 Hz), with the upper sideband again being filtered out. The resulting 20-Hz-wide band centred on 700 Hz was recorded on the other channel of the tape recorder. The particular stimulus conditions were then created by digitally filtering the analog output of the VCR/PCM digital tape system. The two channels of the tape recorder were passed through two independent digital filters. Noise stimuli were presented continuously at a pressure spectrum level of approximately 50 dB.

Procedure. Thresholds were determined using a 3AFC three-down, one-up adaptive procedure, estimating the 79.4% detection threshold (Levitt, 1971). An initial step-size of 8 dB was reduced to 4 dB after two reversals, and further reduced to 2 dB after two more reversals. A threshold run was stopped after 12 reversals, and the average of the last eight reversals was taken as the threshold for a run. Four threshold runs were averaged to compute the final threshold, unless the range of the runs was greater than 3 dB; in that case, a fifth run was obtained and included in the average. Each trial was preceded by a 300-msec warning light. Each interval was marked by a 400-msec light. The inter-stimulus interval was 300 msec. Visual feedback was provided after each response. Stimuli were delivered to the right ear by means of a TDH 49 earphone. Subjects were seated in a double-walled sound-attenuating booth.

Results and Discussion

Figure 1 shows average results for three listeners for conditions in which the signal resulted in an energy increment. For the sake of clarity, results are graphed separately in terms of whether the flanking bands most proximal to the signal frequency were 100 Hz (left panel) or 200 Hz (right panel) away from the signal frequency. The dashed line indicates the threshold for the 700-Hz masker band alone, and CMR is defined as a reduction in threshold (in dB) from this baseline. For the case of one or two flanking bands, the data show a proximity effect, with larger CMRs occurring for flanking bands located relatively close to the signal frequency (e.g. CMRs from about 3 to 5 dB for 200-Hz spacing, but from about 7 to 8 dB for 100-Hz spacing).

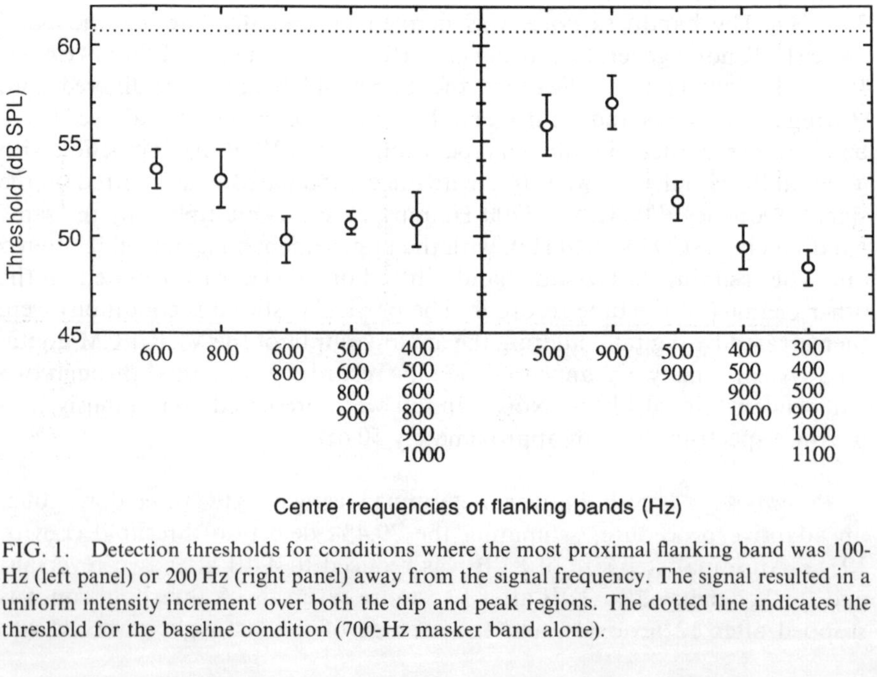

FIG. 1. Detection thresholds for conditions where the most proximal flanking band was 100-Hz (left panel) or 200 Hz (right panel) away from the signal frequency. The signal resulted in a uniform intensity increment over both the dip and peak regions. The dotted line indicates the threshold for the baseline condition (700-Hz masker band alone).

When more than three flanking bands were present, the effect of proximity was small or absent. In general, the results show an increase in CMR with increasing numbers of flanking bands present, with a maximum CMR of about 10–12 dB for six flanking bands present. This result indicates that the differences between data for the case where the signal causes a uniform increment over envelope peak dip regions of the envelope, and the case where the signal causes an increment only in the peak regions of the envelope are not related to the number of flanking bands present: when a relatively large number of flanking bands are present, large CMRs occur for a signal that causes a uniform increment, whereas no CMR or a negative CMR occurs when the signal results in an increment only in the peak regions of the envelope (Grose & Hall, 1989; Moore et al., 1990). Considering these factors alone, the most parsimonious interpretation of the present results is that only that part of the signal occurring in the dip regions of the envelope contributes to the CMRs observed.

Figure 2 shows average results for three listeners for conditions in which the signal resulted in an energy decrement. Again, results are graphed separately in terms of whether the flanking bands most proximal to the signal frequency were 100 Hz (left panel) or 200 Hz (right panel) away from the signal frequency. The most striking difference between these results and those shown in Figure 1 (level increment) is that CMR shows no apparent increase

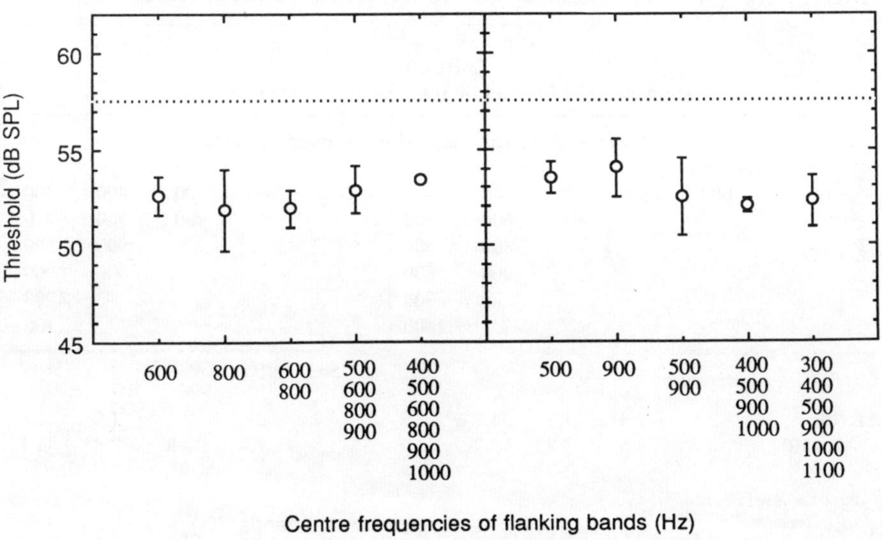

FIG. 2. Detection thresholds for conditions where the most proximal flanking band was 100-Hz (left panel) or 200 Hz (right panel) away from the signal frequency. The signal resulted in a uniform intensity decrement over both the dip and peak regions. The dotted line indicates the threshold for the baseline condition (700-Hz masker band alone).

as the number of flanking bands increases. However, in all cases where flanking bands were present, positive CMRs occurred. This result is somewhat paradoxical when viewed along with the results of Moore et al. (1990). They found that when the signal resulted in a decrease in level in either the peak or the dip of the envelope, no CMR was obtained. We will return to this issue in the general discussion.

The main finding of this experiment was that substantial CMRs occurred both for uniform increments and uniform decrements in level for the context of multiple comodulated flanking noise bands. However, a comparison of the CMR magnitudes for the two cases (level increment versus level decrement) is also of some interest. In Table 1, the data are presented in terms of the level change in dB (increment or decrement) associated with detection threshold. The relatively poor level discrimination in the baseline condition (4.9 dB ΔL for an increment and -6.6 dB ΔL for an intensity decrement) is consistent with previous studies employing narrowband noise stimuli (Bos & de Boer, 1966; Hall & Grose, 1988). The CMRs shown in Table 1 are calculated by subtracting the ΔL in the experimental condition from the ΔL in the baseline condition. This method of calculating CMR is atypical but is useful for comparing CMRs resulting from level increments versus level decrements. For the case of a single flanking band present, the CMRs are larger for the decrement case; however, when more than one flanking band was present, CMRs were similar for increments or decrements. Future research on stimuli

TABLE 1
Change in Level Caused by the Signal at Threshold (ΔL)

	Centre Frequency(ies) of Noise Band(s) (Hz)									
	600	800	600 800	500 600 800 900	400 500 600 800 900 1000	500	900	500 900	400 500 900 1000	300 400 500 900 1000 1100
Case of a level increment										
ΔL (dB)	2.5	2.4	1.7	1.8	1.9	3.2	3.5	2.1	1.6	1.5
CMR (dB)	2.4	2.5	3.2	3.2	3.0	1.8	1.4	2.8	3.4	3.4
Case of a level decrement										
ΔL (dB)	−3.1	−2.8	−2.8	−3.3	−3.5	−3.5	−3.2	−3.1	−2.9	−3.0
CMR (dB)	3.5	3.8	3.8	3.3	3.1	3.1	3.4	3.5	3.7	3.6

Note: CMR is calculated re ΔL in the baseline condition (4.9 dB increment, or 6.6 dB decrement).

similar to the above but also employing typical Profile Analysis parameters would be of interest from the standpoint of exploring commonalities between CMR and Profile Analysis.

The depiction of the data in terms of level change (Table 1) shows that the level discrimination was generally better for level increments. The literature is relatively sparse on the question of the relative sensitivity of the auditory system to increments versus decrements in level. Forrest and Green (1987) found that the just-detectable change in level was very similar for increments and decrements, whereas the data of Irwin and Purdy (1982) suggest that increments in a noise band are more detectable than are decrements.

PRELIMINARY EXPERIMENTS ON THE DETECTION OF SIGNALS IN ENVELOPE PEAK REGIONS

We conducted two preliminary experiments that investigated further the behaviour of CMR for signals presented in envelope peak regions. Moore et al. (1990) suggested that the reason no CMR was obtained when signals were added in the peak region of an AM stimulus might be that detection performance in the baseline condition (no flanking band present) was already quite good for such stimuli—that is, the detection of an increment in a regular, sinusoidally modulating stimulus is sufficiently fine that little room is left for improvement due to the addition of comodulated flanking bands. We therefore attempted to test the possibility of obtaining CMR for envelope peak regions using noise maskers, rather than regular sinusoidal AM maskers. Our aim was to maintain the paradigm of Experiment 1—that is, the same stimulus was used as both the signal and the baseline (on-signal) masker, such that the signal always added in phase with the masker. Both preliminary experiments indicated an absence of CMR when the signal occurred only during the peaks of the masker envelope. However, each of the two procedures presented certain limitations.

Preliminary Study 1 Frozen Noise Stimuli

Method

Three bands of noise were digitally generated using additive synthesis with 0.5-Hz spectral spacing. The sampling rate was 2500 Hz, and the duration of each waveform was 2 sec. The centre frequencies of the noisebands were 500, 700, and 900 Hz, and each had a bandwidth of 20 Hz. In generating the first noiseband, each sinusoid had its amplitude drawn from a Rayleigh distribution and its phase from a rectangular distribution. For the remaining two noisebands, the same amplitude and phase spectra were employed (but shifted up in frequency). The resultant triplet of Gaussian noisebands therefore had comodulating envelopes. The two signal conditions were derived from the noiseband centred at 700 Hz. In the "peak" condition, the original 700-Hz band was stripped of segments in which the amplitude of the envelope fell below 50% of the peak value by setting these segments to zero amplitude. The temporal locations and fine structure of the remaining portions were identical to the original noiseband. Similarly, in the "dip" condition, only those portions of the original 700-Hz noiseband that had envelope amplitudes less than 25% of the peak amplitude were retained. Again the temporal locations and fine structures of these segments were unchanged from the original waveform.

The two signal conditions were presented in each of two masker conditions. One masker consisted of the triplet of comodulating noisebands, the other consisted of the 700-Hz noiseband alone. In each condition, the masker and signal waveforms were output synchronously and continuously through two channels of a DAC, resulting in a 0.5-Hz periodicity. After lowpass filtering at 1000 Hz, the parallel analog waveforms were fed into two identical digital filters that were set to pass 30-Hz wide bands centred on the frequency(ies) of interest; that is, either 700 Hz alone, or 500 + 700 + 900 Hz. The sampling rate of the filters was 2500 Hz, with 512 taps per filter. The purpose of the filters was to remove energy "splatter" in the signal due to the abrupt transitions of the nulled segments in the waveform. The outputs from the filters were then lowpass filtered at 1000 Hz and, after appropriate attenuation, mixed and sent to one earphone of a TDH 49 headset. The masker pressure spectrum level was 50 dB.

Masked threshold for the signal was measured according to the 3AFC procedure described previously. The duration of each interval in the forced-choice procedure was 500 msec. During the target interval, the signal waveform was gated on for 500 msec, including a 50-msec cosine-squared rise/fall time. Because the gating sequence was not synchronized to the periodicity of the cyclical noise, the portion of the signal waveform that was presented in any target interval varied randomly. Also, as the maximum duration of signal waveform that was devoid of energy was 431 msec, it was possible on rare occasions for a target interval to contain minimal signal energy. Three listeners with normal hearing participated in the preliminary study. All were experienced in psychoacoustic listening tasks.

Results

The pattern of results was the same for all three listeners and showed two distinct effects: (1) with the placement of the signal only in the peaks of the masker, there was essentially no difference in threshold between the single-band masker and the 3-band comodulated masker (mean CMR = 0.8 dB); (2)

with the placement of the signal in the dips of the masker, threshold was markedly lower in the 3-band comodulated masker than in the single-band masker (mean CMR = 9.3 dB). However, the intensity increment at threshold for the peak placement of the signal in the single-band masker was only about 2 dB, which was rather better than the 5 dB threshold observed for intensity discrimination in continuous random noise. (The intensity increment at threshold for the dip placement of the signal in the single-band masker was about 1.5 dB.) This suggested that perhaps performance for peak placement was sufficiently exquisite in the single-band masker that further improvement with comodulation cues was not possible. The low threshold may have been due to slight spectral cues resulting from the marginal energy splatter passed by the digital filter centred on the signal. However, another possibility arises from the listeners' observation that the temporal pattern of the cyclical noise became increasingly familiar with practice, such that slight intensity deviations from it became more salient.

In an effort to circumvent the possible learning effect associated with the use of frozen noise, it was decided to repeat the general paradigm but to use continuous random noise in the generation of the stimuli.

Preliminary Study 2
Multiplied Analog Noise Stimuli

Method

A triplet of comodulating narrow bands of (non-Gaussian) noise was generated by multiplying a single lowpass noise (0–20 Hz) by pure tones of 500, 700, and 900 Hz. The two masking conditions consisted of either the three bands presented together or the band centred at 700-Hz presented alone. In either case, the band centred at 700-Hz was also used as the signal but was only presented during peaks in the waveform envelope. Thus the 700-Hz noiseband was only added to itself in phase during the peaks of the waveform. This selective presentation was achieved by synchronously rectifying the lowpass noise (which defined the waveform envelope) and adjusting its level such that only the major peaks in the waveform were of sufficient magnitude to trigger an electronic gate through which the 700-Hz noiseband signal was channelled.

In all other respects the procedure was the same as that reported for the first preliminary study. Three listeners with normal hearing participated.

Results

The results for the three listeners exhibited the same trend: thresholds for the peak placement of the signal were not consistently different between the single-band masker and the three-band masker. This would suggest an absence of CMR when the signal, derived from a random noise, is added to itself only in the peaks of the stimulus. However, this conclusion must be moderated in the present preliminary study because of the marked intrasubject variability. This variability appeared to be due to the random occurrence of the signal within the target interval—that is, the occurrence of a waveform peak (and hence the presentation of the signal) was completely random with respect to the occurrence of the target interval, and, in some instances, the signal did not occur during a target interval. Because of this limitation a third stimulus configuration was constructed to address the question of whether a CMR exists for peak placement of the signal.

EXPERIMENT 2

Detection of Tone Burst Signals as a Function of their Placement in the Envelope Cycle of Modulated Masking Noise

The two preliminary studies described above gave some suggestion of an absence of CMR when the signal occurred only in the peaks of a modulated masking noise. However, those techniques proved limited because of the learning effect associated with periodic frozen noise and because of the sporadic occurrence of the signal in ongoing random noise. In order to overcome these limitations, a third technique was developed whereby a train of tone bursts was placed in either the peaks or the dips of a square-wave modulated noise and threshold measured as a function of the bandwidth of the noise.

Method

A continuous train of tone bursts centred on 700 Hz was generated by outputting a single digitally-generated burst repetitively through one channel of a DAC. The duration of the burst at the half-amplitude points was 25 msec with a cosine-squared rise/fall time of 25 msec, and the inter-burst interval was 50 msec. This resulted in a burst-to-burst periodicity of 10 Hz. The stimulus was generated at a sampling rate of 5000 Hz and anti-alias filtered at 2000 Hz. On the second channel of the DAC, a single cycle of a 10-Hz square wave was synchronously output. The square wave was used to modulate a broadband noise (0–5000 Hz), which was subsequently filtered to the desired bandwidth by means of a digital filter (IHR Universal). The bandwidths investigated were 100, 250, and 2500 Hz. The 100-Hz bandwidth was chosen because it is approximately the same as the equivalent rectangular bandwidth (ERB) of the auditory filter at 700 Hz (Moore & Glasberg, 1983). Therefore thresholds obtained with this masker would be accounted for entirely by within-band effects. The bandwidths of 250 Hz and 2500 Hz were chosen because they were considerably wider than the ERB at 700 Hz; therefore comparisons between thresholds for these maskers with the threshold for the 100-Hz wide masker would provide an indication of the across-frequency effect (CMR). By varying the phase relation between the digital square wave and the tone burst cycle, the train of tone bursts could be presented either in the peaks or in the dips of the modulated noise. As a comparison to the peak-placement and dip-placement results of the tone-burst train, a parallel set of conditions was also run where the signal was a 700-Hz pure tone. The pure tone had the same peak amplitude as the tone burst. Finally, to provide a reference for the thresholds in modulated noise, conditions were also constructed where the two signal types were presented in unmodulated noise.

In all other respects the procedure was the same as that described previously. The presentation intervals of the 3AFC were 400 msec in duration, including a 50-msec rise/fall time. Three listeners experienced in psychoacoustic tasks participated.

Results and Discussion

Figure 3 summarizes the masked threshold results. The results across the three subjects were very similar, so average data are shown along with standard deviations (error bars). First consider the data for the 400-msec pure tone signal, presented in either unmodulated noise (open squares) or modulated noise (closed squares). As expected, for the unmodulated case

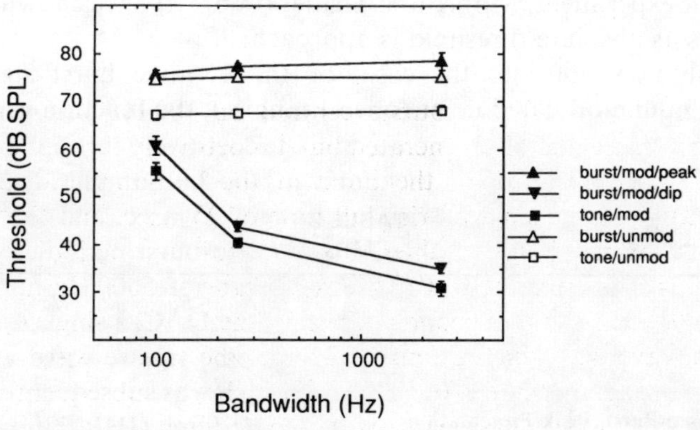

FIG. 3. Mean threshold as a function of masker bandwidth. Error bars show plus and minus one standard deviation. Parameters are signal type (triangles = 25-msec bursts, squares = 400-msec pure tones); masker type (filled symbols = modulated noise, unfilled symbols = unmodulated noise); and signal temporal position (non-inverted triangle = peak region, inverted triangle = dip region).

threshold changes negligibly as bandwidth increases (since the narrowest bandwidth is approximately the same as the ERB at the signal frequency). In the modulated noise case, the tone threshold was lower than for the unmodulated case even for the 100-Hz bandwidth (by about 12 dB). Because the noise bandwidth is approximately the same as the ERB, the lower threshold in modulated noise must be due to within-channel "listening in the dips" rather than to CMR (Carlyon et al., 1989; Hall & Grose, 1989). However, the figure shows that the modulated noise threshold decreases appreciably as the masker bandwidth increases beyond the ERB, this effect apparently being due largely to across-frequency processing. We take as a measure of CMR the threshold in modulated noise for the 100-Hz bandwidth minus the threshold in modulated noise for the 250-Hz bandwidth and the 2500-Hz bandwidth. This results in CMRs of 14.9 dB and 24.4 dB, respectively (see Table 2). In the terminology of Carlyon et al. (1989), this measure of CMR is defined as $NOCUE_{mod} - CUE_{mod}$. Carlyon et al. (1989) used a similar approach but defined CMR as the difference in thresholds between the unmodulated and modulated wideband noise conditions ($CUE_{unmod} - CUE_{mod}$), adjusted by the difference between the unmodulated and modulated thresholds in the narrow-band condition ($NOCUE_{unmod} - NOCUE_{mod}$). In the present case this would have yielded approximately the same measure of CMR as the CUE_{unmod} threshold and the $NOCUE_{unmod}$ threshold were very similar. The present CMRs are markedly larger than those found by Carlyon et al. (1989) for an 11-Hz modulation rate. Two reasons may underlie this. First, their "ERB-width" masker was 400 Hz wide (centred at 4000 Hz), which was likely to have rendered the dips more clearly defined in within-channel analysis. Second, their masker spectrum level was 30 dB lower than the present experiment; Moore and Shailer (in press) have shown that CMR diminishes as absolute threshold is approached.

We will now consider the case for the 25-msec burst signal. When presented in unmodulated noise (open triangles), the function is parallel but

TABLE 2
CMRs

	Noise Bandwidth (Hz)	
	250	2500
25-msec Burst, Peak Presentation	−1.7	−2.7
25-msec Burst, Dip Presentation	17.2	25.7
400-msec Tone, Modulated noise	14.9	24.4

CMRs = threshold in modulated noise for 100-Hz bandwidth minus threshold in modulated noise for 250-Hz and 2500-Hz bandwidths.

approximately 7 dB higher than that for the 400-msec pure tone in unmodulated noise. This difference is probably related to the temporal integration property of the ear. Considering now the thresholds in modulated noise for the 25-msec bursts presented in the dip portions (inverted, filled triangles), it can be seen that the functions are again roughly parallel but higher (by about 5 dB) than the function for the 400-msec pure tone signal. Thus the CMR is again substantial for the 25-msec burst case, when bursts are presented in the masker dips. However, the function of greatest importance to the present study is that for the 25-msec bursts presented in the masker peaks (non-inverted filled triangles). The figure indicates that there was no hint of a masking release for this function. In fact, the thresholds for the 25-msec bursts presented in the masker peaks were actually higher than for the unmodulated noise case—that is, as in the data of Moore et al. (1990), there was some evidence of a negative CMR for the case of signals presented in masker peaks.

GENERAL DISCUSSION

The Role of Energy in Masker Peak and Dip Regions

A consistent finding of the present study was that CMR fails to occur for signals presented in the peak regions of the masker envelope, even though noise maskers were used to remove the possibility of an excessively low baseline threshold. As noted previously, the dip listening model (Buus, 1985) is generally consistent with the above result, whereas the correlation model and EC model are not. However, the dip listening model does not predict the finding of Experiment 1 that substantial CMRs can occur when the S/N ratio is no better in the dip regions than in the peak regions—that is, information provided by the flanking bands about the location of noise dips could not effectively improve the S/N ratio, and thus no CMR would be predicted by the dip-listening hypothesis. In order to account for all of the present data, it would have to be assumed that it is the dip regions that provide the information resulting in CMR, but that it is an across-frequency comparison of information contained in the dip regions that results in the CMR, rather than a simple integration of energy within the dip portions of the on-signal band (as proposed by the dip-listening model). An alternative point of view is that CMR is based upon more than one cue, and that more than one mechanism accounts for CMR. By this account, the CMR obtained in Experiment 1 could be viewed as a special case of CMR where the simple dip listening mechanism does not contribute; here, CMR could be accounted for by envelope subtraction without prior equalization.

It is not immediately obvious why the auditory system fails to obtain a CMR for signals present in the peak region of the masker. One important factor to consider, however, is that the situation where a signal affects only the peak portions of a masker is extremely unlikely to occur in a real-life environment. It is much more likely that a signal will also affect the dip portions of the envelope. Under that circumstance, if a signal is intense enough to alter the masker waveform in the peak portions, the masker waveform will be altered much more substantially in the dip portions. It is therefore possible that the mechanism responsible for CMR has evolved to be sensitive only to those across-frequency differences in envelope that occur in the envelope dip regions. A related possibility is that information in the peak regions of the envelope is available to the CMR mechanism, but is rejected when there are no across-frequency envelope differences also apparent in the dip regions. Both possibilities have the disadvantage of being more processing-intensive than a mechanism that performs a single across-frequency analysis on the entire envelope. That is, the auditory system must identify and limit analysis to the dip regions and/or determine the relation between information in the peak regions with that in the dip regions. The added complexity would, however, result in a possible decrease in false alarms without materially decreasing sensitivity. This is because an apparent change that occurs only in the peak regions of a background masking sound is unlikely to represent the occurrence of a separate sound source, and the S/N ratio is likely to be more favourable in the dip regions in any case.

Another possibility that would account for the lack of CMR for signals occurring only in envelope peak regions was suggested by Moore et al. (1990). They suggested that the poor performance obtained for signals presented in masker peaks might be related to the modulation detection interference (MDI) described by Yost and Sheft (1989). Yost and Sheft found that the threshold for detecting amplitude modulation at one frequency was impaired by the presence of amplitude modulation at a flanking frequency. Moore et al. (1990) suggested that this "across-channel masking" phenomenon might account for the absent or negative CMR occurring in the case where the signal was added to the peak region of the envelope. For example, the energy fluctuations of the flanking bands might actually blunt sensitivity to a fluctuation change in the peak region of the on-signal band. This interpretation receives some support in the present data, as the threshold was slightly higher for the case where the 25-msec bursts were added to the peak regions of the modulated noise than when they were added to continuous noise (see Figure 3).

CMR for Level Decrements

In Experiment 1 it was found that CMRs occurred for cases where the signal resulted in a level decrement at the signal frequency, and it was noted that this result was somewhat difficult to reconcile with the data of Moore et al. (1990). They examined cases where a signal resulted in a level decrement in either the peak region, or in the dip region of the envelope, and found no evidence for a CMR in either case. This result appears inconsistent with the present finding that substantial CMRs exist when a decrement occurs in both the peaks and dips of the on-signal masker. Our first line of reasoning concerning this discrepancy arose from the subjective reports of our listeners as to the salient cue in the decrement detection task. The subjects reported that detection of the decrement in the comodulated condition was unique in that instead of hearing the signal in the signal interval, they heard the pitch of the signal band surface abruptly in the inter-stimulus interval that followed the signal interval. The percept was similar to the emergence of a single component in a complex tone brought about by pulsing it on and off. This report suggested to us that the CMR obtained for signal decrements could be based largely upon a sequential comparison of across-frequency energy (during versus after the signal interval), rather than upon a simultaneous comparison of across-frequency energy (which has been assumed to underlie most CMR effects). Thus the detection of decrements in a CMR paradigm might be a rather special case. The above interpretation is consistent with the fact that no CMR was found by Moore et al. (1990) for the case of level decrements as these investigators used gated maskers that resulted in silent interstimulus intervals. However, a prediction arising from this interpretation is that a CMR would not have been evident in our data if our task also had involved gated maskers. In a brief post-hoc experiment, we put this prediction to the test but observed CMRs of the same magnitude as for the continuous masker; thus this hypothesis was inadequate to reconcile our findings with those of Moore et al. We next considered that a release from suppression may have contributed to our results in the comodulated condition—that is, as the signal band was decremented, its suppression of the comodulated flanking bands would have diminished, and the pitches of the flanking bands may therefore have become more salient. This hypothesis was tested by presenting the flanking bands to the contralateral ear (thereby negating the possibility of a peripheral suppression component), but a substantial (5 dB) masking release continued to be present. Thus the apparent inconsistency between the results of Moore et al. (1990) and those of the present study remains unresolved. Further work is required to deduce the nature of the mechanism(s) underlying the masking release associated with a decrement detection task.

Conclusions

1. Substantial CMRs occur for cases where multiple comodulated flanking bands are present, and the signal results in either a level increment or level decrement at the signal frequency. CMRs obtained in these conditions are not consistent with a dip-listening hypothesis. However, this does not rule

out the possibility that the dip-listening hypothesis accounts for CMR in conditions where the cues for CMR are less impoverished.

2. CMR fails to occur for signals presented in the peak regions of the masker envelope, even when noise maskers are used in order to remove the possibility of an excessively low baseline threshold.

3. The failure to obtain CMR for signals presented in envelope peak regions indicates either that information in peak regions is not included in the across/frequency analysis underlying CMR, or that in order for information in peak regions to be utilized, across-frequency envelope differences must also exist in the dip regions of the envelope.

REFERENCES

Bos, C.E. & de Boer, E. (1966). Masking and discrimination. *Journal of the Acoustical Society of America, 39*, 708–715.

Bregman, A.S. (1978). The formation of auditory streams. In J. Requin (Ed.), *Attention and performance VII*. Hillside, NJ: Lawrence Erlbaum Associates, Inc.

Bregman, A.S., Abramson, J., Doehring, P., & Darwin, C.J. (1985). Spectral integration based on common amplitude modulation. *Perception & Psychophysics, 37*, 483–493.

Bregman, A.S. & Campbell, J. (1971). Primary auditory stream segregation and perception of order in rapid sequences of tones. *Journal of Experimental Psychology, 89*, 244–249.

Buus, S. (1985). Release from masking caused by envelope fluctuations. *Journal of the Acoustical Society of America, 78*, 1958–1965.

Carlyon, R.P., Buus, S., & Florentine, M. (1989). Comodulation masking release for three types of modulator as a function of modulation rate. *Hearing Research, 42*, 37–46.

Cohen, M.F. (1989). Increased CMR resulting from lowered levels of masker band. *Journal of the Acoustical Society of America, 86*, 598.

Cohen, M.F. & Schubert, E.D. (1987). Influence of place synchrony on detection of a sinusoid. *Journal of the Acoustical Society of America, 81*, 452–458.

Dannenbring, G.L. & Bregman, A.S. (1978). Streaming vs. fusion of sinusoidal components of complex tones. *Perception & Psychophysics, 24*, 369–376.

Darwin, C.J. (1983). Auditory processing and speech perception. In H. Bouma & H. Bouwhuis (Eds.), *Attention and performance X*. Hillside, NJ: Lawrence Erlbaum Associates, Inc.

Durlach, N.I. (1963). Equalization and cancellation theory of binaural masking-level differences. *Journal of the Acoustical Society of America, 35*, 1206–1218.

Fletcher, H. (1940). Auditory Patterns. *Reviews of Modern Physics, 12*, 47–65.

Forrest, T.G. & Green, D.M. (1987). Detection of partially filled gaps in noise and the temporal modulation transfer function. *Journal of the Acoustical Society of America, 82*, 1933–1943.

Green, D.M. (1988). *Profile analysis*. New York: Oxford University Press.

Green, D.M., Kidd, G., & Picardi, M.C. (1983). Successive vs. simultaneous comparison in auditory intensity discrimination. *Journal of the Acoustical Society of America, 73*, 639–643.

Green, D.M., Mason, C.R., & Kidd, G.R. (1984). Profile analysis: Critical bands and duration. *Journal of the Acoustical Society of America, 75*, 1163–1167.

Green, D.M., McKey, M.J., & Licklider, J.C.R. (1959). Detection of a pulsed sinusoid in noise as a function of frequency. *Journal of the Acoustical Society of America, 31*, 1446–1452.

Grose, J.H. & Hall, J.W. (1989). Comodulation masking release using SAM tonal complex maskers: Effects of modulation depth and signal position. *Journal of the Acoustical Society of America, 85*, 1276–1284.

Haggard, M.P., Hall, J.W., & Grose, J.H. (1990). Comodulation masking release as a function of bandwidth and test frequency. *Journal of the Acoustical Society of America, 88*, 113–118.

Haggard, M.P., Harvey, A.D.G., & Carlyon, R.P. (1985). Peripheral and central components of comodulation masking release. *Journal of the Acoustical Society of America, 78*, S63.

Hall, J.W. (1986). The effect of across-frequency differences in masking level on spectro-temporal pattern analysis. *Journal of the Acoustical Society of America, 79*, 781–787.

Hall, J.W. (1987). Experiments on comodulation masking release. In W. Yost & C. Watson (Eds.), *Auditory processing of complex sounds*. Hillsdale, NJ: Lawrence Erlbaum Associates, Inc.

Hall, J.W., Cokely, J., & Grose, J.H. (1988). Combined monaural and binaural masking release. *Journal of the Acoustical Society of America, 83*, 1839–1845.

Hall, J.W. & Fernandes, M.A. (1983). The effect of random intensity fluctuation on monaural and binaural detection. *Journal of the Acoustical Society of America, 74*, 1200–1203.

Hall, J.W. & Grose, J.H. (1988). Comodulation masking release: Evidence for multiple cues. *Journal of the Acoustical Society of America, 84*, 1669–1675.

Hall, J.W. & Grose, J.H. (1989). Spectro-temporal analysis in cochlear hearing impairment: Effects of frequency selectivity, temporal resolution, signal frequency, and rate of modulation. *Journal of the Acoustical Society of America, 85*, 2550–2562.

Hall, J.W. & Grose, J.H. (1990). Comodulation masking release and auditory grouping. *Journal of the Acoustical Society of America, 88*, 119–125.

Hall, J.W., Grose, J.H., & Haggard, M.P. (1988). Comodulation masking release for multi-component signals. *Journal of the Acoustical Society of America, 83*, 677–686.

Hall, J.W., Grose, J.H., & Haggard, M.P. (1990). Effects of flanking band proximity, number, and modulation pattern on comodulation masking release. *Journal of the Acoustical Society of America, 87*, 269–283.

Hall, J.W. & Haggard, M.P. (1983). Co-modulation—A principle for auditory pattern analysis in speech. *International Conference on Acoustics*, 69–71.

Hall, J.W., Haggard, M.P., Fernandes, M.A. (1984a). Detection in noise by spectro-temporal pattern analysis. *Journal of the Acoustical Society of America, 76*, 50–56.

Hall, J.W., Haggard, M.P., & Harvey, A.D.G. (1984b). Release from masking through ipsilateral and contralateral comodulation of a flanking band. *Journal of the Acoustical Society of America, 76*, S76.

Irwin, R.J. & Purdy, S.C. (1982). The minimum detectable duration of auditory signals for normal and hearing-impaired listeners. *Journal of the Acoustical Society of America, 71*, 967–974.

Levitt, H. (1971). Transformed up-down methods in psychoacoustics. *Journal of the Acoustical Society of America, 49*, 467–477.

Margolis, R.H. & Small, A.M. (1975). The measurement of critical masking bands. *Journal of Speech and Hearing Research, 40*, 1414–1419.

McAdams, S. (1984). The auditory image: A metaphor for musical and psychological research on auditory organization. In R. Crozier & A. Chapman (Eds.), *Cognitive processes in the perception of art*. Amsterdam: North Holland.

McFadden, D. (1986). Comodulation masking release: Effects of varying the level, duration, and time delay of the cue band. *Journal of the Acoustical Society of America, 80*, 1658–1667.

McFadden, D., Jeffress, L.A., & Ermey, H.L. (1971). Differences of interaural phase and level in detection and lateralization: 250 Hz. *Journal of the Acoustical Society of America, 50*, 1484–1493.

Moore, B.C.J. (1990). Comodulation masking release: Spectro-temporal pattern analysis in hearing. *British Journal of Audiology, 24*, 131–137.

Moore, B.C.J. & Emmerich, D.S. (1990). Monaural envelope correlation perception, revisited:

Effects of bandwidth, frequency separation, duration, and relative level of the noise bands. *The Journal of the Acoustical Society of America, 87*, 2628–2633.

Moore, B.C.J. & Glasberg, B.R. (1983). Suggested formulae for calculating auditory filter bandwidths and excitation patterns. *Journal of the Acoustical Society of America, 74*, 750–753.

Moore, B.C.J., Glasberg, B.R., & Schooneveldt, G.P. (1990). Across-channel masking and comodulation masking release. *Journal of the Acoustical Society of America, 87*, 1683–1694.

Moore, B.C.J., Hall, J.W., Grose, J.H., & Schooneveldt, G.P. (1990). Accounting for the variability in CMR. *Journal of the Acoustical Society of America, 88*, 1694–1702.

Moore, B.C.J. & Schooneveldt, G.P. (1990). Comodulation masking release as a function of bandwidth and time delay between on-frequency and flanking-band maskers. *Journal of the Acoustical Society of America, 88*, 725–731.

Moore, B.C.J. & Shailer, M.J. (in press). Comodulation masking release as a function of level. *Journal of the Acoustical Society of America.*

Patterson, R.D. (1976). Auditory filter shapes derived with noise stimuli. *Journal of the Acoustical Society of America, 59*, 640–654.

Patterson, R.D. & Nimmo-Smith, I. (1980). Off-frequency listening and auditory filter asymmetry. *Journal of the Acoustical Society of America, 67*, 229–245.

Richards, V.M. (1987). Monaural envelope correlation perceptions. *Journal of the Acoustical Society of America, 82*, 1621–1630.

Scharf, B. (1970). The critical band. In J.V. Tobias (Ed.), *Foundations of modern auditory theory*. New York: Academic Press.

Schooneveldt, G.P. & Moore, B.C.J. (1987). Comodulation masking release (CMR): Effects of signal frequency, flanking band frequency, masker bandwidth, flanking band level, and monotic versus dichotic presentation of the flanking band. *Journal of the Acoustical Society of America, 82*, 1944–1956.

Schooneveldt, G.P. & Moore, B.C.J. (1989a). Comodulation masking release (CMR) as a function of masker bandwidth, modulator bandwidth, and signal duration. *Journal of the Acoustical Society of America, 85*, 273–281.

Schooneveldt, G.P. & Moore, B.C.J. (1989b). Comodulation masking release (CMR) for various monaural and binaural combinations of the signal, on-frequency, and flanking bands. *Journal of the Acoustical Society of America, 85*, 262–272.

Spiegel, M.R. & Green, D.M. (1981). The effect of duration on masker profile analysis. *Journal of the Acoustical Society of America, 70*, S86.

Trinder, J.R. (1983). Hardware–software configuration for high performance digital filtering in real time. *Proceedings of the IEEE International Conference on Acoustics and Speech Signal Processing, 2*, 687–690.

Wegel, R.L. & Lane, C.E. (1924). The auditory masking of one pure tone by another and its probable relation to the dynamics of the inner ear. *Physics Review, 23*, 266–285.

Yost, W.A. & Sheft, S. (1989). Across-critical-band processing of amplitude-modulated tones. *Journal of the Acoustical Society of America, 85*, 848–857.

Zwicker, E.B. (1974). On the psychophysical equivalent of tuning curves. In E. Zwicker & E. Terhardt (Eds.), *Facts and models in hearing*. Berlin: Springer-Verlag.

Revised manuscript received 30 November 1990

THE QUARTERLY JOURNAL OF EXPERIMENTAL PSYCHOLOGY, 1991, *43A* (3) 373–399

Spectral, Intensive, and Temporal Factors Influencing Overshoot

Sid P. Bacon and Michael A. Smith
Arizona State University, Tempe, Arizona, U.S.A.

Threshold was measured for a 10-msec, 4.0-kHz signal presented near the onset or in the temporal centre of a 400-msec noise masker. Overshoot, the difference (in dB) between these two thresholds, was seen only for masker bandwidths wider than a critical band. The threshold near masker onset, and hence overshoot, could be reduced by the presence of an additional noise that was presented continuously or gated on and off prior to masker onset. The spectral, intensive, and temporal properties of this effect were studied. When the additional noise was continuous and either bandpass filtered with a variable bandwidth or notch filtered with a variable notchwidth, the results indicated that energy *both* near and remote from the signal frequency contributed to the reduction in overshoot. The effect of this additional noise was highly dependent upon its relative level. When the additional noise was 400 msec in duration and the delay between its offset and the onset of the masker was varied, overshoot "recovered" to its maximum value within about 50 msec. Finally, as the duration of the additional noise was varied from 3 to 400 msec while the time between its offset and masker onset was fixed, the reduction in overshoot was virtually complete for durations of about 25–50 msec. The results are consistent with the notion that overshoot at least partly reflects peripheral adaptation, and that this adaptation is not restricted to the signal frequency channel but, rather, extends in both directions over several channels.

Scientists have been studying auditory masking for more than 100 years (e.g. Mayer, 1876), and the results from such experiments comprise a significant proportion of the literature on audition. Although the majority of studies have been concerned with the effects of intensity and frequency, many have been concerned with the effects of time. The importance of understanding the temporal properties of auditory masking is underscored by the fact that most

---

Requests for reprints should be sent to Sid P. Bacon, Department of Speech and Hearing Science, Arizona State University, Tempe, Arizona 85287–0102, U.S.A.

This work was supported by NIDCD Grant DC00424. We are grateful to David Reiter for his programming expertise. Bob Carlyon, Brian Moore, Gail Takahashi, and an anonymous reviewer provided helpful comments on an earlier version of this paper.

sounds in our natural environment are dynamic or time-varying—that is, they are characterized by rapid changes in amplitude or frequency or both, and thus a complete understanding of masking must include any time-dependent effects.

This paper is concerned with temporal effects that occur in the context of simultaneous masking—that is, masking in which the signal and masker overlap in time. It has been known for many years that the threshold for a brief tonal signal can improve as the onset of that signal is delayed relative to the onset of a longer duration *noise* masker (e.g., Samoilova, 1959; Scholl, 1962; Zwicker, 1965a, 1965b; Elliott, 1965, 1967, 1969; Fastl, 1976). This temporal effect, known as overshoot (Zwicker, 1965a), is most pronounced for signal frequencies above about 1.0–2.0 kHz (Zwicker, 1965a; Fastl, 1976). Although the size of the overshoot effect varies from subject to subject, it can be as large as 10–20 dB. A similar improvement in threshold can be observed when comparing the masking produced by a brief, gated masker with that produced by a continuous masker (Wier, Green, Hafter, & Burkhardt, 1977; Carlyon & Moore, 1986; Carlyon, 1987). Temporal effects in masking have been studied rather extensively of late (e.g. Carlyon, 1987; Moore, Poon, Bacon, & Glasberg, 1987; Carlyon & Sloan, 1987; McFadden, 1988, 1989; Champlin & McFadden, 1989; McFadden & Champlin, 1990; Bacon, 1990). Although this paper is concerned with temporal effects with noise maskers, we note that a considerable amount of attention has been devoted to temporal effects in masking by *sinusoidal* maskers (e.g. Green, 1969; Leshowitz & Cudahy, 1972, 1975; Soderquist, Carstens, & Frank, 1981; Bacon & Viemeister, 1985a, 1985b; Bacon & Moore, 1986a, 1986b, 1987; Kimberley, Nelson & Bacon, 1989; Bacon, Hedrick, & Grantham, 1989). The temporal effects observed for these maskers occur primarily when the masker frequency is greater than the signal frequency.

Green (1969) offered three possible explanations for his results on the difference in masking effectiveness between gated and continuous sinusoidal maskers, and, in general, for the overshoot effect: (1) splatter (or spread) of masker energy resulting from gating; (2) a narrowing of the critical band or auditory filter with time; and (3) neural adaptation. Green suggested that all three could contribute to some degree to his results. We consider each possible explanation below (also see McFadden & Wright, 1990, for a detailed discussion).

The splatter of masker energy can, in fact, elevate thresholds near masker onset when the masker is narrowband and presented away from the signal in frequency (Zwicker & Fastl, 1972; Leshowitz & Cudahy, 1975; Bacon & Viemeister, 1985a), and thus this could explain to some extent why Green's (rectangularly) gated masker produced considerably (up to 40 dB) more masking than his continuous masker. This problem of splatter can be avoided—without eliminating the temporal effect—by appropriately shaping the masker's onset and offset and thereby reducing considerably the amount of spread (Bacon & Viemeister, 1985a). For broadband maskers, splatter of masker energy is not considered a problem because gating does not significantly change the masker's long-term power spectrum.

A critical band or auditory filter that narrows with time would ultimately allow less overall noise power to interfere with the detection of a signal within its passband. There are ample data indicating that psychophysical frequency selectivity can improve with time (e.g. Scholl, 1962; Elliott, 1965, 1967; Bacon & Viemeister, 1985a; Bacon & Moore, 1986b; Kimberley et al., 1989; Carlyon, 1989; Wright, 1989; cf. Moore et al., 1987), and thus this explanation could account for at least some of the temporal effect observed in simultaneous masking. There are, however, certain aspects of the data on temporal effects that make such an explanation problematic (see McFadden & Wright, 1990). For one, it seems unlikely that the critical band could change by the factor of 10 that would be necessary to account for the 10-dB improvement in threshold that is often observed when a brief signal is moved from near the beginning to near the temporal centre of a noise masker.

Clearly the most popular explanation for overshoot is that it reflects short-term adaptation in auditory-nerve fibres tuned near the signal frequency (Smith & Zwislocki, 1975; Smith 1979). The response of most auditory-nerve fibres to a gated stimulus is characterized by an initial high probability of discharge followed by a rapid and then a more gradual decline to an asymptotic or steady-state value (e.g. Kiang, Watanabe, Thomas, & Clark, 1965). This gradual decline is referred to as "short-term adaptation." Smith and Zwislocki (1975) and Smith (1979) have shown that the response of an auditory-nerve fibre to a "masker" adapts over time, but that the response to a superimposed "signal" does not adapt; hence the neural signal-to-masker ratio—and presumably signal detectability—improves with time during masker presentation.

At present, a complete understanding of the auditory processing that underlies the temporal effects observed in simultaneous masking does not exist, nor is it even clear whether the same processing can account for the effects observed with both broadband and narrowband maskers. Nevertheless, it does seem likely that peripheral adaptation (Smith & Zwislocki, 1975; Smith, 1979) is involved. Of importance now in our efforts to understand overshoot is to determine whether additional processing is also involved, and if it is, to determine the nature of that processing.

One approach to studying overshoot involves presenting an *additional* noise stimulus either simultaneously with the noise masker or gated on and off prior to masker onset. Several studies have revealed that the presence of an additional noise can reduce or eliminate overshoot by lowering the threshold for a signal presented near the beginning of the masker (Zwicker, 1965a; Elliott, 1969; Carlyon, 1987; McFadden, 1989). Assuming that the auditory processing that is responsible for this improvement in threshold, or masking release, is the same processing that is responsible for the improvement in threshold that occurs during the course of masker presentation (i.e. for the overshoot effect), it should be possible to manipulate various aspects of this additional stimulus in order to characterize certain properties of overshoot. This, in turn, could provide insight into the mechanisms underlying the effect.

Zwicker (1965a) used a continuous broadband noise as an additional stimulus and examined the effect of the level of this noise on the threshold for a brief tone presented near the onset of a broadband masker. The background noise had little or no effect when its level was 20 dB or more below the level of the gated masker. For smaller differences in level, however, threshold declined and finally reached its steady-state value (i.e. the one obtained for a signal positioned well after masker onset) when the level difference reached 2.5 dB. Zwicker's finding that the effectiveness of the additional background noise was dependent upon its relative level is consistent with the idea that the additional stimulus induced adaptation, as most adaptation effects are highly level-dependent.

More recently, Carlyon (1987) studied the effects of a continuous background noise on the threshold for a brief tone masked by a brief bandpass masker; the background noise consisted of a single band centred at the 6.5-kHz signal frequency (bandpass noise) or two flanking bands, one on either side of 6.5 kHz (notched noise). He found that the level of the background noise had to be within about −20 to +5 dB relative to the level of the masker in order to reduce the masked threshold. Carlyon argued that the continuous noise induced adaptation in the frequency region of the masker and signal, and that this adaptation was responsible for lowering masked threshold. He also showed that the notched noise lowered threshold more than did the bandpass noise, a result that led him to suggest that some mechanism other than adaptation, such as peripheral suppression or central inhibition, may be involved.

By gating the background noise on and off prior to the onset of the masker, it is possible to evaluate the temporal characteristics of this masking release. This was done originally by Zwicker (1965a) and Elliott (1969). They measured the threshold for a brief tone presented at various times after the cessation of a temporal gap in an otherwise continuous broadband noise. For gaps 5 msec or less (Zwicker, 1965a), thresholds were similar to those in the presence of a continuous masker, but for longer gap durations, masked thresholds increased (Zwicker, 1965a; Elliott, 1969), presumably because the auditory system had had sufficient time to "recover" from the prior stimulation.[1] (Note that here "recover" refers to an *increase* in threshold.) Recovery was almost complete for gap durations of 50 msec.

---

[1] Both Zwicker (1965a) and Elliott (1969) interpreted their data to indicate that the excitation produced by the preceding stimulus declined as a function of time following stimulus offset. Thresholds were lower with short gaps because the excitation produced by the preceding

Included among the series of experiments conducted by Carlyon (1987) was an experiment in which the offset of a notched noise preceded the onset of a brief bandpass masker and sinusoidal signal. He observed that signal threshold was lowest for short delays between the notched noise and bandpass masker, and that it increased as the delay increased up to values of about 160 msec, where threshold was approximately equal to that obtained without a preceding noise stimulus. Carlyon noted the similarity between the time required for complete (or nearly complete) recovery in his experiment and the time required for a comparable recovery in forward-masking experiments (e.g. Jesteadt et al., 1982; Moore & Glasberg, 1983a), a similarity that may be consistent with an adaptation-based explanation for his results (Harris & Dallos, 1979; cf. Relkin & Turner, 1988).

McFadden (1989) recently performed some experiments similar to those described above. Instead of using a broadband noise as a masker, however, and inserting silent periods or gaps in the entire band of noise—as had been done by Zwicker (1965a) and Elliott (1969)—McFadden used a masker that consisted of three independent bands whose centre frequencies were below, at, and above the signal frequency. Surprisingly, he found that it was *not* the band centred at the signal frequency that controlled the recovery, but rather it was the flanking bands: It was necessary to insert a temporal gap in (at least one of) the two flanking bands in order to observe the recovery effect; a gap in only the band centred at the signal frequency had no effect. This result emphasizes the importance of energy remote from the signal frequency for overshoot, and, as noted by McFadden, indicates that the common physiological explanation for overshoot needs to be extended to incorporate adjacent frequency regions. In McFadden's experiments, most of the recovery occurred within 100–200 msec, but recovery was not necessarily complete within 300 msec. This prolonged recovery led McFadden to suggest that overshoot may be based on physiological processing at a site central to the auditory nerve.

Although the studies reviewed above are generally consistent with the hypothesis that overshoot reflects an adaptation process, several aspects of the data cast doubt on whether overshoot can be accounted for entirely by adaptation of auditory-nerve fibres, and in particular, by adaptation of those fibres tuned to the signal frequency. Some of the data even suggest that other (possibly central) mechanisms may play an important role in accounting for

---

stimulus had not decayed completely, and thus the gated masker was more like a continuous masker whose level had been temporarily reduced (during the gap) just prior to signal presentation. Thresholds were higher with long gaps because the decay of excitation was complete, or nearly so, by masker onset. An interpretation based upon decaying excitation is similar to the original interpretation of forward masking (Plomp, 1964), although now forward masking is usually described in terms of recovery from adaptation (e.g. Harris & Dallos, 1979; Jesteadt, Bacon, & Lehman, 1982; cf. Relkin & Turner, 1988).

overshoot. In most of the experiments reported here, overshoot was measured in the presence of an additional noise that was presented continuously or was presented such that its offset preceded masker onset by some duration. These experiments were designed to provide additional information on the spectral, intensive, and temporal parameters underlying overshoot in an effort to determine further to what extent the psychophysical data resemble adaptation effects observed physiologically at the auditory nerve.

Method

Subjects. Five subjects participated; four were female. They ranged in age from 21 to 27 years, with a mean age of 23 years. Each subject's absolute thresholds were not worse than 10 dB HL (ANSI, 1969) at any of the octave frequencies from 0.25 to 8.0 kHz, and each had a minimum of 10 hours of listening experience in overshoot experiments (they were subjects S1–S5 in Bacon, 1990). Subject S5 (the second author) was tested individually, and the other four subjects were usually tested in pairs in a double-walled sound-attenuating chamber. Subjects S1–S4 were paid for their participation.

Apparatus and Stimuli. The noise masker was generated by a waveform synthesizer (Hewlett-Packard, 8904A). The noise was bandpass filtered using four Kemo VBF25.01 filters in series (two highpass and two lowpass, each with an attenuation rate of 135 dB/oct). It was presented at a spectrum level of 20 (S1–S4) or 40 dB SPL (S5).[2] Masker bandwidth was varied in the first experiment but was fixed at 8.0 kHz (0.05–8.05 kHz) in the remaining experiments.

The 4.0-kHz sinusoidal signal was digitally generated and produced (DT2801-A) at a 20-kHz sampling rate. The output of the digital-to-analog converter was lowpass filtered at 4.5 kHz (Kemo VBF25.01, 135 dB/oct). The level of the signal was varied adaptively (Wilsonics, PATT).

The additional noise stimulus was a notched noise or a bandpass noise. The notched noise was generated by two separate random noise generators (GENRAD, 1381). The low-frequency band was filtered by three Kemo VBF25.01 filters (one highpass and two lowpass, each with 135 dB/oct attenuation rate); the high-frequency band (which also served as the bandpass noise) was filtered by four Kemo VBF25.01 filters (two highpass and two lowpass, each with 135 dB/oct attenuation rate). The bands were attenuated

[2] Most of the data reported here for S5 were collected prior to those for subjects S1–S4. At that time, we expected overshoot to be near its maximum for all subjects for a masker spectrum level of 40 dB SPL (as it was for S5). For the other four subjects, however, the overshoot was small or absent at that masker level. Their overshoot was near its maximum for a masker spectrum level of 20 dB SPL (see Bacon, 1990), and thus we chose that level for those subjects.

separately (Wilsonics, PATT) before being added together; they were then led to an electronic switch (Wilsonics, BSIT). The level of the additional noise ranged from −40 to +10 dB relative to the level of the masker.

All stimuli were added together before being amplified, attenuated, and then led to a TDH-49P headphone mounted in an MX/51 cushion.

The noise masker had a total duration (0-voltage points) of 400 msec, with a 5-msec $\cos^2$ rise/fall time. The sinusoidal signal had a total duration of 10 msec, with a 5-msec $\cos^2$ rise/fall time. The onset of the signal occurred near the beginning of the masker (1-msec delay) or in the temporal centre of the masker (195-msec delay). The additional noise, when present, was continuous or was gated with a $\cos^2$ rise/fall time (5 msec unless stated otherwise). The duration of the additional noise and the delay between its offset and masker onset were varied systematically in separate experiments.

All stimulus timing was controlled by a micro-computer (Compaq 386/20) and checked using a digital storage oscilloscope (Tektronix, 2230). Other stimulus parameters were verified with a signal analyser (Hewlett-Packard, 3561A).

Procedure

Thresholds were measured using an adaptive two-interval forced-choice procedure with a decision rule that estimates the 79% correct point on the psychometric function (Levitt, 1971). Lights were used to indicate when the signal might occur and to provide correct-answer feedback. The two observation intervals were separated by 650 msec.

A run started with the signal level well above the estimated threshold value. Signal level was decreased following three correct responses and increased following one incorrect response. The transition from increasing to decreasing level, and vice versa, defined a reversal. The initial step size was 4 dB and was reduced to 2 dB following the second reversal. Each run consisted of 60 trials. The first two or three reversals were discarded (two if the total number of reversals was even, three if it was odd) and the remaining reversals were averaged to obtain the threshold estimate for that run. Runs were discarded on the rare occasions when the standard deviation of the reversals was greater than 5 dB or when there were fewer than 8 total reversals. Each threshold reported is the mean of the estimates from at least three runs, obtained over at least two days. When the standard deviation of the three estimates exceeded 3 dB, an additional estimate was obtained, and all estimates were averaged. This continued until the standard deviation of the estimates was less than 3 dB or until six estimates were obtained. Most (229/248) of the thresholds reported here had standard deviations less than 3 dB; all had standard errors less than 3 dB.

SPECTRAL EFFECTS

Some of the psychophysical data reviewed in the Introduction suggest that overshoot for broadband noise maskers cannot be explained solely by adaptation of auditory-nerve fibres tuned to the signal frequency (e.g. McFadden, 1989). McFadden suggested that energy below and (perhaps especially) above the signal frequency may be more important than energy contained within the critical band centred at the signal frequency. These more recent data are consistent with one of Zwicker's (1965b) seemingly forgotten experiments, where he showed that the masker bandwidth had to be wider than one critical band in order to observe overshoot.[3]

The first set of experiments was designed to examine which frequency regions are most important for overshoot. In particular, they were designed to examine the importance of energy in various spectral regions and to determine whether overshoot depends primarily on energy near the signal frequency.

EXPERIMENT 1

Effects of Masker Bandwidth

The purpose of the first experiment was to replicate Zwicker's (1965b) experiment on the effect of masker bandwidth on overshoot. Overshoot was measured for a wide range of masker bandwidths.

Method

Conditions. Threshold for the 10-msec, 4.0-kHz signal was measured at a delay of 1 or 195 msec relative to the onset of the 400-msec masker. The masker was (approximately) centred arithmetically at 4.0 kHz; its relative bandwidth (bandwidth/signal frequency) was 0.1, 0.2, 0.4, 0.8, 1.2, 1.6, or 2.0 (absolute bandwidth of 0.4, 0.8, 1.6, 3.2, 4.8, 6.4, or 8.0 kHz).

Initially, complete data from all subjects were obtained at a masker spectrum level of 40 dB SPL. Because overshoot was generally small at that level for subjects S1–S4 (see Footnote 2), the masker was reduced to 20 dB SPL for those four subjects for all experiments. Although complete data exist for all five subjects on the other experiments to be reported, scheduling conflicts did not allow complete testing of all subjects on this experiment.

---

[3] The width of the masker in terms of number of critical bands was based upon experiments that had employed signal durations considerably longer than the 2-msec signal used by Zwicker (1965b). Consequently, because the width of the critical band may increase with decreases in signal duration (see Scharf, 1970, for a review), the bandwidth of the maskers used by Zwicker may not have been as wide—in terms of number of critical bands—as was reported.

Complete data from S1 and S3 at 20 dB SPL and from S5 at 40 dB SPL are presented here.

Results

The results are shown in Figure 1. The data are plotted as S/M_0 in dB (i.e. as the signal level at threshold relative to the spectrum level of the noise masker) as a function of relative masker bandwidth. Triangles represent the 1-msec

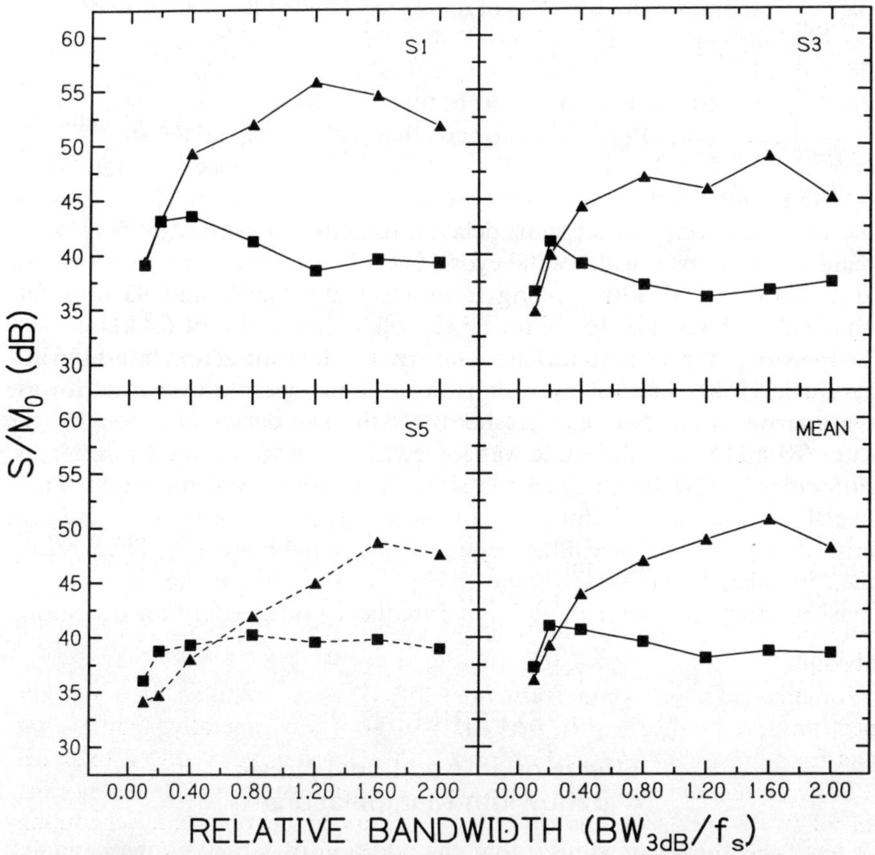

FIG. 1. Threshold for a 10-msec, 4.0-kHz signal presented with a 1-msec (triangles) or a 195-msec (squares) delay within a 400-msec noise masker. Threshold is plotted as the signal level at threshold relative to the spectrum level of the masker, as a function of the relative bandwidth of the noise masker. Relative bandwidth is defined here as the bandwidth (measured from the 3-dB down points) divided by the signal frequency (f_s). The masker was centred at the 4.0-kHz signal frequency. In this and the remaining figures, the data from S5 are connected with a dashed line (compared to a solid line) to emphasize the fact that he was tested at a masker spectrum level of 40 dB SPL, whereas the other subjects were tested at 20 dB SPL.

signal delay, and squares represent the 195-msec signal delay. The data from S5 are connected by a dashed (rather than a solid) line to remind the reader that S5 was tested at a different masker level. First consider the results for the 195-msec delay. Threshold increased as the relative masker bandwidth increased from 0.1 to 0.2 (absolute bandwidths of 0.4 to 0.8 kHz), but then remained relatively constant or even declined a few decibels as the bandwidth was increased further. These results are consistent with other bandwidening experiments (e.g. Fletcher, 1940), and they indicate that the critical band at 4.0 kHz is between 0.4 and 0.8 kHz. This value is reasonably close to the classical estimate (about 0.7 kHz) of the critical bandwidth at 4.0 kHz obtained via masking and loudness experiments (see Scharf, 1970, and Zwicker & Terhardt, 1980), as well as to more recent estimates (about 0.5 kHz) obtained using a notched-noise masking procedure (e.g. Moore & Glasberg, 1983b; Glasberg & Moore, 1990). This suggests that the short signal duration did not appreciably affect the estimate of the critical bandwidth (see Footnote 3).

The results for the 1-msec delay are significantly different from those at the 195-msec delay. At the short delay, threshold increased with increases in relative masker bandwidth well beyond 0.2. Threshold reached an asymptote at a relative bandwidth ranging from about 0.8 for S1 and S3 (absolute bandwidth of 3.2 kHz) to 1.6 for S5 (absolute bandwidth of 6.4 kHz).

The size of the overshoot effect is determined by subtracting threshold at a long delay from threshold at a short delay. There was no overshoot for the two narrowest bandwidths: thresholds for the two delays were roughly the same (S1 and S3), or threshold was somewhat lower (S5) at the 1-msec delay. For wider bandwidths, however, a sizeable overshoot was measured. Thus, overshoot was seen only for masker bandwidths considerably wider than the critical band (or auditory filter) centred at the signal frequency. These results are consistent with the results reported by Zwicker (1965b); they indicate that masker energy remote from the signal frequency is necessary for overshoot.

EXPERIMENT 2

Effects of an Additional Noise: Bandwidth Manipulations

It has been shown previously that the addition of a continuous bandpass noise can lower the threshold for a brief signal presented shortly after masker onset (Zwicker, 1965a; Carlyon, 1987). Zwicker's additional noise was broadband and Carlyon's had a bandwidth that was 0.3 times the 6.5-kHz signal frequency. No one has systematically varied the bandwidth of such an additional noise in an effort to determine which frequency components of the noise are most important for the masking release. In addition, although one might not expect the additional noise to affect the threshold for a brief signal presented well after masker onset, no one has explicitly examined this.

Method

Conditions. Threshold for the 10-msec, 4.0-kHz signal was measured at a delay of 1 or 195 msec relative to the onset of the 400-msec masker. In this and the remaining experiments to be reported here, the masker had a bandwidth of 8.0 kHz (0.05–8.05 kHz). The additional noise was presented continuously; it was bandpass filtered and centred arithmetically at 4.0 kHz. The relative bandwidth of the additional noise was 0.1, 0.2, 0.4, 0.8, or 1.2 (absolute bandwidth of 0.4, 0.8, 1.6, 3.2, or 4.8 kHz); its level was −10 dB relative to the masker level.

Results

The results are shown in Figure 2. Triangles represent a 1-msec signal delay, and squares represent a 195–msec signal delay; open symbols represent thresholds in the absence of the additional noise, whereas filled symbols represent thresholds in the presence of the continuous background noise. In the absence of the additional noise, the size of the overshoot ranged from 7.7 (S3) to 15.2 dB (S4), with a mean value of 11.3 dB. These values are consistent with values obtained previously by others (e.g. Zwicker, 1965a; Elliott, 1965; McFadden, 1989).

Although the additional noise had little or no effect on the threshold at a 195-msec delay (compare open and filled squares), it had a very clear effect on the threshold for a short signal delay. In general, the additional noise reduced threshold by about 3 dB at the narrowest bandwidth (0.4 kHz); from there, threshold continued to decline with further increases in bandwidth. Threshold at the short delay reached the threshold at the long delay (except for S1) by the time the bandwidth had reached its largest value (4.8 kHz); in other words, the continuous noise generally eliminated overshoot. The data presented here indicate that although energy in the additional noise immediately around the signal frequency region can reduce threshold at masker onset, energy in adjacent frequency regions is necessary to reduce threshold to its steady-state value. It is interesting that bandwidths of 0.4 and 0.8 kHz can reduce overshoot (this experiment), but that masker bandwidths of 0.4 and 0.8 kHz do not yield overshoot (Experiment 1). It implies on the one hand that energy near the signal frequency is necessary for maximum overshoot, but on the other hand that such energy is not sufficient to produce (any) overshoot.

EXPERIMENT 3

Effects of an Additional Noise: Notchwidth Manipulations

In the previous experiment, the continuous background noise always had energy around the signal frequency, and the effects of systematically adding

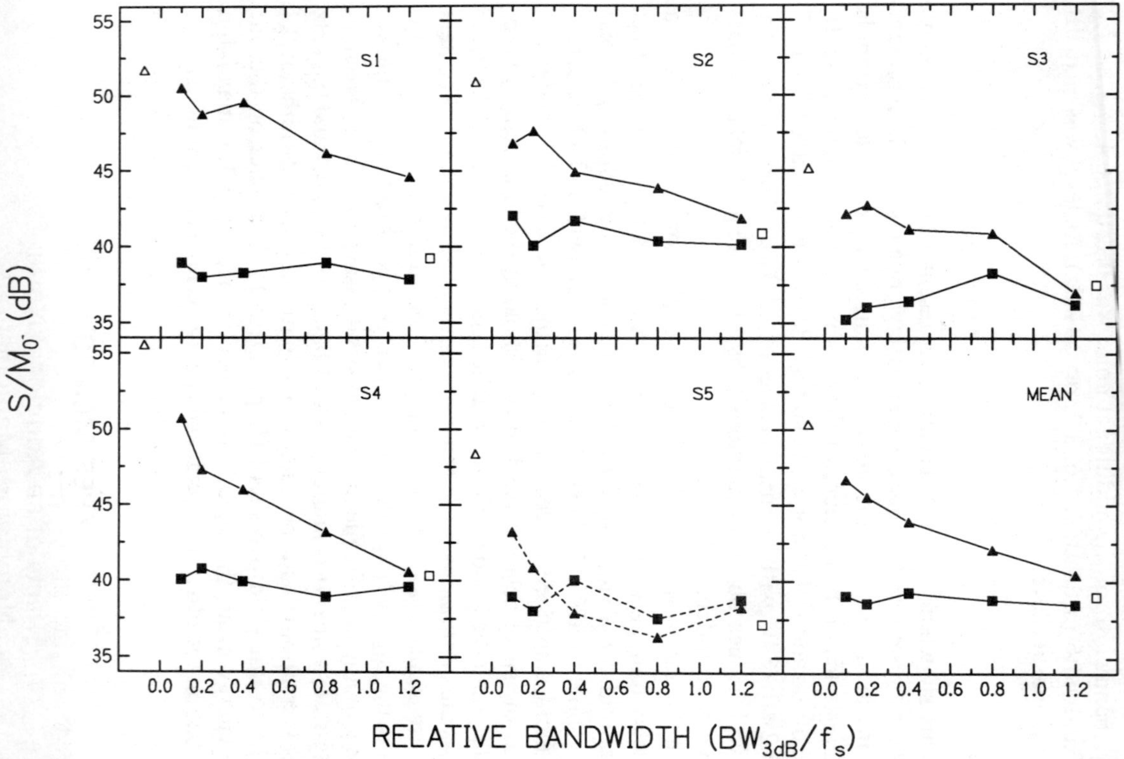

FIG. 2. Masked threshold as a function of the relative bandwidth of an additional noise. The additional noise was centred at 4.0 kHz and was presented continuously. The 10–msec, 4.0-kHz signal was presented 1 msec (triangles) or 195 msec (squares) after the onset of the 400-msec noise masker. Masker bandwidth was 8.0 kHz. Open symbols represent thresholds in the absence of the additional bandpass noise. Masker spectrum level was 20 (S1–S4) or 40 dB SPL (S5); the relative level of the additional noise was − 10 dB.

energy outside that region were studied. In this experiment, a notch centred at the signal frequency was created in a broadband noise, and the effectiveness of that notched noise in reducing overshoot was determined as a function of notchwidth.

Method

Conditions. Because the continuous background noise had no effect on the long-delay condition in the previous experiment, thresholds in this and the remaining experiments were measured only at a 1-msec delay. The continuous noise extended from 0.05 to 8.05 kHz (i.e. it covered the same frequency range as did the masker); the notch was centred arithmetically at 4.0 kHz. The relative notchwidth was 0.1, 0.2, 0.4, 0.8, or 1.2 (absolute notchwidth was 0.4, 0.8, 1.6, 3.2, or 4.8 kHz). The level of the notched noise in its passband was −10 dB relative to the level of the masker. The depth of the notch (i.e. the difference between the level of the notched noise in its upper or lower passband and the level of the noise at 4.0 kHz) was 13, 21, 26, 31, and 33 dB for the relative notchwidths of 0.1, 0.2, 0.4, 0.8, and 1.2, respectively.

Results

The functions relating threshold to relative notchwidth are given in Figure 3. There was a consistent trend for threshold to increase with increases in notchwidth. For the narrowest notchwidth, thresholds were somewhat (2–5 dB) higher than the steady-state thresholds (open symbols to the left), indicating—consistent with the results with a continuous bandpass noise—that energy in the frequency region immediately surrounding the signal was at least somewhat important for lowering threshold. As notchwidth increased threshold increased and reached an asymptote at a relative notchwidth of about 0.8 (absolute notchwidth of 3.2 kHz). The asymptotic threshold was about equal to the threshold obtained at the same 1-msec delay but in the absence of the continuous noise (open symbols to the right)—except for S1, whose threshold was inexplicably 5.5 dB higher at the widest notchwidth. Because threshold increased for relative notchwidths considerably larger than 0.1 to 0.2 (absolute notchwidths wider than 0.4 to 0.8 kHz), these data are consistent with those from the first two experiments in indicating that energy relatively remote from the signal frequency is important for overshoot.

The effectiveness of the additional noise at a relative notchwidth of 0.2 can be compared with the effectiveness of Carlyon's (1987) additional noise, which was fixed at a relative notchwidth of 0.2. The notched noise presented here reduced threshold by an average of 5 dB, whereas Carlyon's notched noise reduced threshold by about 1–6 dB (see his Figs. 1–3). Thus, despite

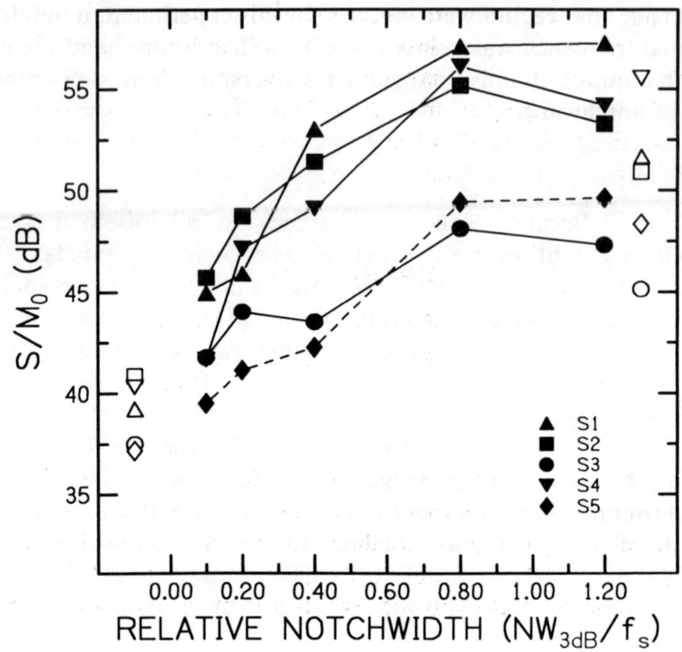

FIG. 3. Masked threshold as a function of the relative notchwidth of an additional background noise. The notched noise was presented continuously, and its notch was centred at 4.0 kHz. The 10-msec, 4.0-kHz signal was presented 1 msec after the onset of the 400-msec noise masker. Masker bandwidth was 8.0 kHz. Open symbols represent thresholds in the absence of the additional notched noise, in which case the signal was presented with a 195-msec (left side) or 1-msec (right side) delay. Masker spectrum level was 20 (S1–S4) or 40 dB SPL (S5); the relative level of the background noise was −10 dB.

several differences in the stimuli across the two studies (e.g. this study used a broader masker and a different signal frequency), the threshold reduction was about the same.

INTENSIVE EFFECTS

If the effect of the continuous background noise reflects some type of adaptation, then that effect should be level-dependent. Using a broadband masker and background, Zwicker (1965a) found that the reduction in overshoot for a 5.0-kHz signal was highly dependent upon the relative level of the background noise. Carlyon (1987) showed that the threshold for a brief 6.5-kHz tone masked by a brief bandpass masker depends upon the relative level of the background noise; the most effective relative level was −5 dB when the background was bandpass noise and 5 dB when it was notched noise. Carlyon also examined the effect of relative level for a notched-noise background centred at signal frequencies of 1.0 and 3.0 kHz. The effect was significantly less pronounced at these lower frequencies. Indeed, threshold generally changed relatively little at the lower frequencies for relative levels ranging from −20 to 0 dB. This raises the question as to whether the effects observed in Experiments 2 and 3 for a signal frequency of 4.0 kHz will depend upon relative background level.

EXPERIMENT 4

Effects of an Additional Noise: Level Manipulations

Method

Conditions. Threshold was measured at a delay of 1 msec relative to the onset of the 400-msec masker. Masker bandwidth was 8.0 kHz. The continuous background was a bandpass noise centred at 4.0 kHz, with a relative bandwidth of 1.2, or was a notched noise that extended from 0.05 to 8.05 kHz and had a relative notchwidth of 0.2 centred at 4.0 kHz. The level of the additional noise relative to the level of the masker ranged from −40 to 10 dB.

Results

The results for the bandpass and notched noise are shown in Figures 4 and 5, respectively. First consider the results for the bandpass noise. For relative levels of −40 to −30 dB, the continuous noise had little or no effect on threshold. As the level was increased, however, threshold decreased and was within a few decibels of the steady-state threshold (open symbols to the right) for a relative level of −10 dB. The finding that S5 alone showed a significant reduction in threshold at −30 dB may be due to the fact that he was tested at a higher overall level. For all subjects, as the noise level was increased above −10 dB, threshold increased, presumably because the additional noise was masking the signal. The finding that threshold was lowest for a relative noise level of −10 dB is consistent with Carlyon's (1987) results at 6.5 kHz.

The results for the notched noise are shown in Figure 5. As was seen for the bandpass noise, the low levels did not significantly change masked threshold (and hence overshoot), but as the noise level was increased, threshold declined and reached (or went slightly below) the steady-state threshold at relative levels of 0 to 10 dB. Comparing the results from Figures 4 and 5, the most effective notched noise reduced threshold on the average by 3.5 dB more than did the most effective bandpass noise (see also Carlyon, 1987). This is presumably due to the fact that the notched noise can be presented at a higher level—and thus produce a larger effect (albeit off

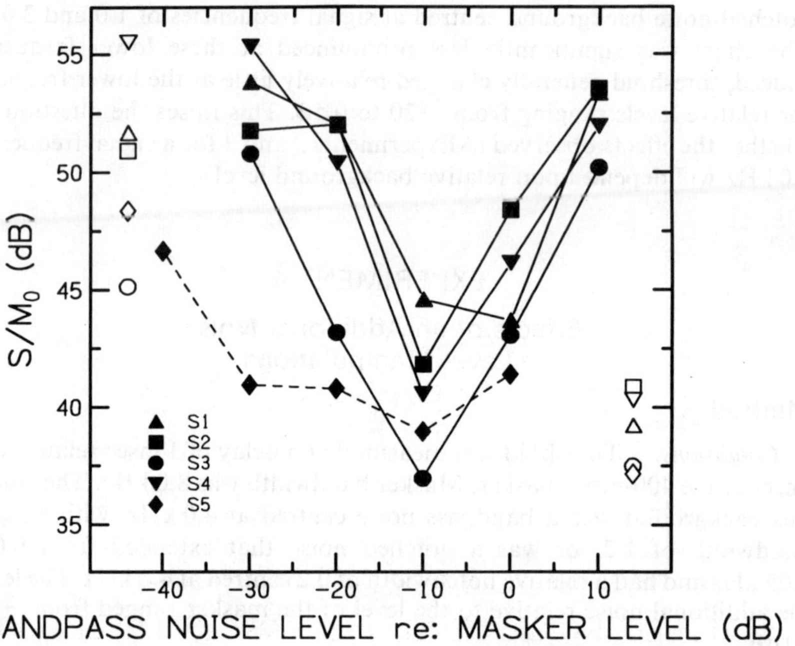

FIG. 4. Masked threshold as a function of the relative level of an additional bandpass noise (relative bandwidth of 1.2, centre frequency of 4.0 kHz). The 10-msec, 4.0-kHz signal was presented 1 msec after the onset of the 400-msec noise masker. Masker bandwidth was 8.0 kHz. Open symbols represent thresholds in the absence of the additional bandpass noise, in which case the signal was presented with a 1-msec (left side) or 195-msec (right side) delay.

frequency)—before producing significant masking at the signal frequency. When both background noises were at a relative level of −10, however, the bandpass noise was, on the average, about 5 dB more effective than the notched noise. A similar, but smaller, effect can be seen in Carlyon's (1987) data. This suggests, consistent with the results from Experiments 2 and 3, that frequency components near the signal frequency are important for overshoot.

The level-dependence observed in this experiment strongly suggests that the background noise is, in fact, inducing a certain amount of adaptation in the auditory system, which reduces signal threshold near masker onset.

TEMPORAL EFFECTS

A continuous background noise does not allow one to measure the temporal characteristics of the masking release observed in Experiments 2–4. Moreover, with a continuous background, one cannot rule out the possibility that the effect of the additional noise is mediated by other mechanisms such as

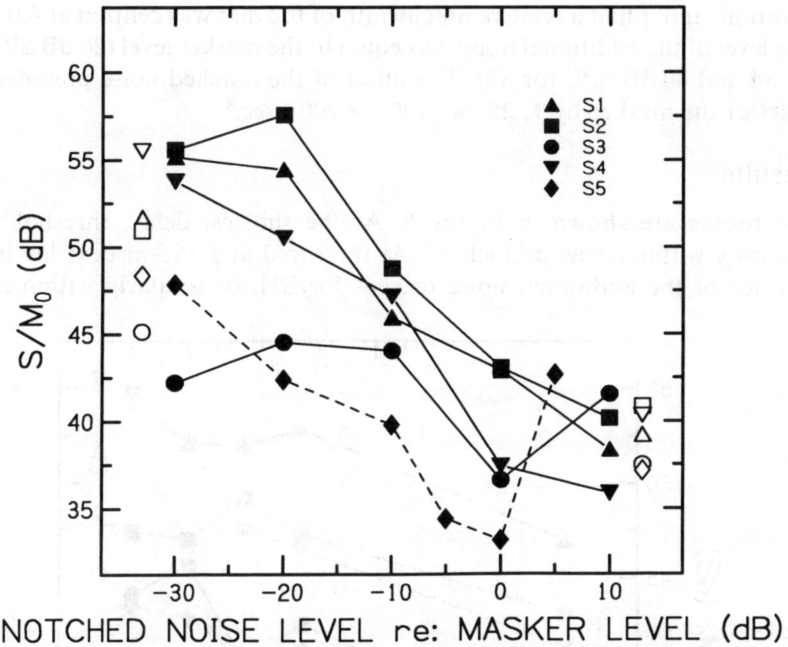

FIG. 5. Masked threshold as a function of the relative level of an additional notched noise (relative notchwidth of 0.2 centred at 4.0 kHz). The 10-msec, 4.0-kHz signal was presented 1 msec after the onset of the 400-msec noise masker. Masker bandwidth was 8.0 kHz. Open symbols represent thresholds in the absence of the notched noise, in which case the signal was presented with a 1-msec (left side) or 195-msec (right side) delay.

suppression (e.g. Sachs & Kiang, 1968; Arthur, Pfeiffer, & Suga, 1971; Houtgast, 1972; Shannon, 1976; Javel, Geisler, & Ravindran, 1978), which operate only when stimuli are presented simultaneously. Indeed, Carlyon (1987) suggested that some of his data might be accounted for by suppression effects. The main purpose of the last two experiments was to measure the recovery and growth of the masking release in order to relate those temporal characteristics to the recovery and growth of adaptation observed in auditory-nerve fibres. The secondary purpose was to provide insight into whether suppression influenced the results in Experiments 2–4.

EXPERIMENT 5

Recovery Method

Conditions. Threshold was measured at a delay of 1 msec relative to the onset of the 400-msec masker. The additional noise was 400 msec in duration, and it had a relative notchwidth of 0.2 that was centred at 4.0 kHz. The level of the additional noise was equal to the masker level (20 dB SPL for S1–S4 and 40 dB SPL for S5). The offset of the notched noise preceded the onset of the masker by 1, 25, 50, 100, or 200 msec.[4]

Results

The results are shown in Figure 6. At the shortest delay, threshold was generally within a few decibels of the threshold at a 195-msec delay in the absence of the additional noise (except for S1), or similarly within a few

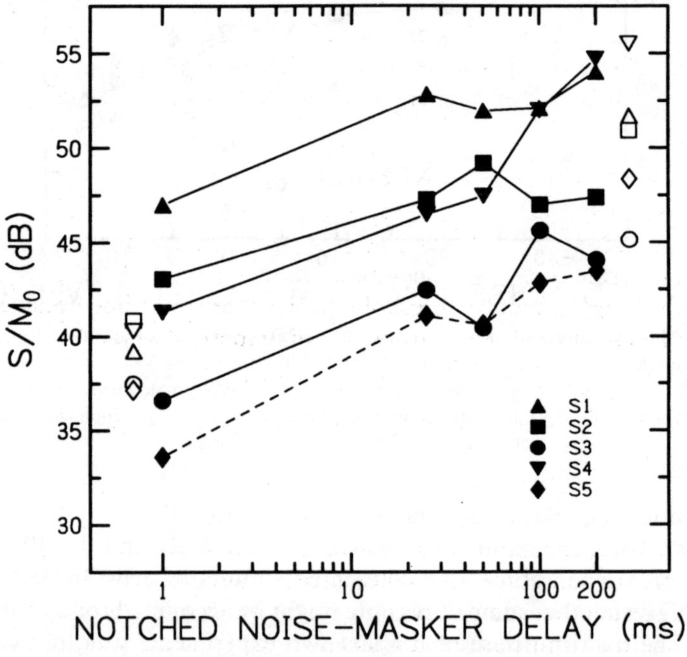

FIG. 6. Masked threshold as a function of the delay between the offset of a 400-msec notched noise and the onset of a 400-msec broadband masker (see Footnote 4). The notched noise had a relative notchwidth of 0.2 (centred at 4.0 kHz) and was presented at a relative level of 0 dB. Masker bandwidth was 8.0 kHz. The 10-msec, 4.0-kHz signal was presented 1 msec after the onset of the masker. Open symbols represent thresholds in the absence of the notched noise, in which case the signal was presented with a 195-msec (left side) or 1-msec (right side) delay.

---

[4] Due to a calibration/programming error, the actual delays between the offset of the additional noise and the onset of the masker were 4 msec less than the reported delays (i.e. the actual delays were −3, 21, 46, 96, or 196 msec). As a result, there was some overlap between the additional noise and the masker at the shortest delay. Subsequent data collection confirmed that this minimal overlap did not influence the results: thresholds with a delay of −3 msec were virtually the same as those obtained with a delay of 1 msec.

decibels of the threshold in the presence of the continuous additional noise (see Fig. 5), suggesting that suppression probably did not influence thresholds in the presence of the additional noise. Threshold increased as the delay between noise offset and masker onset increased, consistent with previous results (Zwicker, 1965a; Elliott, 1969; Carlyon, 1987, 1989; McFadden, 1989). Most of the increase in threshold (recovery) occurred as the delay increased to 25 msec, where threshold increased by an average of 5.7 dB. Threshold changed only gradually, if at all, for delays from 25–200 msec (except for S4, who showed a steeper increase in threshold at delays between 25 and 200 msec). Recovery was essentially complete (threshold within 3 dB of the threshold in the absence of the additional noise) for all subjects except S5. It is unclear whether this protracted recovery for S5 reflects merely an individual difference, or whether it can be accounted for by the fact that he was tested at higher levels, where long-term effects may be more likely.

EXPERIMENT 6

Growth

The results from the last experiment indicate that a 400-msec noise is sufficiently long to reduce threshold to a value near that obtained under steady-state conditions. The purpose of this experiment was to determine the growth of this effect.

Method

Conditions. Threshold was measured for a signal at a delay of 1 msec relative to the onset of the 400-msec masker. Masker bandwidth was 8.0 kHz. The additional noise was presented at a relative level of 0 dB; it had a relative notchwidth centred at 4.0 kHz of 0.2. The duration of the notched noise was 3, 6, 12, 25, 50, 100, or 200 msec; its rise/fall time was 1 msec (for durations of 3, 6, 12, and 25 msec) or 5 msec (for durations of 25, 50, 100, and 200 msec). Thus, both rise/fall times were used when the noise duration was 25 msec. The offset of the notched noise preceded the onset of the masker by 1 msec.[5]

---

[5] As a result of the error noted in Footnote 4, the delay between the offset of the notched noise and the onset of the masker was −3 msec when the rise/fall was 5 msec. The delay was 1 msec, however, when the rise/fall was 1 msec. The similarity between the results obtained with a 1-msec rise/fall and those obtained with a 5-msec rise/fall when the notched-noise duration was 25 msec supports the finding noted in Footnote 4 that the minimal temporal overlap between the notched noise and the masker did not significantly influence the results reported here.

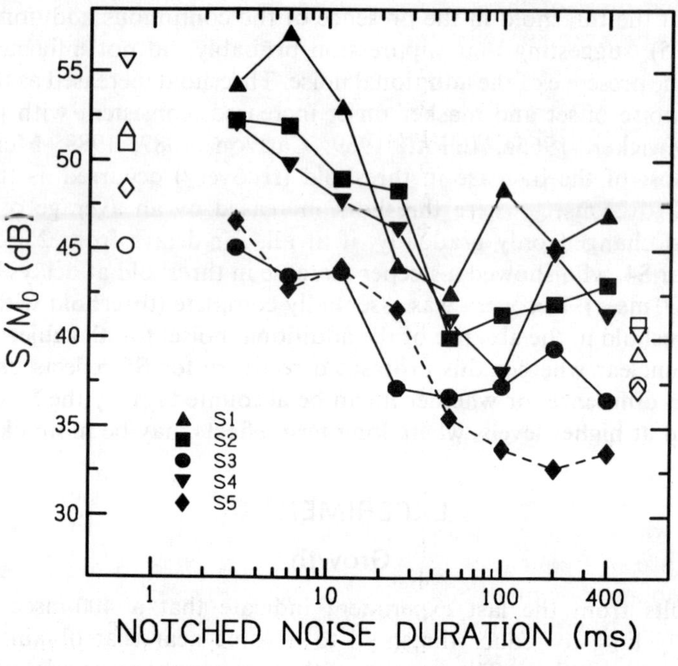

FIG. 7. Masked threshold as a function of the duration of a notched noise (relative notch-width of 0.2 centred at 4.0 kHz, and a relative level of 0 dB), whose offset preceded the onset of a 400-msec broadband masker by about 1 msec (see Footnote 5). The 10-msec, 4.0-kHz signal was presented 1 msec after the onset of the masker. Open symbols represent thresholds in the absence of the notched noise, in which case the signal was presented with a 1-msec (left side) or 195-msec (right side) delay.

Results

The results are shown in Figure 7. The thresholds given for the 25-msec noise are those obtained with a 5-msec rise/fall time. Thresholds were essentially the same (except for S3, whose threshold was 6 dB higher) for the 1-msec rise/fall time.

Despite individual differences, there was a clear general trend for thresholds to decrease as noise duration was increased from 3 msec to a value somewhere around 50–100 msec. Thresholds declined at a rate between 6.1 (S3) and 8.5 dB/decade (S2). These results are consistent with the fact that most of the improvement in threshold that occurs as a brief signal is moved in time through a longer duration masker occurs during the first 20–50 msec (Zwicker, 1965a). These results do, however, differ from those presented by Carlyon (1987), who measured threshold for a brief 6.5-kHz signal masked by a bandpass masker as a function of the duration of a notched noise that was gated on before the masker and usually gated off with the masker. He found that most of the improvement in threshold occurred for preceding durations between 80–160 msec.

DISCUSSION

As discussed in the Introduction, overshoot is usually attributed to adaptation of auditory-nerve fibres tuned near the signal frequency. In particular, it is typically assumed that the initial high rate of response to the masker (i.e. the neural onset response) interferes with (i.e. masks) the detection of the signal. Although the results presented here, particularly those with regard to intensive and temporal characteristics, are consistent with an adaptation-based explanation for overshoot (see below), the experiments on the spectral characteristics indicate that overshoot cannot be explained solely by adaptation at or near the signal frequency. Overshoot for broadband maskers is governed *both* by frequency components remote from, as well as by frequency components near, the signal frequency. The importance of remote frequencies is clear from the finding that overshoot exists only for a noise masker whose bandwidth is wider than about a single critical band. The importance of frequencies near the signal frequency is highlighted by the results obtained with an additional noise: energy in the additional noise contained only within approximately a critical band of frequencies produced some reduction in overshoot (Figure 2), and conversely, removing energy from that frequency region reduced the effect (Figure 3). Thus, energy near the signal frequency contributes to overshoot, even if it does not itself yield overshoot.

The importance of energy both near and remote from the signal frequency is *suggested* in the data reported by McFadden (1989, his Fig. 2). In his experiments, he asked subjects to detect a 6-msec, 2.5-kHz signal that was presented 4 msec after the cessation of a temporal gap in an otherwise continuous noise. The noise consisted of three independent bands, one centred at the signal frequency and one on either side of that centred band. Thresholds were low for short gaps, presumably because the auditory system had not recovered from the preceding stimulation, but thresholds usually increased as the gap duration increased. McFadden observed complete recovery (with a 300-msec gap) when all three bands were gapped, only partial recovery when the flanking bands alone were gapped, and little or no recovery when only the centre band was gapped. Thus, although gapping the centre band was not sufficient to produce recovery, it was necessary in order to produce *complete* recovery. Whether the important factor was the gapping of the components within the critical band centred at the signal frequency or those just outside the critical band is not known, however, because the centre band was about 2.5 times wider than one critical band.

McFadden (1989) described the results from a pilot experiment designed to determine whether the low- and high-frequency flanking bands were equally effective in producing the recovery. His results led him to conclude that both regions are important, but that the high-frequency region may be more important. This issue was examined here as well in a supplementary experiment. Threshold at masker onset was measured in the presence of a continuous notched noise (relative notchwidth of 0.2 centred at 4.0 kHz) with a relative level of 0 dB. For all subjects, when both the high- and low-frequency sides were present, threshold for a signal near masker onset was reduced significantly relative to the condition without the notched noise (see Figure 5). The effect of just the high or the low side was subject-dependent, although for all subjects two bands were more effective than one. Subjects S1 and S2 showed no reduction in threshold (and hence no reduction in overshoot) with a single band; for S3, both bands were about equally effective, whereas for S4 and S5 the high band was more effective. From these data it is not possible to say in general whether one side or the other is more important, though it is possible to say that stimulation of both sides results in a larger masking release than stimulation of either side alone. Moreover, for the subjects tested here, when there was a difference between the high and low side, the high side was more effective. In passing, we note that data currently being collected from our laboratory using somewhat different stimulus conditions suggest that although both sides are important, the high side may be somewhat more important.

As noted above, it is unlikely that overshoot can be accounted for by adaptation confined to auditory-nerve fibres tuned to the signal frequency. It has even been suggested (e.g. Carlyon, 1987; McFadden, 1989) that overshoot represents, in part, processing at levels higher than the auditory nerve. Before addressing the issue of central processing, it may be constructive to consider to what extent the effects observed here might be explained by adaptation in auditory-nerve fibres.

The recovery functions (Figure 6) are generally similar to those observed in auditory-nerve fibres. For example, Harris and Dallos (1979, their Figure 3) measured the firing rate of single auditory-nerve fibres in response to a fixed-level, short-duration signal presented in isolation or after some delay following a longer duration "adaptor". The onset response to the signal was virtually absent for short adaptor-signal delays (1–5 msec), was present but reduced at somewhat longer delays (10–20 msec), and was *near* its unadapted level for delays longer than 50 msec. Assuming that the recovery of the neural onset response to the masker presented here follows a similar time course, the physiological data are consistent with the fact that the majority of the recovery observed here (a recovery that results in higher thresholds for a signal near masker onset) occurred for delays between 1 and 25 msec. The physiological data are similarly consistent with psychophysical data presented by Zwicker (1965a), Elliott (1969), and Carlyon (1987). Zwicker and Elliott both measured threshold for a brief signal presented shortly after the cessation of a temporal gap in an otherwise continuous broadband noise.

Recovery of overshoot was nearly complete for gap durations of 50 msec. Carlyon's experiment was similar to the one performed here. He measured the threshold for a brief 6.5-kHz tone masked by a brief bandpass noise as a function of the delay between the offset of a 320-msec notched noise and the onset of the masker and signal. Recovery was nearly complete within 160 msec, and, as can be seen in his Figure 6, most of the recovery occurred during the first 20–40 msec. Whether the fairly protracted recovery functions observed in the gapping experiments reported by McFadden (1989) can be accounted for by recovery from *long-term* adaptation in auditory-nerve fibres (e.g. Kiang et al., 1965), or instead by complex neural interactions occurring across cells located central to the auditory nerve, as suggested by McFadden (1989), is certainly unclear at this point.

The growth functions shown in Figure 7 seem consistent with properties of auditory-nerve responses. Harris and Dallos (1979, their Figure 13) examined the effect of adaptor duration on the firing rate of an auditory-nerve fibre in response to a fixed-level, short-duration signal presented 5 msec after adaptor offset. The onset response to the signal was reduced even for a 2-msec adaptor, and it was reduced further with increases in adaptor duration up to about 50 msec; there was no additional effect of adaptor duration for increases beyond 100 msec. The psychophysical growth functions follow a similar time course: most of the growth occurred for durations between 3 and 50–100 msec.

Although the similarities between the masking release observed here and adaptation effects observed by others at the level of the auditory nerve strongly suggest that peripheral adaptation is involved, the importance of frequency components remote from the signal frequency requires additional explanation, for it indicates that overshoot cannot be accounted for entirely by adaptation of those fibres tuned to the signal frequency. One must explain why onset responses *outside* the signal channel interfere with signal detection.

In their articles examining the effects of temporary hearing loss on overshoot, Champlin and McFadden (1989) and McFadden and Champlin (1990) suggested that under normal conditions the onset responses from a group of fibres to a broadband stimulus may be combined at a location central to the auditory nerve. When those onset responses are synchronized (with one another), the summed response will exhibit a large onset response followed by a fairly flat steady-state response; when they are not synchronized, the summed response will be relatively flat throughout the duration of stimulation. Thus, assuming that this summation occurs over a fairly large number of fibres, this scheme could account for why spectrally distant onset responses could interfere with the detection of the onset response to a brief signal.

To account for the data presented here and elsewhere (e.g. Zwicker, 1965b; McFadden, 1989), this summation must occur over a fairly wide range of frequencies. And, *if* it is the case that frequencies above the signal frequency are more important than those below, then the summator must either be receiving input disproportionately from higher frequency fibres, or those higher frequency fibres must be better synchronized (and hence contribute more) than the lower ones. This latter notion is at least consistent with the fact that, in response to a brief stimulus, the firing of high-frequency fibres is more synchronized than is the firing of low-frequency fibres (due to the fact that the travelling wave slows down as it moves from the base to the apex of the cochlea), though it is unclear whether the relatively small differences in the velocity of the travelling wave just on either side of the 4.0-kHz place are sufficient to account for the psychophysical results (e.g. Teas, Eldredge, & Davis, 1962; Zerlin, 1969).

Related temporal effects observed psychophysically (e.g. Zwicker, 1964; Viemeister, 1980; Viemeister & Bacon, 1982; Summerfield, Haggard, Foster, & Gray, 1984; Summerfield, Sidwell, & Nelson, 1987; Bacon & Blake, 1990) may also be accounted for by some type of a pooled response from an array of differentially adapted auditory-nerve fibres (see McFadden & Wright, 1990, for a detailed discussion). However, the fairly long time courses observed in some of these experiments (e.g. Viemeister, 1980) suggest that additional (probably central) processing may also be involved (McFadden, 1989).

Finally, it is interesting to note that this *pooled, synchronized response* is a plausible explanation for the fact that overshoot is observed almost exclusively (1) at high frequencies (Zwicker, 1965a), where the onset responses to the masker would be highly synchronized across fibres, and (2) for short signals (Zwicker, 1965a), where, because onset responses to the signals are likely to be important, onset responses to the masker are potentially most interfering.

REFERENCES

ANSI (1969). Specifications for audiometers (ANSI S3.6–1969). New York: American National Standards Institute.

Arthur, R.M., Pfeiffer, R.R., & Suga, N. (1971). Properties of "two-tone inhibition" in primary auditory neurons. *Journal of Physiology*, *212*, 593–609.

Bacon, S.P. (1990). Effect of masker level on overshoot. *Journal of the Acoustical Society of America*, *88*, 698–702.

Bacon, S.P. & Blake, P.E. (1990). Temporal effects in simultaneous masking by vowels and consonant-vowels. *Journal of Speech and Hearing Research*, *33*, 38–44.

Bacon, S.P., Hedrick, M.S., & Grantham, D.W. (1989). Temporal effects in simultaneous pure-tone masking in subjects with high-frequency sensorineural hearing loss. *Audiology*, *27*, 313–323.

Bacon, S.P. & Moore, B.C.J. (1986a). Temporal effects in simultaneous pure-tone masking: Effects of signal frequency, masker/signal frequency ratio, and masker level. *Hearing Research*, *23*, 257–266.

Bacon, S.P. & Moore, B.C.J. (1986b). Temporal effects in masking and their influence on psychophysical tuning curves. *Journal of the Acoustical Society of America*, *80*, 1638–1645.

Bacon, S.P. & Moore, B.C.J. (1987). Transient masking and the temporal course of simultaneous tone-on-tone masking. *Journal of the Acoustical Society of America, 81*, 1073–1077.

Bacon, S.P. & Viemeister, N.F. (1985a). Simultaneous masking by gated and continuous sinusoidal maskers. *Journal of the Acoustical Society of America, 78*, 1220–1230.

Bacon, S.P. & Viemeister, N.F. (1985b). The temporal course of simultaneous tone-on-tone masking. *Journal of the Acoustical Society of America, 78*, 1231–1235.

Carlyon, R.P. (1987). A release from masking by continuous, random, notched noise. *Journal of the Acoustical Society of America, 81*, 418–426.

Carlyon, R.P. (1989). Changes in the masked thresholds of brief tones produced by prior bursts of noise. *Hearing Research, 41*, 223–236.

Carlyon, R.P. & Moore, B.C.J. (1986). Detection of tones in noise and the "severe departure" from Weber's law. *Journal of the Acoustical Society of America, 79*, 461–464.

Carlyon, R.P. & Sloan, E.P. (1987). The "overshoot" effect and sensory hearing impairment. *Journal of the Acoustical Society of America, 82*, 1078–1081. See also *Journal of the Acoustical Society of America, 83*, 1193.

Champlin, C.A. & McFadden, D. (1989). Reductions in overshoot following intense sound exposures. *Journal of the Acoustical Society of America, 85*, 2005–2011.

Elliott, L.L. (1965). Changes in the simultaneous masked threshold of brief tones. *Journal of the Acoustical Society of America, 38*, 738–746.

Elliott, L.L. (1967). Development of auditory narrow-band frequency contours. *Journal of the Acoustical Society of America, 42*, 143–153.

Elliott, L.L. (1969). Masking of tones before, during, and after brief silent periods in noise. *Journal of the Acoustical Society of America, 45*, 1277–1279.

Fastl, H. (1976). Temporal masking effects: I. Broad band noise masker. *Acustica, 35*, 287–302.

Fletcher, H. (1940). Auditory patterns. *Reviews of Modern Physics, 12*, 47–65.

Glasberg, B.R. & Moore, B.C.J. (1990). Derivation of auditory filter shapes from notched-noise data. *Hearing Research, 47*, 103–138.

Green, D.M. (1969). Masking with continuous and pulsed sinusoids. *Journal of the Acoustical Society of America, 46*, 939–946.

Harris, D.M. & Dallos, P. (1979). Forward masking of auditory nerve fiber responses. *Journal of Neurophysiology, 42*, 1083–1107.

Houtgast, T. (1972). Psychophysical evidence for lateral inhibition. *Journal of the Acoustical Society of America, 51*, 1885–1894.

Javel, E., Geisler, C.D., & Ravindran, A. (1978). Two-tone suppression in auditory nerve of the cat: Rate-intensity and temporal analyses. *Journal of the Acoustical Society of America, 63*, 1093–1104.

Jesteadt, W., Bacon, S.P., & Lehman, J.R. (1982). Forward masking as a function of frequency, masker level, and signal delay. *Journal of the Acoustical Society of America, 71*, 950–962.

Kiang, N.Y.-S., Watanabe, T., Thomas, E.C., & Clark, L.F. (1965). *Discharge patterns of single fibers in the cat's auditory nerve.* Cambridge, MA: MIT Press, Research Monograph Number 35.

Kimberley, B.P., Nelson, D.A., & Bacon, S.P. (1989). Temporal overshoot in simultaneous-masked psychophysical tuning curves from normal and hearing-impaired listeners. *Journal of the Acoustical Society of America, 85*, 1660–1665.

Leshowitz, B. & Cudahy, E. (1972). Masking with continuous and gated sinusoids. *Journal of the Acoustical Society of America, 51*, 1921–1929.

Leshowitz, B. & Cudahy, E. (1975). Masking patterns for continuous and gated sinusoids. *Journal of the Acoustical Society of America, 58*, 235–242.

Levitt, H. (1971). Transformed up-down methods in psychoacoustics. *Journal of the Acoustical Society of America, 49*, 467–477.

McFadden, D. (1988). Absence of overshoot in a dichotic masking condition. *Journal of the Acoustical Society of America, 83*, 1685–1687.

McFadden, D. (1989). Spectral differences in the ability of temporal gaps to reset the mechanisms underlying overshoot. *Journal of the Acoustical Society of America, 85*, 254–261.

McFadden, D. & Champlin, C.A. (1990). Reductions in overshoot during aspirin use. *Journal of the Acoustical Society of America, 87*, 2634–2642.

McFadden, D. & Wright, B.A. (1990). Temporal decline of masking and comodulation detection differences. *Journal of the Acoustical Society of America, 88*, 711–724.

Mayer, A.M. (1876). Research in acoustics. *Philosophical Magazine, 11*, 500–507.

Moore, B.C.J. & Glasberg, B.R. (1983a). Growth of forward masking for sinusoidal and noise maskers as a function of signal delay: Implications for suppression in noise. *Journal of the Acoustical Society of America, 73*, 1249–1259.

Moore, B.C.J. & Glasberg, B.R. (1983b). Suggested formulae for calculating auditory-filter bandwidths and excitation patterns. *Journal of the Acoustical Society of America, 74*, 750–753.

Moore, B.C.J., Poon, P.W.F., Bacon, S.P., & Glasberg, B.R. (1987). The temporal course of masking and the auditory filter shape. *Journal of the Acoustical Society of America, 81*, 1873–1880.

Plomp, R. (1964). Rate of decay of auditory sensation. *Journal of the Acoustical Society of America, 36*, 277–282.

Relkin, E.M. & Turner, C.W. (1988). A reexamination of forward masking in the auditory nerve. *Journal of the Acoustical Society of America, 84*, 584–591.

Sachs, M.B. & Kiang, N.Y.-S. (1968). Two-tone inhibition in auditory nerve fibers. *Journal of the Acoustical Society of America, 43*, 1120–1128.

Samoilova, I.K. (1959). Masking of short tone signals as a function of the time interval between masked and masking sounds. *Biofizika, 4*, 550–558. (English translation: *Biophysics, 4*(5), 44–52.)

Scharf, B. (1970). Critical bands. In J.V. Tobias (Ed.). *Foundations of modern auditory theory* (Vol. 1, pp. 159–202). London: Academic Press.

Scholl, von H. (1962). Das dynamische Verhalten des Gehors bei der Unterteilung des Schallspektrums in Frequenzgruppen. *Acustica, 12*, 101–107.

Shannon, R.V. (1976). Two-tone unmasking and suppression in a forward-masking situation. *Journal of the Acoustical Society of America, 59*, 1460–1470.

Smith, R.L. (1979). Adaptation, saturation, and physiological masking in single auditory-nerve fibers. *Journal of the Acoustical Society of America, 65*, 166–178.

Smith, R.L. & Zwislocki, J.J. (1975). Short-term adaptation and incremental responses in single auditory-nerve fibers. *Biological Cybernetics, 17*, 169–182.

Soderquist, D.R., Carstens, A.A., & Frank, G.J.H. (1981). Backward, simultaneous, and forward masking as a function of signal delay and frequency. *Journal of Auditory Research, 21*, 227–246.

Summerfield, Q., Haggard, M.P., Foster, J., & Gray, S. (1984). Perceiving vowels from uniform spectra: phonetic exploration of an auditory after-effect. *Perception and Psychophysics, 35*, 203–213.

Summerfield, Q., Sidwell, A., & Nelson, T. (1987). Auditory enhancement of changes in spectral amplitude. *Journal of the Acoustical Society of America, 81*, 700–708.

Teas, D.C., Eldredge, D.H., & Davis, H. (1962). Cochlear responses to acoustic transients. An interpretation of whole nerve action potentials. *Journal of the Acoustical Society of America, 34*, 1438–1459.

Viemeister, N.F. (1980). Adaptation of masking. In G. Van den Brink & F.A. Bilsen (Eds.), *Psychophysical, physiological, and behavioural studies in hearing* (pp. 190–199). The Netherlands: Delft University Press.

Viemeister, N.F. & Bacon, S.P. (1982). Forward masking by enhanced components in harmonic complexes. *Journal of the Acoustical Society of America, 71*, 1502–1507.

Wier, C.C., Green, D.M., Hafter, E.R., & Burkhardt, S. (1977). Detection of a tone burst in continuous- and gated noise maskers; Defects [sic] of signal frequency, duration, and masker level. *Journal of the Acoustical Society of America, 61*, 1298–1300.

Wright, B.A. (1989). Auditory-filter shapes at three test frequencies with a burst and a fringed notched-noise masker. *Journal of the Acoustical Society of America, 86* (Supplement 1), S121.

Zerlin, S. (1969). Traveling-wave velocity in the human cochlea. *Journal of the Acoustical Society of America, 46*, 1011–1015.

Zwicker, E. (1964). "Negative afterimage" in hearing. *Journal of the Acoustical Society of America, 36*, 2413–2415.

Zwicker, E. (1965a). Temporal effects in simultaneous masking by white-noise bursts. *Journal of the Acoustical Society of America, 37*, 653–663.

Zwicker, E. (1965b). Temporal effects in simultaneous masking and loudness. *Journal of the Acoustical Society of America, 38*, 132–141.

Zwicker, E. & Fastl, H. (1972). On the development of the critical band. *Journal of the Acoustical Society of America, 52*, 699–702.

Zwicker, E. & Terhardt, E. (1980). Analytical expressions for critical-band rate and critical bandwidth as a function of frequency. *Journal of the Acoustical Society of America, 68*, 1523–1525.

Revised manuscript received 3 November 1990

THE QUARTERLY JOURNAL OF EXPERIMENTAL PSYCHOLOGY, 1991, *43A* (3) 401–421

Effects of Phase Changes in Low-numbered Harmonics on the Internal Representation of Complex Sounds

J. Denis McKeown and C. J. Darwin

University of Sussex, U.K.

A series of experiments investigated the effect of phase changes in low-numbered single harmonics in target sounds that were either synthesized steady-state vowels or periodic signals having only a single formant. A matching procedure was used in which subjects selected a sound along a continuum differing in first formant frequency in order to get the best match with the target sound; perceptual effects of the phase manipulations in the target were detected as a change in the matched first formant frequency. Stimuli had to contain at least three harmonics to produce the effect, but it did not require a particular starting phase of the components. A suppression phenomenon is discussed, in which phase changes alter the phase-locking characteristics of auditory fibres tuned to low-numbered harmonics.

Listeners can detect a change in the phase of a single harmonic of a complex periodic sound, particularly when the harmonic is high-numbered and unresolved by the auditory system (Goldstein, 1967; Mathes & Miller, 1947). The mechanisms that could be responsible for the detection of such phase changes have been well reviewed recently (Moore & Glasberg, 1989; Patterson, 1987). The proposed mechanisms differ in whether they invoke the known non-linearities of the ear.

A linear model can be regarded as consisting of a bank of bandpass filters, each tuned to a different frequency. High-numbered, unresolved harmonics add within an auditory filter, giving a complex waveform at their output. The particular shape of this waveform varies with the relative phase of the individual components. Harmonic components that are more widely spaced

---

Requests for reprints should be sent to Denis McKeown, Applied Psychology Unit, 15 Chaucer Road, Cambridge CB2 2EF, U.K.

This research was supported by grants from the SERC to the second author. Drs R. B. Gardner and R. P. Carlyon provided considerable help and discussion.

in frequency than the auditory filter bandwidth are separately resolved by the filterbank into simple tones. Consequently, changes in the relative phases of these components will *not* change the waveform shape emerging from a single auditory filter. It will, however, change the relative phase of the waveforms emerging from the different filters. Such a model can readily explain the easier detectability of phase changes in high- than in low-numbered harmonics by postulating that changes that result in a change of waveshape at the output of a single filter are easier to detect than are phase changes across different filters.

A different type of explanation of phase sensitivity invokes the non-linearity of the ear. This explanation is able to account for our sensitivity to phase changes in low-numbered harmonics, without having to invoke across-filter mechanisms. Two tones (with frequencies f_1 and f_2) whose patterns of neural activity ("excitation patterns": Moore, 1986) overlap sufficiently will generate tones at other frequencies as distortion products, most significantly at a frequency of $2f_1$–f_2 (the cubic distortion tone). The phase of the cubic distortion tone varies with the relative phases of the two primary tones (Goldstein, 1967; Zwicker, 1981). Consequently, if there is a third primary tone present at the same frequency as the distortion tone, these two tones will add to give a resultant whose amplitude varies with the relative phase of the primaries. A phase change in one harmonic is thus detected as an intensity change in a lower harmonic (Buunen, 1975; Buunen & Bilsen, 1974; Buunen, Festen, Bilsen, & van den Brink, 1974; Buunen, ten Kate, Raatgever, & van den Brink, 1977).

If auditory non-linearities can produce changes in the subjective intensity of low-numbered harmonics in response to changes in their relative phase, then such phase changes might result in a change in the phonetic quality of a speech sound. The reason for this is that the phonetic quality of, for example, vowel sounds depends in part on the first formant frequency. The first formant frequency in turn is related to the relative intensities of the (generally low-numbered) harmonics around the first formant peak (Assmann & Nearey, 1987; Darwin & Gardner, 1985). Any change in the relative intensities of these low-numbered harmonics could therefore cause a shift in the apparent frequency of the formant peak.

In this paper, we look for such shifts in perceived formant frequency, by using a matching procedure, where the matching continuum varies in formant frequency. If phase changes *do* lead to changes in the subjective intensity of the low-numbered harmonics, we might be able to detect such changes in terms of a shift in the matched formant frequency. The advantage of using this method is that other changes in the subjective quality of a sound produced by phase changes (for instance timbral changes that are not related to formant frequency) should not produce any consistent shift along the formant-matching continuum.

We already have some evidence from a vowel identification task that phase changes do produce phonetically relevant changes (Darwin & Gardner, 1986, Experiment 3). With suitably placed higher formants, the distinction between /ɪ/ and /ɛ/ can be made by simply varying the first formant frequency. The experiment estimated a subject's phoneme boundary between /ɪ/ and /ɛ/ along a continuum of synthesized steady-state vowels differing in F1. The phoneme boundary was at an F1 frequency of around 440 Hz. When the phase of the fourth harmonic (500 Hz) was changed, the phoneme boundary shifted by about 15 Hz. Phase changes had not previously been shown to influence perceived formant frequencies.

These phoneme boundary changes could, in principle, have arisen via the generation of combination tones as described above. But the size of the phoneme boundary shift appears too large for this explanation, judged by the measured levels of combination tones for appropriate frequencies and frequency spacings (Zwicker, 1981).

An alternative suggestion exploits another aspect of the auditory system's non-linearity—synchrony suppression. The extent to which auditory nerve fibres phase-lock to a particular frequency in complex sounds can be influenced by the relative phases of the components (Palmer, Winter, Gardner, & Darwin, 1987). If the perceived intensity of a harmonic in the auditory system is signalled by the extent to which the auditory nerve synchronizes to its frequency (Palmer, Winter, & Darwin, 1986; Young & Sachs, 1979), then phase-sensitive synchrony suppression could reduce the extent of that synchrony and hence produce a change in the perceived intensity of that component. This change would in turn alter the perceived first formant frequency.

The experiments reported in this paper extend the earlier findings, but use a matching rather than a labelling task. Matching paradigms need not use speech sounds, and so allow a wider range of sounds to be investigated. First we wished to examine whether phase changes in "target" vowels could be mapped onto differences in first formant frequency in a continuum of "matching" vowels. One particular concern was whether any perceptual effect of advancing the phase of a harmonic was equivalent to altering its intensity; if so, advancing the phase of a component lying below the first formant peak should produce the opposite effect to the same manipulation of a component lying above the formant peak. We use the matching paradigm also to establish that an effect of phase requires at least three harmonics; finally, we investigate how it depends on the starting phases of the component sounds.

On each trial of the following experiments the subject hears a pair of sounds on demand; the first is the target, and the second is one from the matching continuum. The subject adjusts the position of the second sound along the continuum to produce the best match (Figure 1). The sounds from

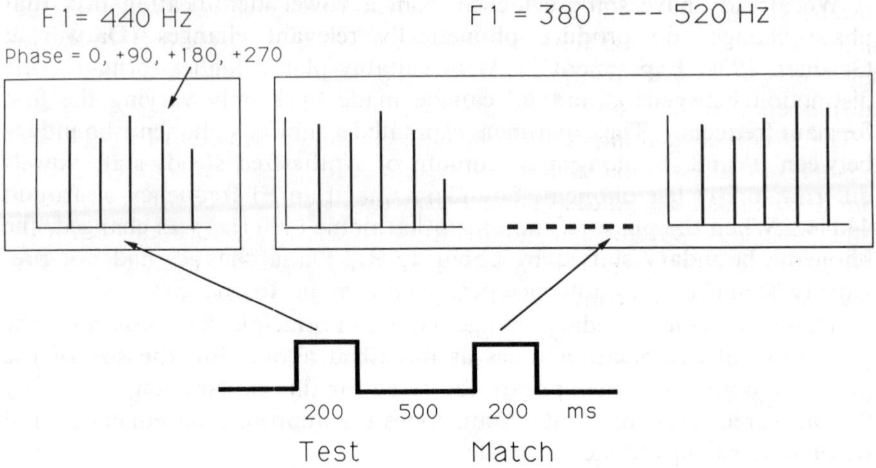

FIG. 1. Stimulus matching procedure used in the experiments. Schematic spectra of the first formant region of the test (or "target") sound and of the matching sound are shown. The matching sound is taken from a continuum of sounds differing in first formant frequency.

the matching continuum differ in their first formant frequency, and so have different relative intensities of their low-numbered harmonics. If a phase change between the components of the target sound changes the perceived relative intensities of the harmonics, then subjects should change their preferred match position along the (F1) continuum.

We first demonstrate that this matching paradigm does indeed produce a consistent phase effect for sounds like those used in the previous labelling experiment. We then examine in greater detail, using smaller numbers of subjects, how the effect varies with changes to different parameters of the stimulus.

EXPERIMENT 1

The first experiment attempts to replicate with a matching paradigm the changes in perceived first formant frequency of a vowel with the phase of a harmonic close to the formant peak found by Darwin and Gardner (1986).

Method

Stimuli and Procedure. Following Darwin and Gardner (1986), four-formant vowels were synthesized by adding together sine waves at harmonic frequencies with the amplitudes and phases given by the transfer function produced by a software formant synthesizer (Klatt, 1980) in serial mode. The Klatt synthesizer produces phase spectra that are close to those of natural vowels. The resonators of the synthesizer give large changes in the relative phases of the individual harmonics around F1. Stimuli were 200 msec in duration, with 16 msec rise and fall times. The frequency spacing (fundamental frequency) of harmonics was 125 Hz.

The 20 sounds making up the matching continuum varied in F1 from 350 to 540 Hz in 10-Hz steps, giving /ɪ/-like sounds at low F1 values and /ɛ/-like sounds at higher F1 values. The frequencies of the higher formants were 2300, 2900, and 3800 Hz. The bandwidths of the first four formants were 90, 110, 170, and 1000 Hz, respectively. Figure 2 shows the power spectrum of a vowel sound from the continuum close to the /ɪ/–/ɛ/ phoneme boundary.

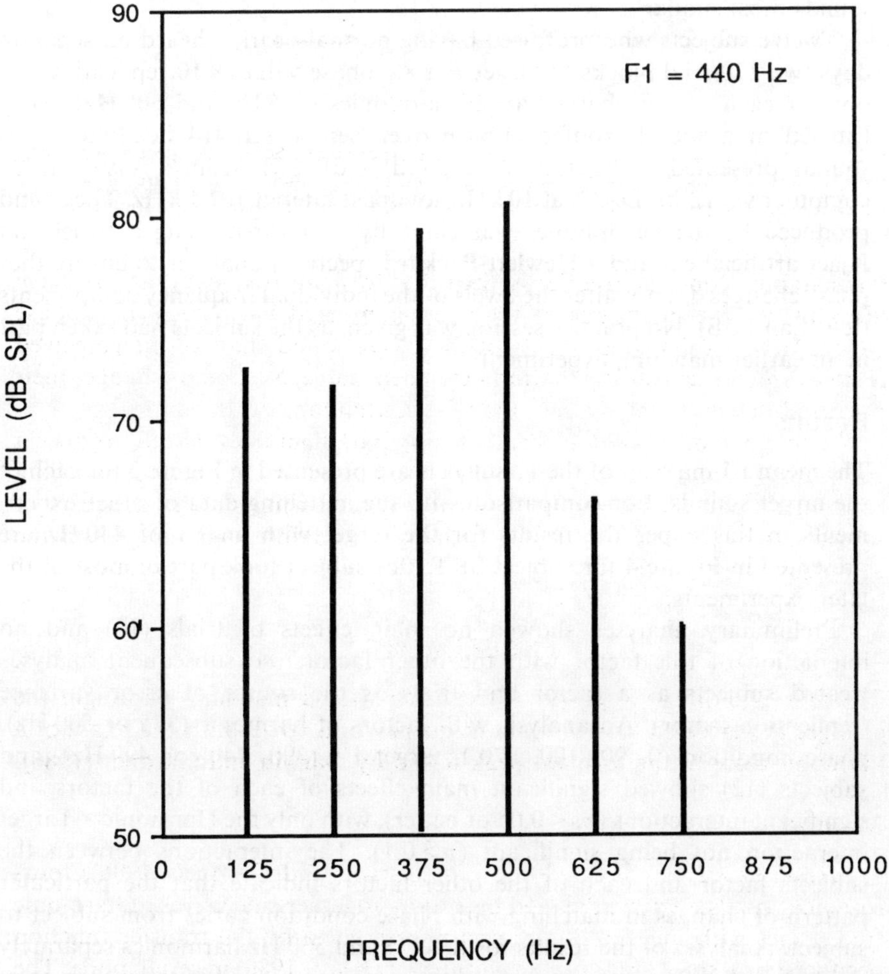

FIG. 2. Schematic spectrum of the low-frequency region of vowel-type used in Experiment 1.

Comparison ("target") sounds had the same amplitude spectra, but their phase spectra were changed by advancing the phase of either the 375-Hz harmonic or the 500-Hz harmonic by 0, 90, 180, or 270° relative to the phase of the vowel's transfer function. Three F1 values were used for the targets, at 390, 440 and 490 Hz (identical to the 5th, 10th, and 15th members of the continuum, respectively). A trial consisted of a target sound followed after 500 msec by a sound from the continuum. Subjects could then select alternative sounds from the continuum to find the best match using keyboard keys to move different numbers of steps in either direction. An instruction sheet advised subjects to bracket the target before making their final selection. The instructions included the phrase to "match to the vowel that sounds most similar".

Twelve subjects who professed having normal-hearing heard on separate days two 120-trial blocks (3 target F1s × 4 phase values × 10 replications)—one for each of the phase-changed harmonics (375 Hz and 500 Hz). They listened in a sound-proofed cubicle over Sennheiser 414 headphones to sounds presented monaurally at around 70 dB SPL from a VAX-11/780 computer via 12-bit DACs at 10 kHz, low-pass filtered at 4.5 kHz. The sound produced by the headphones was carefully monitored using a Bruel and Kjaer artificial ear and a Hewlett-Packard spectrum analyser to ensure that phase changes did not alter the levels of the individual frequency components (less than 1 dB). No practice session was given, as the subjects had taken part in an earlier matching experiment.

Results

The mean F1 matches of the 12 subjects are presented in Figure 3 for each of the target sounds. For comparison with the matching data of other experiments in this paper the results for the target with an F1 of 440 Hz are presented in Figure 4 for subject SRT; this subject took part in most of the later experiments.

Preliminary analyses showed no main effects of trials (10) and no interaction of this factor with the other factors, so subsequent analyses treated subjects as a factor and trials as the source of error variance (replication factor). An analysis with factors of harmonic (375 or 500 Hz), phase condition (0, 90, 180, 270°), target F1 (390, 440, or 490 Hz), and subjects (12) showed significant main effects of each of the factors and significant interactions (ps < 0.05 or better), with only the Harmonic × Target interaction not being significant ($p > 0.1$). The interactions between the subjects factor and each of the other factors indicate that the particular pattern of changes in matching with phase condition varies from subject to subject. Analyses of the results for the 375 and 500 Hz harmonics separately showed main effects of phase condition, target, and subjects in each case; interactions were highly significant (all ps < 0.01).

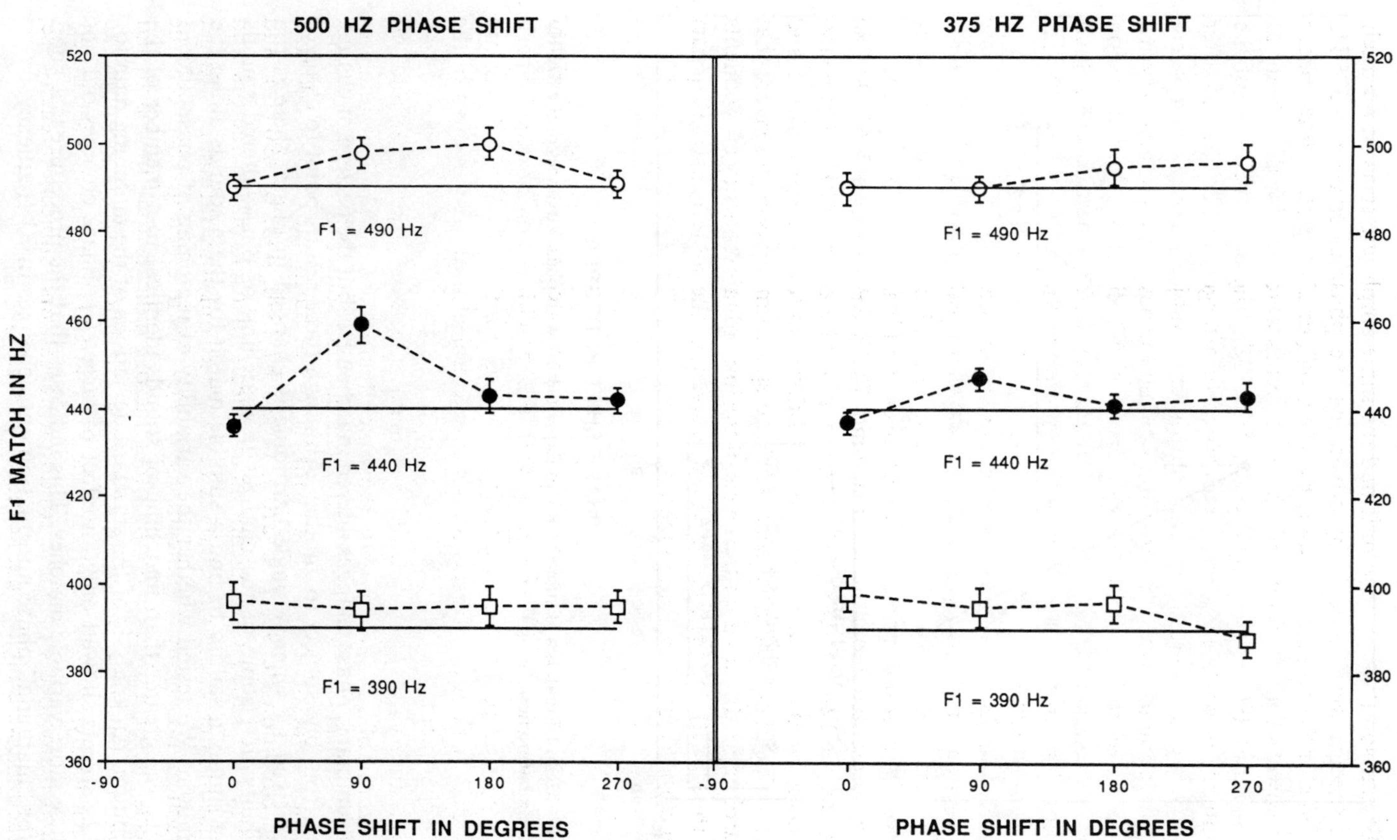

FIG. 3. F1 matches averaged over the 12 subjects in Experiment 1, when the 500-Hz harmonic (left), or 375-Hz harmonic (right) was advanced in phase. Vertical bars are standard errors over 10 trials.

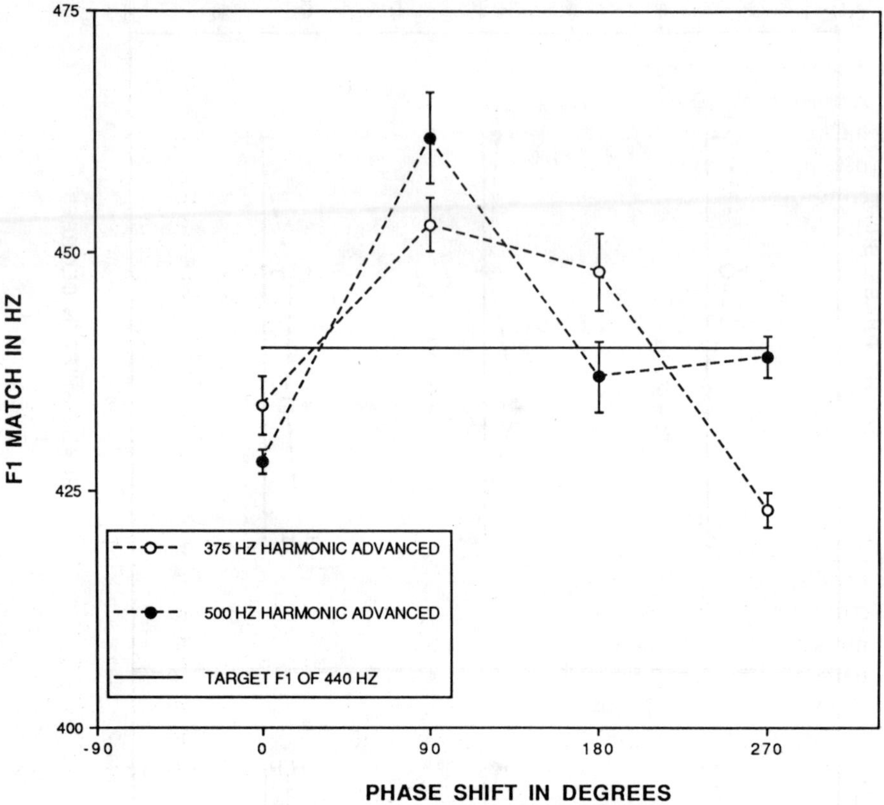

FIG. 4. Mean F1 matches of subject SRT in Experiment 1 with phase advances of the 375-Hz or 500-Hz harmonics.

In summary, phase changes altered matched F1, but the pattern of change varied from one subject to another. Although these results point to changes in perceived F1 when a single harmonic is changed in phase, there is the possibility that some of the changes in matching of phase-altered sounds reflect simply a failure to find a suitable match for these sounds along the continuum. We tested whether the variability of matching of phase-altered sounds was greater than matching of sounds identical to a member of the continuum. An analysis of the standard deviations of the matching data for the 12 subjects showed only an effect of target F1. Phase changes did not produce more variable matches. This indicates that the procedure is a good one for "mapping" phase information onto changes in F1 frequency.

Discussion

The first experiment has replicated with a matching paradigm the result reported by Darwin and Gardner (1986) that the relative phase of a harmonic near F1 changes apparent F1 frequency. The present experiment uses a wider range of conditions than the earlier one, but replicates common conditions closely. The largest effect in the previous experiment was produced by a 90° phase advance in the 500-Hz component, which lowered the phoneme boundary by about 15 Hz from 445 to 430 Hz. A lower phoneme boundary corresponds to a higher perceived formant frequency. In the present experiment the F1 target at 440 Hz was matched to a 20-Hz higher F1 when the phase of the 500-Hz harmonic was advanced by 90°. The matching result is thus quantitatively similar to that found earlier.

The other conditions show smaller changes, with considerable variability across different subjects. Variability between subjects in the extent of auditory non-linearities has been reported by Zwicker (1981). A consistent feature in Figure 3, however, is that the changes produced by shifting the 375-Hz component, although smaller, are in the same direction as those produced by changing the phase of the 500-Hz component. As these two components are always on opposite sides of the formant frequency, it is unlikely that the phase change is making the changed component more perceptually prominent (Kubovy & Jordan, 1979). If it were, then phase changes to the two harmonics should have given shifts in opposite directions.

The following experiments exploit the matching paradigm to examine phase effects on perceived formant frequency for sounds that are simpler than the vowels used in the first experiment.

EXPERIMENT 2

Experiment 2 uses 2- and 3-component sounds shaped by a formant filter, with the higher component changing in phase. If the effects found in the first experiment are due to a cubic difference tone adding to a third frequency (Buunen et al., 1974), then we should not expect to find any shift in matched F1 when only two components are used. The experiment also includes two different fundamental frequencies.

Method

Stimuli and Procedure. Sounds with either two or three harmonics were produced using the same software synthesizer as in the first experiment. There were four separate test blocks in this experiment, which differed in fundamental frequency (80 or 125 Hz) and in number of harmonics (2 or 3). For stimuli with a fundamental of 80 Hz, the two- and three-component sounds were 400 and 480 Hz, and 320, 400, and 480 Hz. For stimuli with a fundamental of 125 Hz they were 375 and 500 Hz, and 250, 375, and 500 Hz. The matching continua differed in F1, as before, and contained the same number of harmonics as the target sound. Four subjects, each with audiometrically normal hearing, were tested with the four test blocks on four separate days. The targets had an F1 of 450 Hz, with the phase of the highest harmonic (480 or 500 Hz) advanced by 0, 90, 180, or 270°. The stimuli sounded vowel-like, and as in Experiment 1, subjects were instructed to "match to the vowel that sounds most similar".

Results

Figure 5 shows the four subjects' data for a fundamental of 125 Hz. There was little evidence of any effect of a phase change in two-component sounds, but three-component sounds did show significant effects. There were differences among subjects in the pattern of matching. Thus some subjects showed matching to higher F1 values at 90° and 180° shifts, others matching to lower F1 values at 270° shifts. Phase effects were not markedly different according to whether the fundamental frequency used was 80 or 125 Hz.

An analysis of variance with factors of component (2 or 3), fundamental frequency (80 or 125 Hz), phase condition (0, 90, 180, or 270°) and subjects showed a significant effect of components, of fundamental frequency, of phase condition, and of subjects (*p*s < 0.05 or better); the Components × Phase condition interaction was significant ($p < 0.001$), but there was no significant interaction with subjects. Further analyses were performed on two- and three-component data separately, with factors of fundamental frequency, phase condition, and subjects. First, for three-component stimuli, there were significant main effects of each factor (*p*s < 0.05 or better), a significant Fundamental × Phase Condition interaction ($p < 0.01$), but no interactions with subjects. For two-component stimuli there were no main effects of fundamental frequency or of phase condition, and no interactions (*p*s > 0.1).

Discussion

Experiment 2 has found a consistent effect across subjects of the phase of low-frequency harmonics on matched F1 frequency when sounds had at least three harmonic components. Although the magnitude of the changes is larger for some subjects (JDM, CBS) than for others (SRT, AMB), the generally convex *pattern* of the changes is consistent across all four subjects. It is also clear that the standard errors of the individual data points in Figure 5 are no larger in the phase-shifted conditions than in the unshifted condition. These two points argue for the matching procedure we have used reflecting real changes in perceived formant frequency rather than simply an idiosyncratic strategy for coping with changes in dissimilar perceptual dimensions.

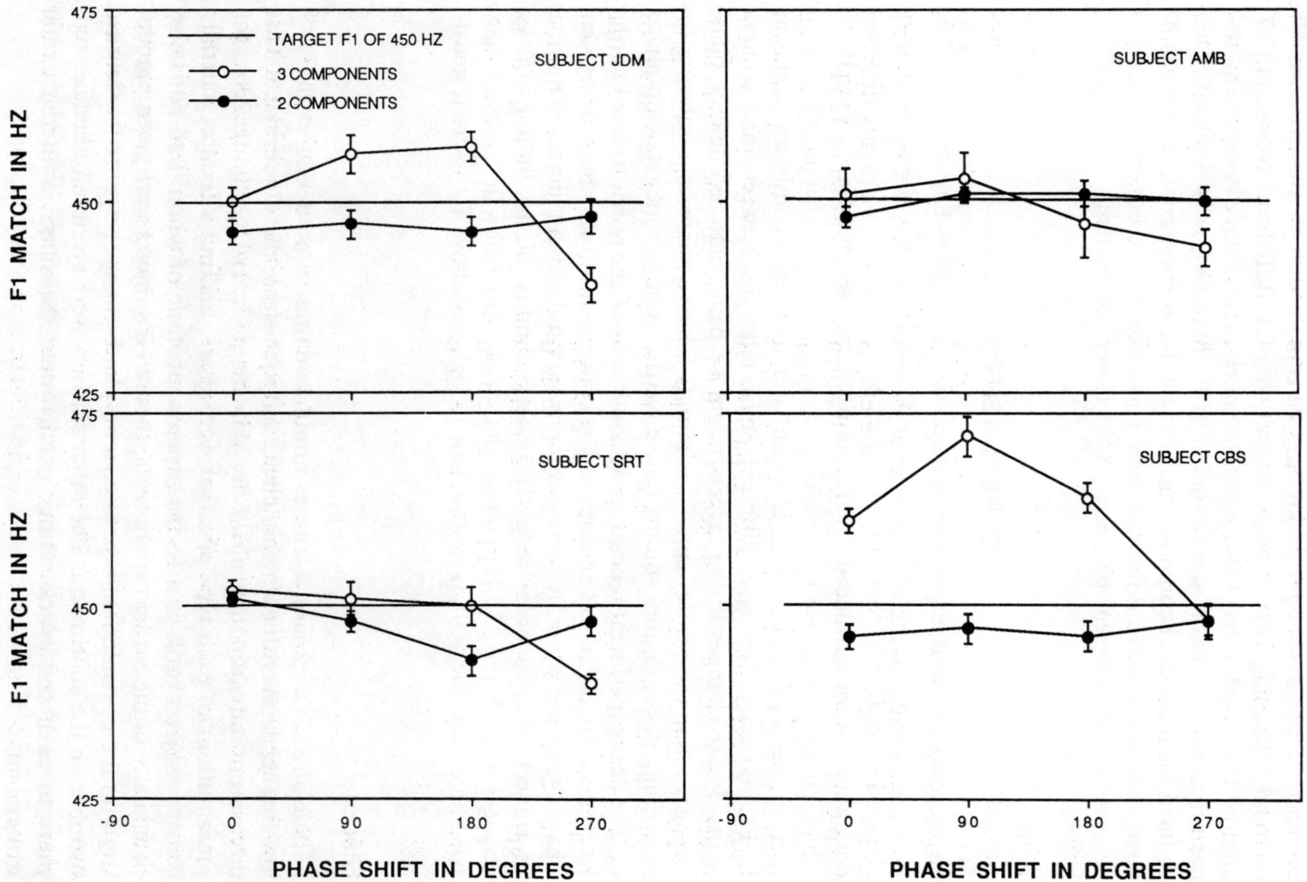

FIG. 5. Mean F1 matches for each of the 4 subjects in Experiment 2 to stimuli with 3 or 2 harmonics and the 500- or 480-Hz component advanced in phase.

We find large and consistent effects when there are three harmonics present, but when the target sound has only two harmonics there is very little evidence of phase changes giving any detectable shift in the matched F1 boundary. The single exception is the shift subject SRT shows between the 0° and the 180° conditions. This exception apart, at least three components are needed to give a reliable shift in matched F1 frequency as a result of phase shifts in the individual components. That finding is compatible with the shift being due to the cubic difference tone generated by the upper two components adding in different phases with the lower component.

EXPERIMENT 3

In the two previous experiments there was a confounding variable. The relative phases of the different sounds along the matching continuum changed according to their formant frequency. The sounds of the matching continuum were produced by formant filters (second-order resonators) which change the phase of a particular component by around 180° as the formant peak passes across it. Different sounds from a continuum differing in F1 frequency thus have different phase relations between their components. Phase changes in the targets might be being matched against phase changes along the continuum. To eliminate relative phase as a criterion for matching, all continuum sounds now have the same (cosine) starting phase.

The next experiment repeats some conditions of the previous one in order to control for the phase artefact in the continuum; it also both introduces phase changes in other frequency components and uses an increased number of subjects (12) in order to extend the generality of the findings. Phase changes in both the 375-Hz component (which lies below F1 in the targets used here) and the 500-Hz component (which lies above F1) were tested.

Method

Stimuli and Procedure. Target stimuli had three components at 250, 375, and 500 Hz, with cosine starting phase and with either the 375- or the 500-Hz component advanced in phase by 45, 90, 135, 180, 225, or 270°. Six presentations of each type of target were given, making a total of 42 trials. Twelve subjects took part in the experiment, four of whom had not taken part in any of the earlier experiments; these four subjects were given practice trials until they could reliably match a no-phase-change target to its identical member on the continuum. The other subjects were given ten practice trials prior to each test block. Other details were the same as in the earlier experiments.

Results

As in Experiment 1, a first analysis of variance used subjects as the source of error variance (replication factor) with factors of component advanced (375 or 500 Hz), phase condition (0, 45, 90, 135, 180, 225, or 270°) and trials (6). The analysis showed neither a main effect of trials nor any interaction of trials with the other factors. Further analyses used trials as the replication factor. An analysis with factors of subjects, component advanced, and phase condition showed a highly significant effect of subjects ($p<0.001$), but neither a main effect of component advanced nor phase condition ($ps>0.1$); however, there were significant interactions of subjects with each of these factors, and a highly significant three-way interaction ($p<0.001$).

The data for the two components were analysed separately. First, for phase changes of the 375-Hz component, there was a highly significant effect of subjects ($p<0.001$), a significant effect of phase ($p<0.05$), and a highly significant interaction between these two factors ($p<0.001$). For the 500-Hz component, there was a highly significant effect of subjects ($p<0.001$), no main effect of phase ($p>0.1$), but a highly significant interaction ($p<0.001$).

The effect of phase thus differs very significantly across subjects, although individual subjects have been found to give replicable data in both this experiment and in the others in the series. Data for the 12 subjects are shown in Figure 6, illustrating the different effect of phase changes to the two different components. Note that different phase shift conditions, progressing from 0° through to 270°, show a fairly regular W-shaped pattern with vowel matches following the phase shift. Although the "starting point" of this regular pattern differed from subject to subject, it was seen in most cases. Also apparent is that phase shifts of the 500-Hz component show a pattern that generally differs from the pattern obtained for phase shifts of the 375-Hz component.

This experiment has eliminated the confounding variable of the phase of sounds along the matching continuum. Clear changes in matching are obtained when all continuum sounds had cosine starting phases. Second, the pattern of the matching is different according to the choice of the harmonic advanced in phase (375 or 500 Hz).

EXPERIMENT 4

Experiment 3 controlled for phase changes along the matching continuum and demonstrated a change in the pattern of shifts produced by introducing the phase change in different frequency components. In the next experiment we keep the phase of the matching continuum and the component that receives the phase change constant, but vary the baseline starting phases of the components. We have chosen three different starting phases, which give

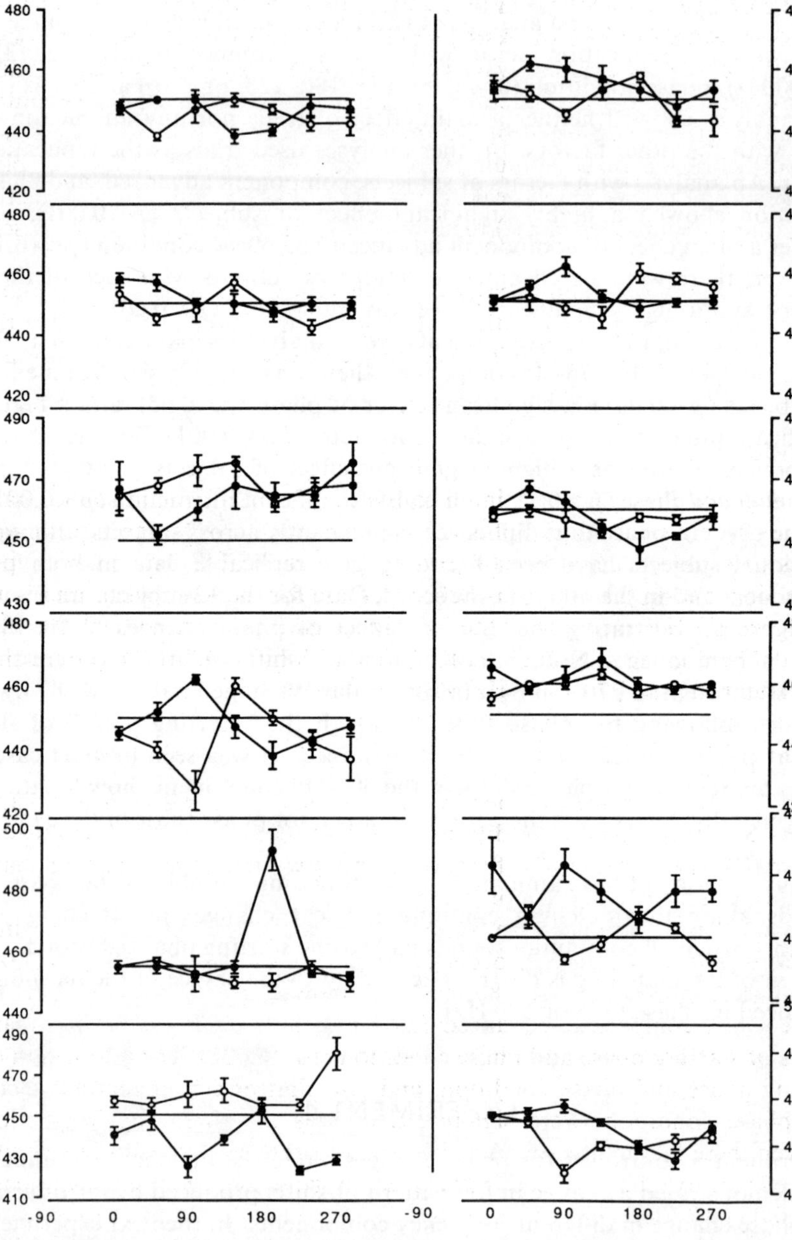

FIG. 6. Mean F1 matches for each of the 12 subjects in Experiment 3 for phase shifts of the 375-Hz (open circles) and 500-Hz (filled circles) components. The targets had an F1 frequency of 450 Hz.

different peak factors in the overall envelope of the sound, and also in the sound after it has been filtered by the cochlea.

Cosine stimuli have a markedly peaky waveform envelope (a high peak factor), both in the original waveform and after auditory filtering. Stimuli with an optimally low peak factor in the original waveform can be computed with an algorithm suggested by Schroeder (Schroeder, 1970). We used two types of Schroeder-phase stimuli; both have a low peak factor, but one (plus Schroeder phase) has a high peak factor after auditory filtering, whereas the other (minus Schroeder phase) maintains a lower peak factor (Kohlrausch, 1988).

As in the previous experiment, in a particular starting phase condition all continuum members had identical starting phases. Phase shifts of both the 375-Hz component and the 500-Hz component were tested in single-formant sounds.

Method

Stimuli and Procedure. Stimuli consisted of single-formant sounds having the first eight harmonics of a 125-Hz fundamental. The experiment was run as six separate test blocks (40 trials per block), consisting of three types of starting phases (cosine, plus Schroeder, or minus Schroeder), and with either the 375-Hz harmonic or the 500-Hz harmonic advanced by 0, 90, 180, or 270° from the phase given in a particular condition. All targets in this experiment had an F1 of 440 Hz. There were two subjects.

Results

Figure 7 shows the results of the two subjects for the cosine and the plus- and minus- Schroeder phase conditions. The two subjects show a consistent pattern of results, with clear differences both between the three starting phase conditions and the two harmonic conditions.

An analysis of variance with factors of subjects (2), starting phase (cosine, plus Schroeder or minus Schroeder), component advanced (375 or 500 Hz), and phase condition (0, 90, 180, or 270°) showed neither a main effect of subjects nor component advanced ($ps > 0.1$), but highly significant main effects of starting phase and phase condition ($ps < 0.001$). The interaction of starting phase and phase condition, and also that of component advanced and phase condition, were significant, as was the three-way interaction between these factors ($ps < 0.01$ or better). Separate analyses showed significant effects for the 375 and 500 Hz component for each starting phase ($ps < 0.05$ or better).

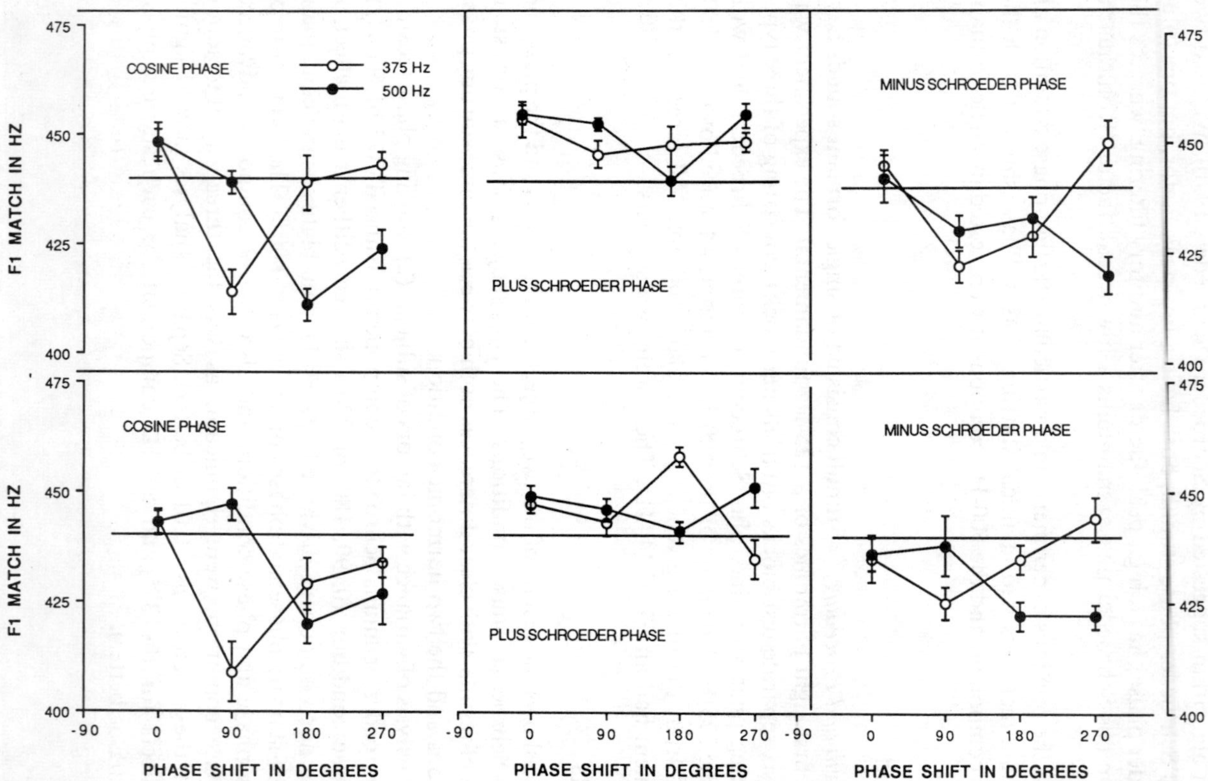

FIG. 7. Mean F1 matches for each of the two subjects in Experiment 4 for cosine starting phase (left), plus Schroeder phase (middle) and minus Schroeder phase (right). The upper half of the figure are the results for subject JDM and the lower half for subject SRT.

Discussion

This experiment varied the starting phases of the components and showed similarity in the pattern of matching across three different starting phase conditions; the W- or V-shaped pattern observed in the other experiments was observed in both subjects' data, and the pattern obtained for the harmonic below the formant peak differed from that found for the harmonic above the formant peak. The two subjects showed similar matching patterns. The particular starting phases chosen are ones reported to govern phase sensitivity in high-numbered unresolved harmonics, with more peaky waveforms showing larger phase effects (Goldstein, 1967). Although the starting phases chosen in the present experiment were ones differing in the peakiness of the waveform envelope, there was only moderate evidence that this envelope characteristic significantly affected the size of the phase effects in the low-numbered (imperfectly-) resolved harmonics used here. Peaky stimuli did not show larger effects, however. Thus, the plus Schroeder phase stimulus (high peak factor after auditory filtering) showed slightly smaller effects than did the other two stimulus types, which were very similar to one another.

GENERAL DISCUSSION

Summary of Findings

1. Advancing the phase of a single harmonic near F1 in steady-state vowels shifts the matched F1 position. The shift can be as much as 35 Hz (in Experiment 4, for example), depending on the subject and the particular experimental conditions.
2. Phase changes in single-formant sounds consisting of the 3 harmonics nearest to F1 produced shifts in matched formant frequency similar to those found in the four-formant vowels, but there was little evidence for such shifts in two-component sounds.
3. The shift in matched F1 is still found when the phase of all the components in the matching continuum is held constant.
4. Different starting phases altered the pattern of shift in matched F1, but starting phases that minimized the peak factor of the waveform envelope did little to reduce the size of the shift compared with cosine starting phases.

In other experiments not reported here (McKeown & Darwin, 1989) we have shown in addition that:

5. A detectable effect of phase on matched F1 can be found with a harmonic spacing (F0) as large as 250 Hz for harmonics around 500 Hz.

It is clear both from these data and those reported previously (Darwin & Gardner, 1986) that phase changes amongst low-numbered harmonics change the timbre of a sound in a way that can be matched against a change in formant frequency and so has potential phonetic significance. The significance of our results lies in three directions: (1) The paradigms that we have used—formant-frequency matching (here) and phoneme boundaries (Darwin & Gardner, 1986)—provide a sensitive technique for detecting changes in the internal representation of the relative amplitudes of the components of complex sounds. (2) The existence of these changes as a result of phase manipulations raises theoretical questions about the underlying mechanisms. (3) Phase effects on phoneme boundaries and matched formant frequencies are potential artefacts for research that inadvertently varies phase relations. It would, however, be disingenuous for us to claim that our phase effects had much practical significance in natural speech communication. The size of the effects is quite small compared with inter-vowel differences, and the natural environment of enclosed rooms plays havoc with the phase spectrum of a sound—although phase might be used systematically by hearing-impaired listeners (Rosen & Smith, 1988).

In contrast to the very small within-subject variability in the matching results were noted differences in the pattern of matching from subject to subject. Differences across subjects may have occurred for a number of reasons. The differences may reflect differences in the effective phase spectrum of the sounds due to changes in headphone position; though the similarity in the matching patterns of individual subjects tested on separate days suggests that this factor is of minor importance. More plausible is that the differences reflect the fact that different subjects "adopt" different criteria or strategies in the formant-matching task. Or the differences may be due to differences in the characteristics of non-linearities from subject to subject, as has been noted by Zwicker (1981). The broad pattern of results across subjects was, however, evident in the W- or V-shaped changes of formant matches following the degree of shift in the phase of a harmonic.

There are two ways in which such changes in matching might come about, both of which invoke non-linearities in the cochlea. First, combination tones could act to alter the relative levels of harmonics (Buunen et al., 1974). This explanation is compatible with the finding in Experiment 2 that at least three harmonics are required to obtain the effect. Second, changes in phase-locking induced by changes in the relative phase of components might be responsible (Palmer et al., 1987).

We have no *direct* evidence against the role of combination tones; we can only estimate their likely effect from published data. The most likely candidate combination tone is the 250-Hz tone generated by the 375- and 500-Hz primaries. Using a cancellation technique on a single listener, Zwicker (1981, Figure 2) obtained the level of the $2f_1$–f_2 cubic difference tone as about 36 dB SPL for 70 dB primaries at frequencies of 540 and 660 Hz (Δf= 120 Hz). The combination tone is thus about 34 dB lower in intensity than the primaries. If such a combination tone were generated by the 375- and 500-Hz components of our stimuli, it could alter the level of the 250-Hz component, which is around 4 dB lower in intensity than the 375 Hz component. However, the magnitude of the change is less than ± 0.3 dB. The appropriate intensity difference limen for a pure tone at 250 Hz is about 1 dB (Jesteadt, Wier, & Green, 1977) so it is very unlikely that our listeners could detect phase changes in the 375- or 500-Hz components by listening to the combination-tone-induced intensity changes in the 250-Hz component.

Even if the intensity change produced by the 250-Hz tone were detectable, it would have very little effect on formant frequency matching. In an unpublished experiment (but see Darwin & Gardner, 1985, for supportive evidence using vowel stimuli) we manipulated the levels of individual harmonics in single formant sounds consisting of the first eight harmonics of a 125-Hz fundamental. We found that level changes of 6 dB in the 375- and 500-Hz harmonics produced shifts in F1 matching equivalent to the largest phase effects observed, but that level changes of 6 or 8 dB in the 250- and 625-Hz harmonics produced negligible changes in F1 matching.

A second possible reason for our phase effects is that suppression is sensitive to the relative phase of the harmonic components. Although the relative phase of the primary components does not alter the intensity of the $2f_1$–f_2 cubic difference tone (Buunen et al., 1974), other aspects of cochlear non-linearity might be phase-sensitive. In guinea-pig auditory nerve, the degree of phase-locking (but not the overall rate of firing) to the frequency components of sounds very similar to those used here has been shown to be altered by the relative phases of the frequency components (Palmer et al., 1987).

To amplify these physiological findings, we used a non-linear cochlear model incorporating suppression to see whether we could find changes in phase-locking to harmonics near F1 when a single component is changed in phase, similar to those found physiologically. The stimuli, like those used in Experiment 2, were single-formant sounds consisting of the first eight harmonics of a 125-Hz fundamental. The computer simulation, due to Roy Gardner (Gardner & Uppal, 1986), implemented a version of a band-pass filter model (Cooke, 1986; Pfeiffer, 1970), using a non-linear stage between two band-pass filters (the reader is referred to Gardner & Uppal, 1986, for details of the model that was implemented). The suppression measure used in the model showed changes of a few dB at harmonic frequencies around the formant peak when a single harmonic was advanced in phase. When the suppressive characteristics were removed from the model, the output showed no phase related changes.

In summary, we have confirmed earlier findings of an effect of phase on the internal representation of low-numbered harmonics in the first formant region. The effect requires at least three harmonics and does not require any particular starting phase relationship between the components. It is unlikely to be due to the effect of combination tones, but may reflect an effect of phase on synchrony suppression.

REFERENCES

Assmann, P.F. & Nearey, T.M. (1987). Perception of front vowels: The role of harmonics in the first formant region. *Journal of the Acoustical Society of America, 81*, 520–534.

Buunen, T.J.F. (1975). Two hypotheses on monaural phase effects. *Acustica, 34*, 98–105.

Buunen, T.J.F. & Bilsen, F.A. (1974). Subjective phase effects and combination tones. In E. Zwicker & E. Terhardt (Ed). *Facts and models in hearing* (pp. 344–352). Berlin: Springer-Verlag.

Buunen, T.J.F., Festen, J.M., Bilsen, F.A., & van den Brink, G. (1974). Phase effects in a three-component signal. *Journal of the Acoustical Society of America, 55*, 297–303.

Buunen, T.J.F., ten Kate, J.H., Raatgever, J., & van den Brink, G. (1977). Combined psychophysical and electrophysiological study on the role of combination tones in the perception of phase changes. *Journal of the Acoustical Society of America, 61*, 508–519.

Cooke, M.P. (1986). A computer model of peripheral auditory processing incorporating phase-locking, suppression and adaptation effects. *Speech Communication, 5*, 261–281.

Darwin, C.J. & Gardner, R.B. (1985). Which harmonics contribute to the estimation of the first formant? *Speech Communication, 4*, 231–235.

Darwin, C.J. & Gardner, R.B. (1986). Mistuning a harmonic of a vowel: grouping and phase effects on vowel quality. *Journal of the Acoustical Society of America, 79*, 838–845.

Gardner, R.B. & Uppal, W.K. (1986). A peripheral auditory model for speech processing. *Proceedings of the Institute of Acoustics, 8*, 555–562.

Goldstein, J.L. (1967). Auditory nonlinearity. *Journal of the Acoustical Society of America, 41*, 676–689.

Goldstein, J.L. (1967). Auditory spectral filtering and monaural phase perception. *Journal of the Acoustical Society of America, 41*, 458–479.

Jesteadt, W., Wier, C.C., & Green, D.M. (1977). Intensity discrimination as a function of frequency and sensation level. *Journal of the Acoustical Society of America, 61*, 169–177.

Klatt, D.H. (1980). Software for a cascade/parallel formant synthesizer. *Journal of the Acoustical Society of America, 67*, 971–995.

Kohlrausch, A. (1988). Masking patterns of harmonic complex tone maskers and the role of the inner ear transfer function. In H. Duifhuis, J.W. Jorst, & H.P. Wit (Ed), *Basic issue in hearing* (pp. 339–346). London: Academic Press.

Kubovy, M. & Jordan, R. (1979). Tone-segregation by phase: On the phase sensitivity of the single ear. *Journal of the Acoustical Society of America, 66*, 100–106.

Mathes, R.C. & Miller, R.L. (1947). Phase effects in monaural perception. *Journal of the Acoustical Society of America, 19*, 780–797.

McKeown, J.D. & Darwin, C.J. (1989). Effects of phase changes in low-numbered harmonics on formant frequency matches. *Journal of the Acoustical Society of America, 85* (Supplement 1), S143–144.

Moore, B.C.J. (1986). *Frequency selectivity in hearing*. London: Academic Press.

Moore, B.C.J. & Glasberg, B.R. (1989). Difference limens for phase in normal and hearing-impaired subjects. *Journal of the Acoustical Society of America, 86*, 1351–1365.

Palmer, A.R., Winter, I.M. & Darwin, C.J. (1986). The representation of steady-state vowel sounds in the temporal discharge of guinea-pig cochlear nerve and primarylike cochlear nucleus neurones. *Journal of the Acoustical Society of America*, *79*, 100–113.

Palmer, A.R., Winter, I.M., Gardner, R.B., & Darwin, C.J. (1987). Changes in the phonemic quality and neural representation of a vowel by alteration of the relative phase of harmonics near F1. In M.E.H. Schouten (Ed), *The psychophysics of speech perception* (pp. 371–376). Dordrecht: Martinus Nijhoff.

Patterson, R.D. (1987). A pulse ribbon model of monaural phase perception. *Journal of the Acoustical Society of America*, *82*, 1560–1586.

Pfeiffer, R.R. (1970). A model for two-tone inhibition of single cochlear nerve fibers. *Journal of the Acoustical Society of America*, *48*, 1373–1378.

Rosen, S. & Smith, D.A.J. (1988). Temporally-based auditory sensations in the profoundly hearing-impaired listener. In H. Duifhuis, J.W. Jorst, & H.P. Wit (Ed), *Basic issue in hearing* (pp. 431–439). London: Academic Press.

Schroeder, M.R. (1970). Synthesis of low peak-factor signals and binary sequences with low autocorrelation. *IEEE Transactions on Information Theory*, *16*, 85–89.

Young, E.D. & Sachs, M.B. (1979). Representation of steady-state vowels in the temporal aspects of the discharge patterns of populations of auditory-nerve fibres. *Journal of the Acoustical Society of America*, *66*, 1381–1403.

Zwicker, E. (1981). Dependence of level and phase of the ($2f_1$–f_2)-cancellation tone on frequency range, frequency difference, level of primaries, and subject. *Journal of the Acoustical Society of America*, *70*, 1277–1288.

Revised manuscript received 17 October 1990

THE QUARTERLY JOURNAL OF EXPERIMENTAL PSYCHOLOGY, 1991, *43A* (3) 423–448

The Perception of Back Vowels: Centre of Gravity Hypothesis

Peter F. Assmann

School of Human Development, The University of Texas at Dallas, Richardson, Texas, U.S.A

According to the formant centre of gravity (FCOG) hypothesis, two vowel formants in close proximity are merged during perceptual analysis, and their contribution to vowel quality depends on the centre of gravity of the formant cluster. Findings consistent with this hypothesis are that two formants can be replaced by a single formant of intermediate centre frequency, provided their separation is less than 3–3.5 Bark; and that changes in their relative amplitudes produce systematic shifts in vowel quality. In Experiment 1, listeners adjusted the frequencies of F1 and F2 in a synthesized 6-formant vowel (with the F1–F2 separation fixed at 250 Hz, i.e. less than 3 Bark) to find the best phonetic match to a reference vowel with modified formant amplitudes. Contrary to FCOG predictions, F2 attenuation did not produce lower frequency matches. Raising the amplitude of F2 led to predicted upward shifts in formant frequencies of the matched vowel, but with increased variability of matches for some stimuli. In Experiment 2, listeners identified synthesized vowels with a range of separations of F1 and F2. Formant amplitude manipulations had no effect on listeners' judgements when the fundamental frequency was low (125 Hz). Small shifts in vowel quality appeared for stimuli with a high fundamental (250 Hz), but the shifts were significantly larger for F1–F2 separations *greater* than 3.5 Bark. These effects of formant amplitude are qualitatively different from those observed with single-formant vowels and are generally incompatible with a formant-averaging mechanism.

Requests for reprints should be sent to Peter F. Assmann, School of Human Development, The University of Texas at Dallas, Box 830688, Richardson, Texas 75083, U.S.A.

Portions of this research were reported at the 108th Meeting of the Acoustical Society of America, Minneapolis, 10 October 1984.

This research was based on a doctoral dissertation carried out at the Department of Linguistics, University of Alberta, and was supported by Social Sciences and Humanities Research Council Doctoral Fellowships. The guidance and helpful suggestions provided by Terry Nearey during the course of this research are gratefully acknowledged. I would like to thank Quentin Summerfield, Sarah Hawkins, and Brian Roberts for their detailed and helpful comments on the manuscript, Dwayne Paschall and Joe Strickland for assistance in preparing the figures and Laurie Checkoway for typing the manuscript.

There is converging evidence from many sources that listeners determine the phonetic quality of vowels on the basis of the frequency locations of the lowest two or three formants (e.g. Potter & Steinberg, 1950; Peterson & Barney, 1952; Delattre, Liberman, Cooper, & Gerstman, 1952; Carlson, Fant, & Granström, 1975; Chistovich, 1985). Several models of vowel identification assume an initial stage of processing in which the frequencies of formants are estimated from the locations of peaks in the auditory excitation pattern of the vowel (e.g. Karnickaya, Mushnikov, Slepokurova, & Zhukov, 1975; Carlson et al., 1975). A persistent problem for such models (as well as for physical analyses of speech) has been to estimate the frequencies of formants accurately in situations where the amplitude of a formant is low, relative to adjacent regions of the spectrum, or where the frequency distance between two adjacent formants is too small to resolve them as separate peaks.

This problem is illustrated in Figure 1. The top panel shows the amplitude spectrum of a synthesized vowel similar to [o], with a fundamental frequency (f_0) appropriate for a male voice ($f_0 = 125$ Hz). The spectrum of the vowel was computed in accordance with the cascade formant synthesis model described by Flanagan (1972). The spectrum envelope, estimated using LPC analysis, has been superimposed on the amplitude spectrum to facilitate visual isolation of the formants. In this example, the first and second formants (F1 and F2) are close together in frequency. F2 does not appear as a distinct peak but, rather, as a "shoulder" on the high-frequency skirt of F1. This is a pattern that is commonly observed in back vowels, particularly when f_0 is high (Klatt, 1982a).

The bottom panel of the figure shows the auditory excitation pattern of the vowel, computed using the model described by Moore and Glasberg (1987). The excitation pattern simulates the limited frequency selectivity of the peripheral auditory system and is sometimes regarded as a representation of the internal spectrum of a sound. It displays the output levels of a bank of "auditory filters" as a function of the centre frequency of the filters. The frequency axis is scaled in units of the equivalent rectangular bandwidths (ERBs) of the filters (Patterson & Moore, 1986).

The figure illustrates two distinct problems for a formant estimation procedure: (1) F1 and F2 give rise to a single energy concentration in the excitation pattern, rather than two distinct peaks at the positions indicated by the arrows; (2) this energy concentration contains a number of secondary peaks, which reflect low-frequency resolved harmonics of the vowel, rather than the first and second formants.

The low-frequency harmonics are resolved because auditory filter bandwidths are narrow at low frequencies, relative to the spacing of the harmonics. In front vowels, where F1 and F2 are widely separated, there is evidence that the subjective estimation of F1 frequency involves a weighting of prominent harmonics (Carlson et al., 1975; Darwin, 1984; Darwin &

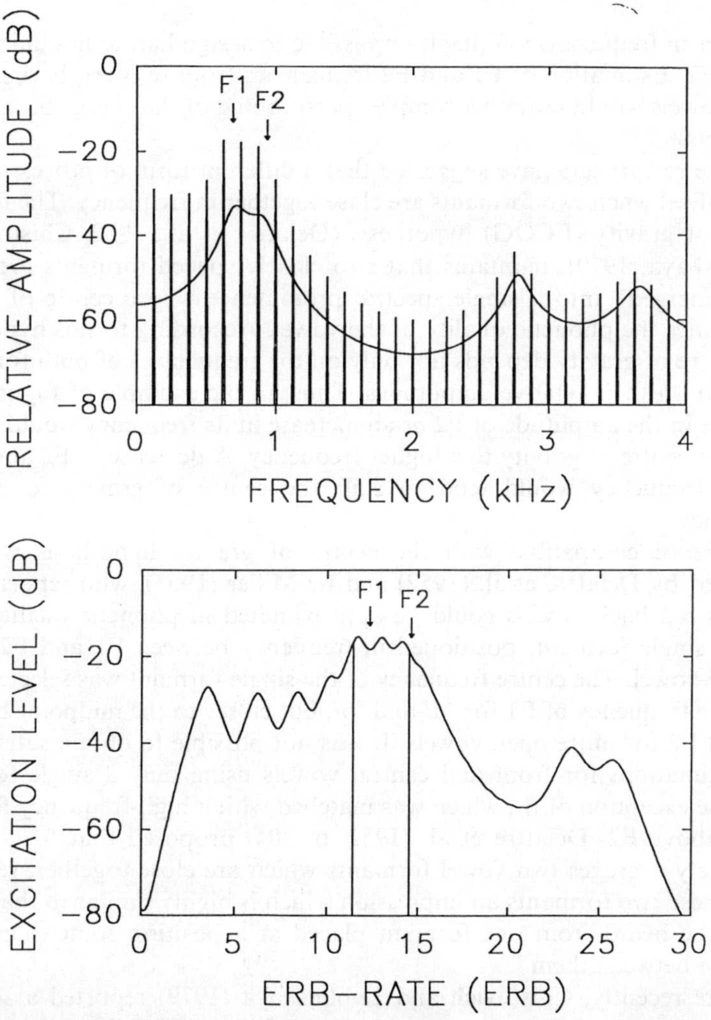

FIG. 1. The top panel shows the amplitude spectrum of a 1024-point Hanning-windowed segment of a synthesized vowel similar to [o]. The continuous line superimposed on the spectrum is the envelope, estimated using LPC analysis. The bottom panel shows the auditory excitation pattern of the vowel. The vertical lines on the excitation pattern indicate a 3-Bark region spanning the most intense harmonics of the vowel. Arrows indicate the frequencies of the first and second formants.

Gardner, 1985; Assmann & Nearey, 1987). F1 frequency in front vowels can be estimated as the weighted mean of the most prominent harmonics (Carlson et al., 1975; Assmann, 1985). However, such a simple strategy will not work in the case of back vowels, because F1 and F2 are often close together in frequency, making it impossible to assign harmonics uniquely to F1 or F2. Estimation of F1 and F2 frequencies from resolved harmonics in back vowels would require a complex partitioning of the energy between the formants.

Some researchers have suggested that a different form of processing may be involved when two formants are close together in frequency. The formant centre of gravity (FCOG) hypothesis (Delattre et al., 1952; Chistovich & Lublinskaya, 1979) maintains that two closely spaced formants are effectively "merged" into a single spectral prominence whose centre of gravity determines the phonetic quality of the vowel. According to this hypothesis, the centre of gravity depends not only on the frequencies of both formants, but also on their relative amplitudes. Thus, in the example of Figure 1, an increase in the amplitude of F2 *or* an increase in its frequency would tend to shift the centre of gravity to a higher frequency. A decrease in F2 amplitude or F2 frequency would tend to shift the centre of gravity to a lower frequency.

Evidence compatible with the centre of gravity hypothesis was first provided by Delattre et al. (1952) and by Miller (1953), who reported that synthesized back vowels could be approximated in phonetic quality using only a single formant, positioned in frequency between F1 and F2 of the natural vowel. The centre frequency of the single formant was selected to be near the frequency of F1 for /u/ and /o/, but closer to the midpoint between F1 and F2 for more open vowels. It was not possible to obtain satisfactory approximations for front and central vowels using only a single formant, with the exception of /i/, which was matched with a high-frequency formant at or above F2. Delattre et al. (1952, p. 204) proposed that "... the ear effectively averages two vowel formants which are close together, receiving from these two formants an impression which is highly similar to that which would be heard from one formant placed at a position somewhere intermediate between them".

More recently, Chistovich and Lublinskaya (1979) reported a series of matching experiments to test predictions of the FCOG hypothesis. They reasoned that if the phonetic quality of back vowels depends on the centre of gravity of the F1–F2 cluster, then a change in the relative amplitudes of F1 and F2 should be perceptually equivalent to the displacement of a *single* formant along the frequency scale. They synthesized single-formant matching stimuli and two-formant reference stimuli. Listeners adjusted the centre frequency of the single formant to find the best match in vowel quality to the two-formant reference. The amplitude of F1 of the reference vowel was either 5 dB lower or 5 dB higher than that of F2, and the frequency separation between F1 and F2 was 350 Hz. Results showed that listeners always chose a single-formant matching stimulus whose centre frequency was intermediate between F1 and F2 of the reference but closer to the more intense formant.

Chistovich and Lublinskaya described a second experiment in which listeners adjusted the amplitude ratio of F1 and F2 in a two-formant vowel to match the phonetic quality of a single formant reference whose frequency was intermediate between F1 and F2. A continuous relationship between the frequency of the single formant and the formant amplitude ratio was reported for small separations of F1 and F2. As the separation between the formants was increased, there was a point beyond which satisfactory matches could not be found. This critical separation of F1 and F2 was estimated to be 3–3.5 Bark.[1]

In a subsequent experiment the relationship between formant amplitude and frequency separation between the formants was investigated using single-formant matches to two-formant vowels. Formant amplitude was manipulated by attenuating either F1 or F2 in steps of 10 dB, relative to its initial level of 75 dB SPL. When the frequency separation of F1 and F2 was small (i.e. less than 3 Bark), a continuous monotonic shift in the frequency of the best single-formant match was found as formant amplitude was adjusted over a range of 40 dB. When the separation between F1 and F2 was large (i.e. greater than 3.5 Bark), a variable distribution of matches was reported. One listener always matched the centre frequency of the single formant so that it coincided in frequency with one of the two formants of the reference stimulus. The other listener matched the single formant to frequencies intermediate between F1 and F2, with a continuous shift in match frequency as a function of formant amplitude. For this subject, the pattern in the means was similar for closely spaced (less than 3 Bark) and widely spaced (greater than 3.5 Bark) formants. However, there was a substantial increase in variability near the middle of the formant amplitude range, where the two formants had similar amplitudes, suggesting a degree of uncertainty in the decision process. Chistovich and Lublinskaya argued that the increased variability and the discontinuity in matching as a function of formant amplitude was evidence that the phonetic quality of vowels with more than a 3.5 Bark separation of F1 and F2 could not be adequately matched by adjusting the frequency of a single formant, and hence that a centre of gravity characterization was not appropriate for such stimuli.

Chistovich and Lublinskaya summarized their main findings as follows: (1) in stimuli with *more* than 3–3.5 Bark separation of F1 and F2, vowel quality is largely independent of changes in the amplitude ratio of the two

[1] The Bark is a unit of critical-band rate, a scale that describes the relationship between auditory critical bands and frequency (Zwicker, 1961; Zwicker & Terhardt, 1980). A difference of 1 Bark corresponds to the width of one critical band. Critical bandwidth is nearly constant at low frequencies (below 500 Hz) and increases roughly as the logarithm of frequency at high frequencies. The Bark scale is closely related to the ERB-rate scale described by Moore and Glasberg (1987).

formants, over a wide range bounded by the detection thresholds for each formant; (2) in stimuli with *less* than the critical separation of F1 and F2, vowel quality can be shifted by changing the relative amplitudes of the formants. These shifts are a continuous function of the formant amplitude ratio, until one formant or the other is so low in amplitude that it is no longer detectable; the stimulus is then effectively a single-formant vowel. Chistovich and Lublinskaya suggested a two-stage mechanism to characterize the auditory processing of vowel spectra: one stage in which the locations of resolved formant peaks are detected, and another in which energy is integrated over a broad region of the spectrum.

The studies reviewed above suggest that formant amplitude may make an important contribution to the phonetic quality of back vowels when F1 and F2 are in close proximity. However, there are several studies indicating only minor effects of formant amplitude in back vowels. Klatt (1982b) synthesized two sets of vowels, one set similar to /æ/ (with a large frequency separation of F1 and F2), and the other similar to /ɑ/ (with closely-spaced F1 and F2). Listeners judged the phonetic similarity between pairs of vowels that differed in one or more stimulus parameters. Results showed that changes in formant bandwidth, formant amplitude, and spectral tilt had little effect on judgements of phonetic quality, despite the fact that each of these manipulations leads to changes in the centre of gravity. Listeners did not show a greater sensitivity to such manipulations for the back vowel. A later study (Klatt, 1985) failed to find evidence for the tradeoff between formant frequency and formant amplitude in back vowels predicted by the FCOG hypothesis. Klatt demonstrated that shifts in vowel quality induced by formant frequency changes could not be cancelled by opposing changes in formant amplitude whose net effect was to maintain a constant centre of gravity.

Ainsworth and Millar (1972) synthesized a continuum of vowels with 8 steps in F1 frequency and 8 steps in F2 frequency and presented the vowels to listeners in an 11-alternative forced-choice identification task. Vowels were presented in conditions where F2 was attenuated by 0, 14, 28, 42, or ∞dB, relative to a fixed level of F1. Analyses of the distribution of responses indicated that each of the 11 vowel response categories dominated a distinct region of the F1 × F2 vowel space. Ainsworth and Millar estimated the centres of these vowel response areas by computing the weighted mean of the response distributions against F1 or F2 frequency. They found that F1 response centres were nearly constant across all conditions of formant amplitude. Even when F1 and F2 were close in frequency, listeners did not compensate for the reduction in F2 amplitude by shifting the response centres toward higher F1 frequencies, as would be predicted by the FCOG hypothesis. F2 centres did not appear to depend substantially upon F2 amplitude either, provided the amplitude difference between F1 and F2 was less than 28 dB. With substantial attenuation of F2, F2 centres drifted from a value appropriate for the vowel category in question towards the mean of the F2 range. Ainsworth and Miller argued in favour of a peak-picking mechanism in vowel perception, on the strength of the evidence that vowel identification was largely unaffected by formant amplitude over a wide (28-dB) range.

Beddor and Hawkins (1990) proposed that formant amplitude may play a more important role in the perception of vowels when the low-frequency region of the vowel has limited spectral contrast—i.e. when the difference between adjacent peaks and valleys that define the formants is small. They reported a matching experiment in which the reference stimuli were nasal vowels whose spectra contain relatively broad, poorly differentiated peaks in the low-frequency region. The matching stimuli were oral vowels differing in F1 frequency. Best-matched vowel pairs were those for which the F1 frequency of the matching stimulus did not coincide with F1 of the reference stimulus but was influenced by the frequency of the nasal formant in a manner suggestive of the centre of gravity effects seen in back vowels.

Beddor and Hawkins reported a further experiment in which the reference stimuli were two-formant approximations to back vowels, with F1 and F2 bandwidths either wider or narrower than those typically found in (non-nasal) spoken vowels. The matching stimuli were two-formant vowels with medium bandwidths. The narrow-bandwidth stimuli were perceived to be similar to medium-bandwidth stimuli with the same formant frequencies; the wide-bandwidth stimuli were perceived to be more similar to medium-bandwidth stimuli that differed in their F1 and F2 frequencies but shared other aspects of spectral shape, such as the amplitudes and frequencies of prominent harmonics in the low-frequency region. Beddor and Hawkins concluded that the relative contribution of formant frequency and formant amplitude may depend on the spectral complexity of the stimuli: formant frequencies may be more important when the spectra have well-defined peaks; formant amplitude and additional aspects of spectral shape may be more important when peaks are poorly defined, as in back vowels, nasal vowels, and vowels with wider-than-normal bandwidths.

The studies reviewed above indicate some disagreement concerning the role of formant amplitude in vowel perception. Two factors that may account for the difference in results are the spectral complexity of the stimuli and the nature of the response task. Data that support the FCOG hypothesis have come mainly from experiments in which a single formant is matched to a two-formant reference vowel. Data that fail to support the hypothesis have used multi-formant vowels and either a vowel identification task (Ainsworth & Millar, 1972) or vowel-similarity judgements (Klatt, 1982b, 1985).

Single-formant vowels resemble natural back vowels in that most of their energy is located in the low-frequency region of the spectrum, but compared to the two-formant reference stimuli there are fewer prominent harmonics in the low-frequency region, the width of the energy concentration is narrower, and the slope of the spectrum on the high-frequency side of the formant peak is steeper. Schwartz and Escudier (1989) have argued that it may be unrealistic to assess the FCOG hypothesis under conditions in which listeners are explicitly instructed to match a "simplified" spectrum to a more "complex" one. Such considerations make it important to test the predictions of the FCOG hypothesis in matching experiments where *both* matching and reference stimuli are multi-formant vowels. In this paper two experiments using multi-formant synthetic vowels are reported: Experiment 1 used a vowel-matching task, and Experiment 2 used vowel identification to evaluate predictions of the FCOG hypothesis and the notion of a 3–3.5 Bark critical distance.

EXPERIMENT 1

Vowel Matching

The FCOG hypothesis makes two predictions about the effects of formant frequency and formant amplitude manipulations in vowels with close spacing of F1 and F2. These predictions are illustrated schematically in the two panels of Figure 2. The upper panel shows the single-formant matching paradigm investigated by Chistovich and Lublinskaya (1979). In this situation, listeners adjust the frequency of a single-formant matching stimulus to compensate for changes in F1 amplitude of a two-formant reference stimulus. When F1 amplitude is lowered, the centre of gravity is increased, and thus the best single-formant match is achieved by increasing the frequency of the single-formant match. When F1 amplitude is raised, the best single-formant match will occur at a lower frequency. The lower panel illustrates a two-formant matching paradigm. Here, listeners adjust the frequencies of *both* formants in a matching stimulus to compensate for changes in F1 amplitude of the reference. An optimal match is expected when the formant centre of gravity of the reference stimulus coincides with the centre of gravity of the matching stimulus, even if this means that the centre frequencies of F1 and F2 in the matching stimulus will no longer be aligned with F1 and F2 in the reference stimulus. When F1 amplitude is lowered, the centre of gravity is increased, and listeners are expected to choose matching stimuli for which one or both of the two formants are higher in frequency. When F1 amplitude is raised, listeners should select matching stimuli with lower formant frequencies.

One difficulty with the two-formant matching paradigm is that there are physical constraints on acceptable formant combinations. For example, the frequency separation between F1 and F2 is rarely less than 200 Hz in natural speech, and formants do not cross one another in frequency. One possibility

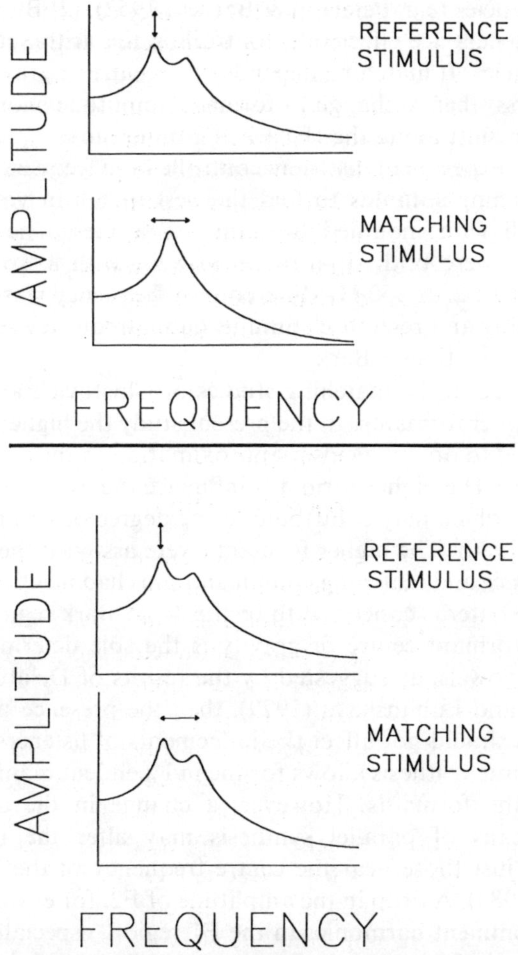

FIG. 2. Schematic amplitude spectra illustrating two different matching paradigms. The top panel shows the single-formant matchings procedure used by Chistovich and Lublinskaya (1979). The bottom panel illustrates a two-formant matching procedure similar to that used in Experiment 1.

is to fix the frequency of one of the formants at a constant value and allow listeners to adjust the frequency of the other formant over a small frequency range. An alternative strategy, adopted in the present experiment, is to *covary* F1 and F2 in the matching stimulus and maintain a constant frequency separation between the formants, as shown in Figure 2.

The decision to covary F1 and F2 in this way can be justified on two grounds: (1) There is a correlation of F1 and F2 frequencies in measurements of natural back vowels: higher F1 frequencies are generally associated with higher F2 frequencies (e.g. Peterson & Barney, 1952). (2) By varying F1 and F2 together, listeners are effectively controlling the arithmetic mean of the formant frequencies. If matching depends on a centre of gravity or formant-averaging process, then a change in formant amplitude should be phonetically similar to a shift along the (F1 + F2)/2 dimension.

In the present experiment, listeners controlled the frequency of the F1, F2 pair in the matching stimulus to find the best match in vowel quality for reference stimuli with modified formant amplitudes. The matching and reference stimuli were both six-formant vowels, with a fixed 250-Hz separation of F1 and F2. A 250-Hz difference in frequency was used to ensure that each matching and reference stimulus had a frequency separation of F1 and F2 that was less than 3 Bark.

The stimuli used in the matching studies of Chistovich and Lublinskaya (1979) lacked higher formants. In the present study the higher formants (F3–F6) were included to obtain a closer approximation to the amplitude spectra of natural vowels. The higher formants influence the overall shape and slope of the spectrum, which may contribute to the degree of naturalness of voice quality[2] (Klatt, 1980). The higher formants were assigned the same frequencies in the reference and matching stimuli and thus had no effect on the centre of gravity, if the latter is conceived to be the 3–3.5-Bark region enclosing F1 and F2. If the formant centre of gravity is the sole determinant of vowel quality in back vowels, as suggested by the results of Delattre et al. (1952) and Chistovich and Lublinskaya (1979), then the presence of a fixed set of higher formants should not affect the judgements of listeners.

Parallel formant synthesis allows for the independent manipulation of the amplitudes of the formants. However, a change in the amplitude of a formant by means of parallel synthesis may alter the levels of *many* harmonics, not just those near the centre frequency of the formant (Fant, 1960; Holmes, 1983). A drop in the amplitude of F2, for example, may lower the levels of prominent harmonics in the F1 region, especially if F1 and F2 are close together in frequency. In front vowels, changes in the amplitudes of harmonics near F1 can lead to shifts in vowel quality (e.g. Assmann & Nearey, 1987) that are unrelated to the FCOG effect, because F1 and F2 are

[2] The centre frequencies of the higher formants (F3–F6) shown in Table 1 were obtained from measured averages of spoken vowels produced by adult males. However, the frequencies of F3 through F6 were *fixed* in each of the reference and matching stimuli used in Experiment 1. It was pointed out by one of the reviewers that a greater degree of naturalness might have been achieved by selecting the frequencies of the higher formants in a way that reflects the natural covariation of the higher formants with F1 and F2. Although the frequencies of F3 and F4 vary somewhat from vowel to vowel in natural speech, the variation in these parameters from talker to talker is considerably greater, and thus it is unclear what sort of covariation would be most appropriate for the matching continuum (which comprises stimuli that do not correspond to any *particular* vowel).

widely separated in frequency. To provide precise control over the frequency ranges affected by changes in formant amplitude, Experiment 1 used additive harmonic synthesis to create the reference and matching stimuli. The amplitude of each harmonic of the vowel was computed using a model of cascade formant synthesis (Flanagan, 1972) and subsequently adjusted, in accordance with a weighting function that either raised or lowered the amplitudes of harmonics above F1. The FCOG model predicts that listeners will select higher-frequency matches when the harmonics above F1 are raised in amplitude, as this manipulation increases the centre of gravity of the F1–F2 cluster. Lower-frequency matches are expected when the amplitudes of these harmonics are lowered, as this decreases the centre of gravity.

Method

Stimuli. The stimuli were generated using digital additive harmonic synthesis. Each stimulus consisted of the lowest 32 harmonics of a constant f_0 of 125 Hz, with amplitude values specified by the cascade formant model (Fant, 1960), and all harmonics were added in sine phase. The contributions of six formants, glottal source and radiation characteristics, and higher-pole correction factor were computed as described by Flanagan (1972). The frequencies and bandwidths of the formants specified as input to the synthesizer are listed in Table 1. All stimuli were 250 msec in duration, with onsets and offsets smoothed using the initial and final half portions of a 30-msec Hamming window. Overall stimulus levels ranged from 79 to 85 dB SPL.

A continuum of matching stimuli was constructed with F1 ranging from 175 to 950 Hz, in steps of 25 Hz. The frequency of F2 was fixed at 250 Hz above that of F1 in both matching and reference stimuli. A difference of 250 Hz corresponds to a separation of F1 and F2 of approximately 2.4 Bark at the low-frequency endpoint of the continuum (F1 = 175 Hz, F2 = 425 Hz) and approximately 1.4 Bark at the high-frequency endpoint (F1 = 950 Hz, F2 = 1200 Hz), as computed by the Bark formula given by Zwicker and Terhardt (1980).

TABLE 1
Formant Frequencies and Formant Bandwidths for the Matching and Reference Stimuli of Experiment 1

F1	(see text)	B1 = 70 Hz
F2 = F1 +	250 Hz	B2 = 90 Hz
F3 =	2750 Hz	B3 = 150 Hz
F4 =	3625 Hz	B4 = 250 Hz
F5 =	4500 Hz	B5 = 300 Hz
F6 =	6000 Hz	B6 = 700 Hz

The reference stimuli were produced by modifying three baseline stimuli drawn from the matching continuum with F1 and F2 frequencies of either 350 and 600 Hz, 450 and 700 Hz, or 550 and 800 Hz. Five amplitude conditions were created for each baseline stimulus by multiplying linear amplitudes of the individual harmonics by a weighting function. Table 2 lists the amplitude increment or decrement, in dB, applied to the harmonics of each reference stimulus by the weighting function. The weights were defined as follows: (1) Harmonics with frequencies less than 125 Hz above the centre

TABLE 2
Amplitude Change Applied to Individual Harmonics of the Reference Stimuli in Experiment 1

Amplitude Condition	*Harmonic Numbers*			Formant Frequencies
	1–3	*4*	*5–32*	
−20 dB	0	−7	−20	
−10 dB	0	−5	−10	F1 = 550 Hz
0 dB	0	0	0	F2 = 800 Hz
+10 dB	0	+7	+10	
+20 dB	0	+16	+20	
	Harmonic Numbers			
	1–4	*5*	*6–32*	
−20 dB	0	−4	−20	
−10 dB	0	−3	−10	F1 = 450 Hz
0 dB	0	0	0	F2 = 700 Hz
+10 dB	0	+5	+10	
+20 dB	0	+13	+20	
	Harmonic Numbers			
	1–5	*6*	*7–32*	
−20 dB	0	−2	−20	
−10 dB	0	−1	−10	F1 = 350 Hz
0 dB	0	0	0	F2 = 600 Hz
+10 dB	0	+3	+10	
+20 dB	0	+9	+20	

Note. Amplitude change in dB.

A value of 0 dB indicates that the harmonic retains its original value, i.e. the value specified by the synthesizer. The frequency of a harmonic is obtained by multiplying its harmonic number by f_0 (125 Hz).

frequency of F1 were not modified. This condition ensured that the two harmonics nearest to the F1 centre frequency were held constant. (2) Harmonics with frequencies above the centre frequency of F2 were adjusted by −20, −10, 0, +10, or +20 dB. (3) Harmonics in the intermediate region were linearly interpolated to avoid discontinuities in the spectrum envelope. In each of the reference stimuli this intermediate region included only one harmonic. Note that the interpolation was performed on a scale of linear amplitude, and thus the effects of amplitude increments and decrements in the intermediate region are asymmetrical when expressed in dB units.

Procedure. Stimuli were presented on-line at a sampling frequency of 16 kHz and 10-bit amplitude quantization, bandpass-filtered (0.068–6.8 kHz, 24 dB/oct spectral rolloff), and presented monaurally to the right channel of a set of TDH-49 headphones.

Stimuli were presented in pairs with a 3-sec intra-pair interval and a 5-sec inter-pair interval. The first member of each pair was one of the 15 reference stimuli, whose order was determined by a randomization list that differed for each listener and for each replication. The second member of the pair was a matching stimulus from the continuum whose F1 frequency was specified by the position of a slide lever adjusted by the listener. The slide lever controlled a potentiometer, which attenuated a 5-V input from a power supply. This signal was sampled and quantized into 25 equal steps, each step specifying a single stimulus on the continuum.

Listeners were presented with vowel pairs and asked to adjust the lever position to find the best match in vowel quality. When satisfied with the match, they pressed a switch, at which time the F1 frequency of the match was recorded automatically, and the next stimulus pair was presented. They were allowed as many trials as needed to arrive at a satisfactory match, but they were instructed to adjust the lever position several times for each reference stimulus. Listeners completed five sessions, each consisting of five replications of the 15 reference stimuli.

Subjects. Five listeners completed the task. All but one had received some prior training in phonetics and had participated in other speech perception experiments. All had normal hearing (pure-tone thresholds lower than 15 dB HL between 125 and 8000 Hz) in the right ear. None reported any difficulty with the task.

Results and Discussion

The data were summarized in terms of the median F1 match frequency, computed separately for each listener and for each reference stimulus. Means and standard deviations of the median matched F1 frequencies are shown in

Figure 3. The dotted lines indicate the nominal F1 and F2 frequencies of the reference stimuli. If formant amplitude had no effect on listeners' judgements, the means would be expected to coincide with the lower of the two dotted lines. There are substantial deviations from these lines in the +10- and +20-dB conditions, indicating that formant amplitude changes did affect matching judgements. An analysis of variance, performed on the

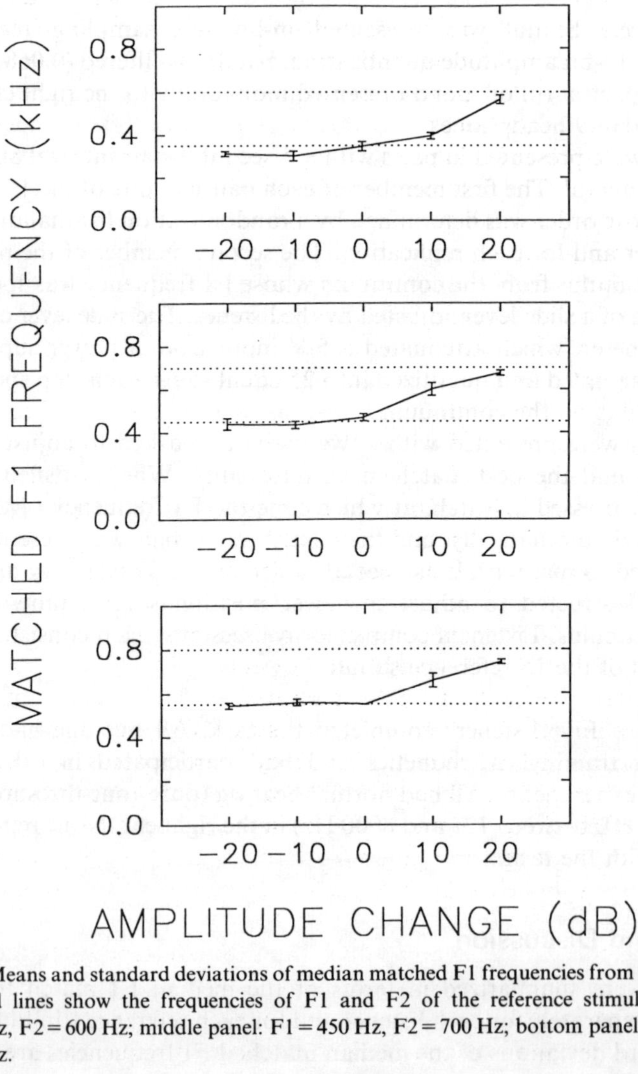

FIG. 3. Means and standard deviations of median matched F1 frequencies from Experiment 1. The dotted lines show the frequencies of F1 and F2 of the reference stimuli. Top panel: F1 = 350 Hz, F2 = 600 Hz; middle panel: F1 = 450 Hz, F2 = 700 Hz; bottom panel: F1 = 550 Hz, F2 = 800 Hz.

median F1 frequencies, revealed a significant interaction of formant amplitude and formant frequency, $F(8, 32) = 3.0$, $p < 0.05$. Dunnett's test indicated significantly higher matched F1s in the +10- and +20-dB conditions relative to the 0-dB condition, but no significant differences emerged in the −10- and −20-dB conditions.

The absence of shifts in the matching data with attenuation of F2 is inconsistent with the FCOG hypothesis. Formant amplitude is clearly influencing matching judgements when the formant amplitudes are boosted, but the variability in the matching histograms for two of the stimuli in the +10-dB condition suggests a degree of uncertainty in listeners' judgements.

Comparisons of the spectra of best-matched pairs (Assmann, 1985) suggests that the most frequently chosen matches are often those for which the frequency of the most prominent harmonic or pair of harmonics of the matching stimulus is aligned with the most prominent harmonics of the reference. Beddor and Hawkins (1990) reported examples of a similar nature in a comparison of the excitation patterns of best-matched pairs of oral and nasal vowels, single- and two-formant vowels, and narrow- and wide-bandwidth vowels.

Figure 4 shows the excitation patterns of two reference stimuli with F1 and F2 frequencies of 550 and 800 Hz (solid lines), along with the modal or most frequently chosen matching stimuli (dotted lines). For the −20-dB amplitude condition (upper panel) a close match is seen in the low-frequency region of the excitation pattern, because the modal matching stimulus has exactly the same F1 frequency as the reference (550 Hz). The excitation patterns of the matching and reference stimuli differ markedly at frequencies higher than 750 Hz. The 750-Hz harmonic appears as a peak in the excitation pattern of the matching stimulus, but only as a shoulder in the reference stimulus. The similarity of the matches for the −20-, −10-, and 0-dB conditions suggests that listeners do not select matching stimuli with lower F1 and F2 frequencies to compensate for the attentuation of F2.

The +20-dB amplitude condition (lower panel) shows a somewhat different pattern. Here, the modal match has an F1 frequency of 725 Hz, close to the nominal F2 of the reference stimulus. Once again, the most prominent harmonic has the same frequency in both patterns (750 Hz). In this case, however, the frequency of the most prominent harmonic was close to F1 in the matching stimulus, but close to F2 in the reference. The discrepancy between the excitation patterns is quite pronounced in the frequency region immediately below and above the most prominent harmonic.

Taken together, these comparisons show that listeners tend to select matches for which the frequencies and relative amplitudes of the most prominent harmonics of the matching stimulus are aligned with those of the reference, regardless of whether these harmonics are close in frequency to the

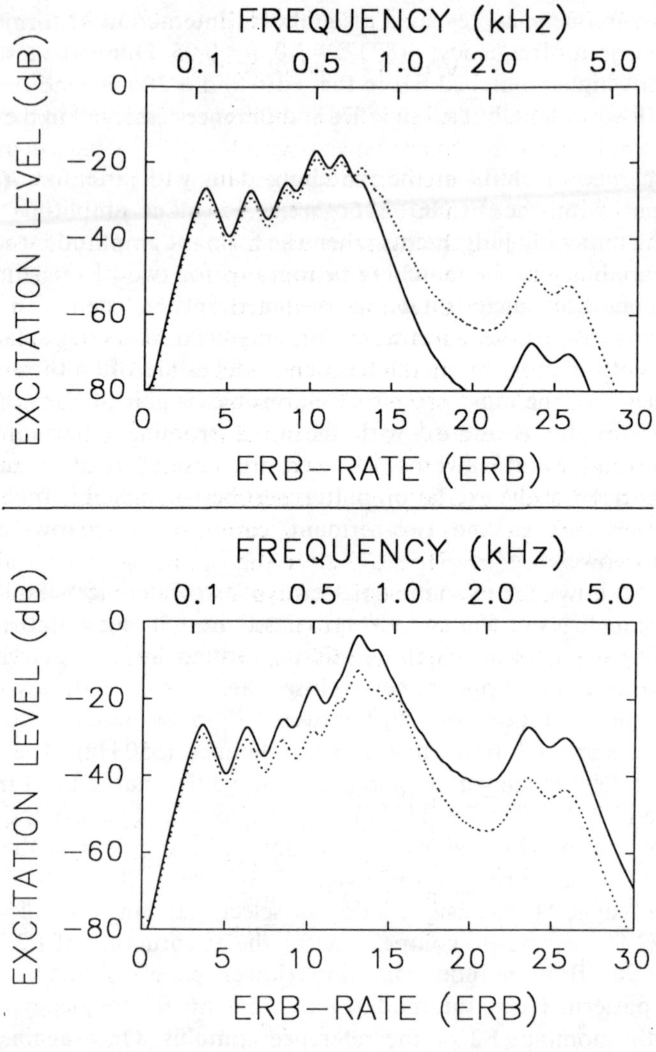

FIG. 4. Auditory excitation patterns of two reference stimuli with F1 and F2 frequencies of 550 and 800 Hz (solid lines) paired with the most frequently chosen matching stimuli (dotted lines). Upper panel: − 20-dB condition; lower panel: + 20-dB condition. The excitation patterns of the matching stimuli have been shifted down by 2 dB to facilitate comparison with the reference stimuli.

nominal F1 or F2. This tendency was not reported in the single-formant matching experiments by Chistovich and Lublinskaya (1979) and suggests that there may be important perceptual differences between single- and multi-formant stimuli.

EXPERIMENT 2

Vowel Identification

Bedrov, Chistovich, and Sheikin (1978) reported an identification experiment that used one- and two-formant vowels with less than 3-Bark separation of F1 and F2. Stimuli were presented to listeners in three conditions: (1) F2 was 5 dB higher in amplitude than F1; (2) F2 was 5 dB lower than F1; or (3) F2 was absent, in which case the stimulus was a single-formant vowel. Identification functions for some of the vowels, plotted as a function of F1 frequency, shifted in the direction predicted by the change in centre of gravity. However, these shifts were not simple linear displacements of the identification functions along the frequency scale; there were also changes in their shapes. This outcome suggests that changes in formant amplitude may not be perceptually equivalent to shifts in the frequencies of the formants.

The experiment of Bedrov et al. used only stimuli with a fixed 350-Hz separation of F1 and F2. The present experiment investigated the effects of formant amplitude changes on the identification of vowels with a range of frequency separations of F1 and F2. If the estimates of critical distance obtained by Chistovich and Lublinsakaya (1979) reflect the limits of a formant integration process, it is predicted that formant amplitude will influence phonetic quality only when F1 and F2 are separated by less than 3–3.5 Bark.

Method

Stimuli. The vowel stimuli formed a two-dimensional continuum, as shown in Figure 5. There were eight steps in F1 (440, 480, 520, 560, 600, 640, 680, and 720 Hz) and three steps in F2 (850, 1000, and 1150 Hz). The synthesis procedure was identical to that used in Experiment 1, except that phase angles were computed using a formula suggested by Schroeder and Merghardt (1982):

$$P_j = (j^2 \pi)/n \quad (1)$$

where P_j is the phase angle, in radians, of the jth harmonic, and n is the total number of harmonics.[3]

Two sets of vowels were produced. The first set was synthesized with an f_0 of 125 Hz, typical of an adult male voice; the second set had an f_0 of 250 Hz, more typical of an adult female voice. In the low-f_0 condition, formant

[3] This formulation avoids the strong peak factor associated with all-sine or all-cosine phases and produces a mellower quality when used as an excitation signal for a source-filter vocoder. Informal listening tests suggest that the difference is relatively small for the stimuli used here.

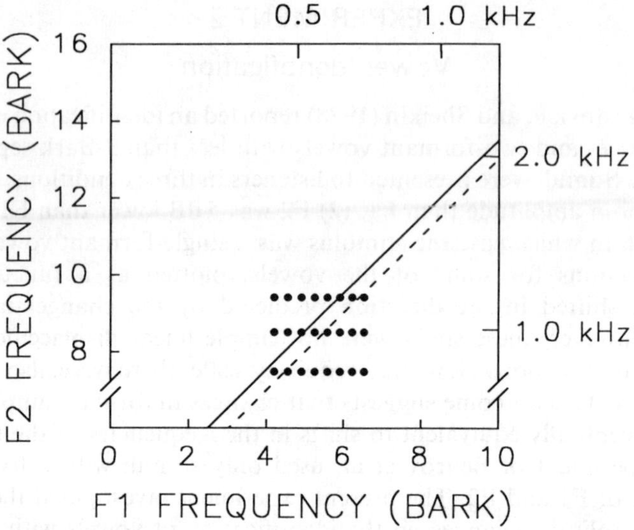

FIG. 5. Formant frequencies (F1 and F2) used in synthesizing the vowels of Experiment 2. Frequencies are plotted on a Bark scale; linear frequencies are shown on opposite axes. The solid diagonal line indicates a difference between F1 and F2 of 3.5 Bark; the dashed line indicates a difference of 3 Bark.

bandwidths and formant frequencies were the same as those listed in Table 1. In the high-f_0 condition, the higher formants F3–F6 were scaled upwards by a factor of 1.2, to take into account the association between f_0 and formant frequencies in natural speech (Peterson & Barney, 1952). Formant bandwidths were identical to those in the low-f_0 condition, as it was found that wider bandwidths did not result in more natural stimuli. For each stimulus from the continuum, three formant amplitude conditions were created. The amplitude modification procedure described in Experiment 1 was used to manipulate the amplitudes of F2 and higher formants relative to the amplitude of F1 in three steps: −6 dB, 0 dB, and +6 dB.

Procedure. Subjects were individually tested in a sound-treated room. Stimulus presentation followed the procedure outlined for Experiment 1, except that the stimuli were presented individually and a multiple-choice switchbox was used by listeners to record their responses. A five-alternative forced-choice task was used. Beside each button was a label with a phonetic symbol and a keyword in standard English orthography:

/u/	/ʊ/	/o/	/ɒ/	/ʌ/
"tool"	"hook"	"boat"	"pot"	"cup"

Each stimulus was repeated, with a 5-sec inter-stimulus interval, until a response button was pressed. If a wrong button was pressed by mistake, listeners could cancel the response by pressing a second button immediately afterwards. Otherwise, the response was recorded and the next item was presented.

Listeners completed four sessions, two for the low-f_0 condition and two for the high-f_0 condition, counterbalanced for order of the f_0 conditions. Each session consisted of 144 stimuli (8 levels of F1, 3 levels of F2, 3 amplitude conditions, and 2 replications). The 144 items were randomized, with a different randomization list for each subject. None of the listeners reported any difficulty with the task.

Subjects. Eight listeners (4 men, 4 women) took part in the experiment. All had received prior training in phonetics and had participated in other speech perception experiments. All had normal hearing and were native speakers of Canadian English.

Results and Discussion

The data were analysed in two ways, discussed separately in the following sections. (1) The effects of amplitude were quantified in terms of shifts of the identification functions within the F1–F2 plane. (2) The size of the amplitude effect was estimated for each vowel and was expressed as a function of the frequency separation between F1 and F2.

Response Centres. An examination of the pooled identification functions for individual vowels revealed that the maxima on these functions often did not exceed 50%. Rather than an analysis in terms of shifts in phoneme boundaries, therefore, the centre of each vowel response area was estimated, and the effects of amplitude were assessed in terms of shifts in response centres (cf. Ainsworth & Millar, 1972). The response centre for a particular vowel was defined as the weighted average of the identification probabilities along a scale of nominal F1 or F2 frequency. (1) Identification responses were pooled across listeners and trials, separately for each vowel response category. (2) For each vowel category and for each amplitude condition, the response centre was computed as follows:

$$C_i = \frac{\Sigma P_i \cdot F_i}{\Sigma P_i} \qquad 2$$

where C_i is the estimated response centre for the *i*th stimulus along either the F1 or F2 dimension, F_i is the frequency value of that formant, and P_i is the number of trials on which the ith stimulus was assigned to the vowel category under consideration. Separate response centres were computed for F1 and F2, and their means are shown in Figure 6.

Consistent with the findings of Ainsworth and Millar (1972), response centres did not change substantially as a function of amplitude. No significant effects of amplitude were found in the low-f_0 condition. In the high-f_0 condition, only F1 centres showed an effect, with a significant Amplitude × Vowel interaction, $F(8, 56) = 2.2$, $p < 0.05$. Dunnett's test indicated a

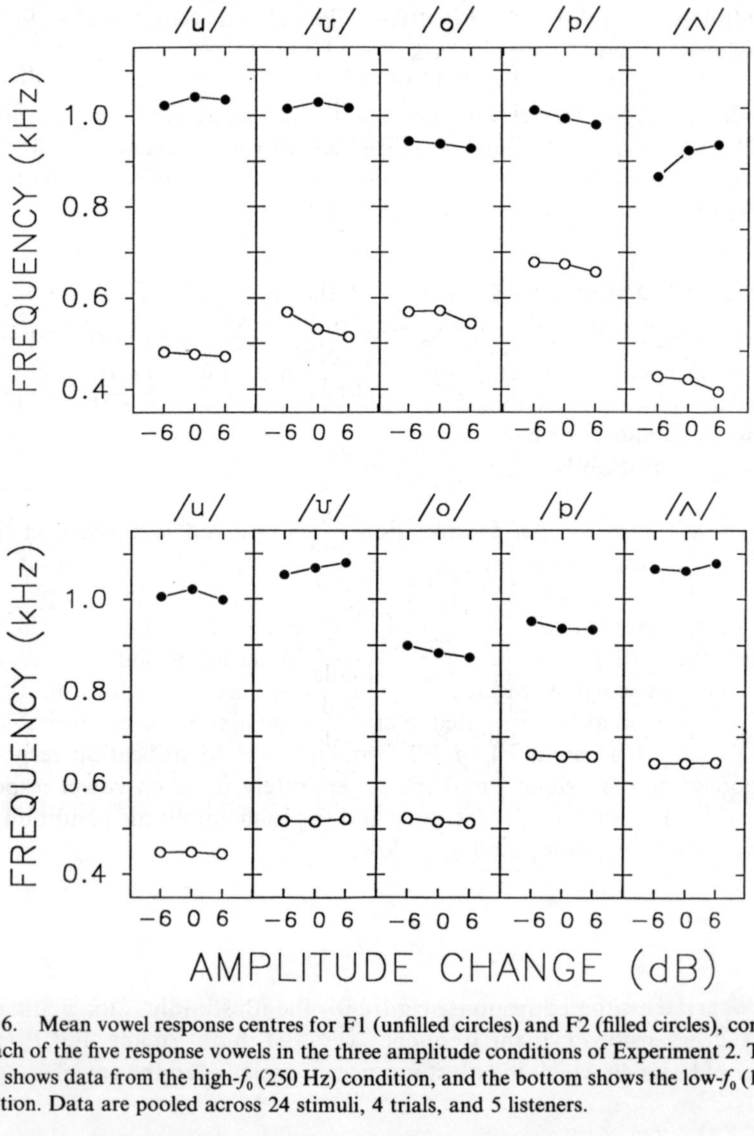

FIG. 6. Mean vowel response centres for F1 (unfilled circles) and F2 (filled circles), computed for each of the five response vowels in the three amplitude conditions of Experiment 2. The top panel shows data from the high-f_0 (250 Hz) condition, and the bottom shows the low-f_0 (125 Hz) condition. Data are pooled across 24 stimuli, 4 trials, and 5 listeners.

significant decreases for /o/ and /ʌ/ in the +6-dB, high-f_0 condition. The observed changes for /o/ and /ʌ/ were in the direction predicted by the centre of gravity hypothesis, but the changes for /ʊ/ were not predicted, as this vowel has more than 3.5 Bark separation of F1 and F2 in Canadian English. Averaging over F1 and F2 centres, both f_0s, and all five vowels, shifts in the +6-dB condition were larger (with a mean upward shift of 17.7 Hz) than shifts in the −6-dB condition (with a mean downward shift of 9.8 Hz).

Amplitude Effects. Response centres can indicate shifts in the identification functions as a function of formant amplitude, but they cannot indicate the size of the effect as a function of the separation between F1 and F2. One measure of the size of the formant amplitude effect is the absolute difference between the identification probabilities for a stimulus in the −6-dB (or +6-dB) conditions and the corresponding stimulus in the 0-dB condition:

$$D_{ij} = |P_{ij} - Q_{ij}| \qquad 3$$

where D_{ij} is an estimate of the size of the amplitude effect, for a given stimulus-response pair, P_{ij} is the number of trials on which listeners assigned the response i to stimulus j in the −6-dB (or +6-dB) condition, and Q_{ij} is the number of trials on which listeners assigned the response i to stimulus j in the 0-dB condition.

Stimuli from the continuum were divided into two classes, depending on whether the separation of F1 and F2 was less than or greater than 3.5 Bark. Distances (D_{ij}) were pooled across response categories and across stimuli within each of these classes. Figure 7 shows the mean formant amplitude effect for stimuli with either less than or greater than 3.5-Bark separation of the formants. Similar results were obtained when a cut-off of 3.0 Bark was used. The FCOG hypothesis predicts large effects of formant amplitude when stimuli have F1–F2 separations smaller than 3–3.5 Bark, and relatively minor effects when the separation of F1 and F2 is larger than 3–3.5 Bark. It is apparent that formant amplitude effects do not show this pattern. In fact, formant amplitude has a *larger* effect on stimuli with more than 3.5-Bark separation of the formants in the high-f_0 condition: −6-dB condition, $t(118) = 3.97$, $p < 0.05$; +6-dB condition, $t(118) = 2.81$, $p < 0.05$). No significant differences were found in the low-f_0 condition.

GENERAL DISCUSSION

The experiments reported above have shown several effects of formant amplitude on the phonetic quality of vowels that are not consistent with the FCOG hypothesis. Unlike the single-formant matching experiments reported by Chistovich and Lublinskaya (1979), Experiment 1 found no

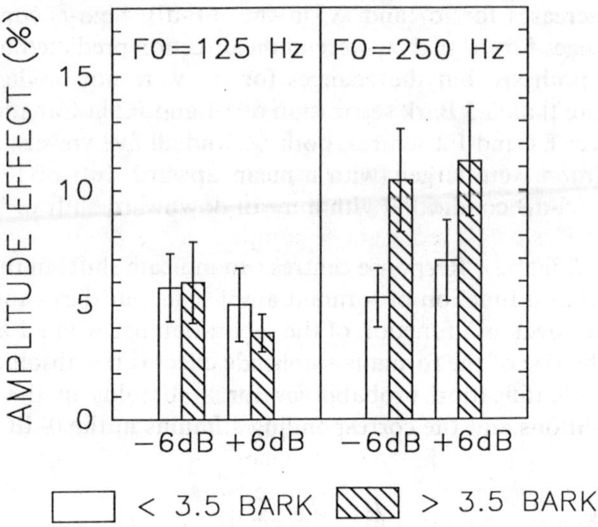

FIG. 7. The size of the formant amplitude effect, in percentages, is expressed in terms of the distance between the identification functions in the −6-and +6-dB conditions with respect to the 0-dB condition. Data are means and standard deviations across the 24 stimuli, 4 trials and 5 listeners.

evidence for a shift in matched formant frequencies with reductions in F2 amplitude. There are three possible explanations for this difference in results: (1) Listeners may not have been able to detect the changes in amplitude of F2 and the higher formants. (2) It is possible that amplitude manipulations did not lower the centre of gravity in the F1–F2 region of the spectrum. (3) Listeners may use a different matching strategy when they control the frequencies of two formants in the low-frequency region, rather than a single formant.

The first two explanations are unlikely to be correct, as the stimuli were similar in many respects to those used by Chistovich and Lublinskaya (1979) to support the FCOG hypothesis. For example, changes in F2 amplitude of −10 and −20 dB lie within the ranges for which Chistovich and Lublinskaya observed continuous shifts in vowel matching as a function of formant amplitude. If the excitation patterns shown in Figure 4 are an accurate reflection of the internal spectra of the vowels, then it seems likely that a 20-dB reduction in the amplitudes of F2 and higher formants would lead to a significant decrease in the centre of gravity. The most plausible explanation is that single- and two-formant matching tasks involve different matching strategies.

When F1 and F2 are close together in frequency, the spectrum may contain two separate peaks, or it may contain a single broad peak close to the centre frequency of the more intense formant, often with a small irregularity or spectral shoulder indicating the presence of the other formant (see Figure 1). In either situation, the overall spectral shape of the F1–F2 cluster is poorly matched by a single formant, because the spectral energy concentration of a single formant has a narrower width and is lower in amplitude. Thus, in single-formant matching experiments, listeners may rely on overall spectral shape cues to minimize the disparity in the low-frequency region. Their best matches may represent a compromise between the conflicting sources of information provided by the two formants of the reference stimulus. This conflict is apt to be minimal when the two formants are close together in frequency.

When two formants are available for matching, listeners appear to adopt a different strategy. The results of Experiment 1 suggest that they often base their matches on an alignment of the frequencies and amplitudes of the most prominent harmonics in the low-frequency region of the matching and reference stimuli. When F2 is reduced in amplitude by 20 dB, the most prominent harmonics are close in frequency to F1; when F2 is increased by 20 dB, the most prominent harmonics have frequencies near F2. The strategy of aligning prominent harmonics has also been observed in matching experiments with front vowels (Assmann & Nearey, 1987).

A second aspect of the FCOG hypothesis, the concept of a critical distance of 3–3.5 Bark, was not supported in the vowel identification data of Experiment 2. Experiment 2 indicated only minor effects of formant amplitude. These effects emerged only when stimuli had a high f_0; no systematic effects of formant amplitude were found in the low-f_0 condition. Moreover, the effects of formant amplitude were larger for stimuli with *greater* than 3.5 Bark separation of the formants. These findings, taken together, suggest that the centre of gravity hypothesis does not provide a comprehensive account of the effects of formant amplitude on vowel quality.

As formant frequency and formant amplitude are correlated in natural speech (Fant, 1956), the latter might function as a supplementary cue to vowel identity. Thus, for example, the relatively low amplitudes of the higher formants in back vowels may serve as an indicator that two formants are present in the low-frequency region. This may be of particular importance when the frequencies of F1 and F2 are close together and only one peak is evident in the low-frequency region.

Figure 8 shows the amplitude spectra of three vowels computed using the cascade synthesis model described above. The top panel shows the spectrum of a front vowel similar to [e], and the middle and bottom panels show amplitude spectra of a back vowel similar to [o]. Vowels shown in the top and middle panels had a high fundamental frequency (f_0=250 Hz), and the vowel shown in the bottom panel had a low fundamental (f_0=125 Hz).

The back vowel shown in the centre panel does not have two separate peaks corresponding to F1 and F2; a simple peak-finding algorithm, applied

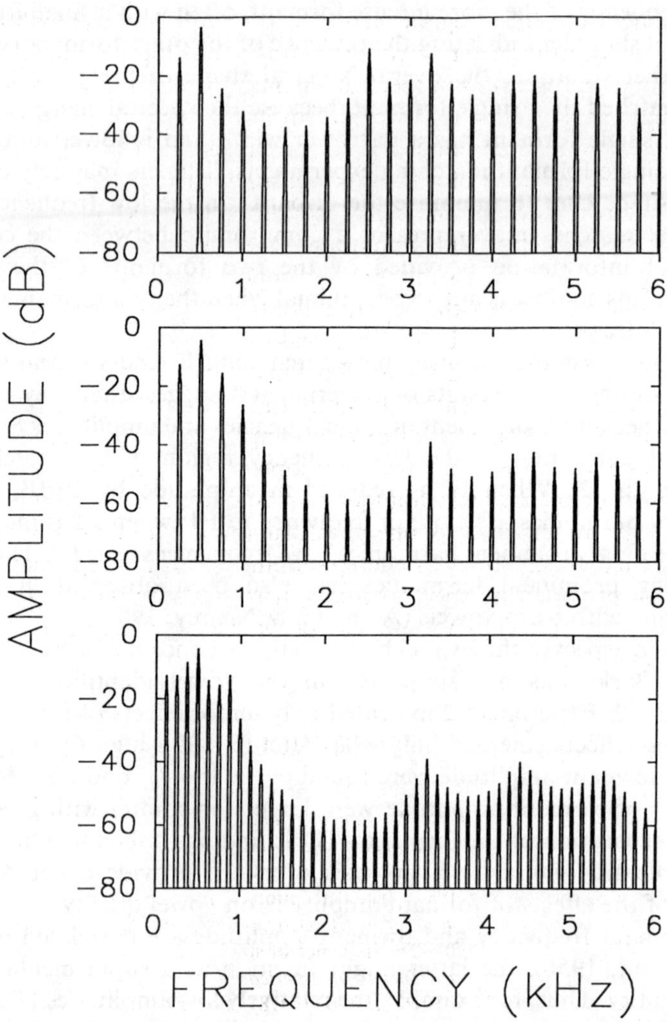

FIG. 8. This figure illustrates the effects on the amplitude spectra of synthetic vowels of changes in f_0 and the frequency separation of F1 and F2. The top panel shows a front vowel with high f_0(f_0 = 250 Hz; F1 = 500 Hz; F2 = 2500 Hz). The bottom panel shows a back vowel with low f_0(f_0 = 125 Hz; F1 = 464 Hz; F2 = 863 Hz). In the middle panel, the same formant pattern is shown with an octave increase in f_0(f_0 = 250 Hz; F1 = 464 Hz; F2 = 863 Hz).

to the amplitude spectrum, would be unable to determine that two formants were present rather than one. By contrast with the front vowel at the top, however, there are several indicators that two formants are present in the low-frequency region. For example, the high-frequency side of the peak representing the F1–F2 cluster is steeper, and the amplitudes of all components in the frequency region between 1 and 6 kHz are reduced. The difference in spectral pattern between the top and middle panels might be described in terms of a shift in spectral balance. Listeners have no difficulty in identifying these vowels: the vowel shown in the top panel is similar to [e], and those shown in the middle and lower panels are heard as high-pitched and low-pitched versions of a back vowel similar to [o].

It is of interest that only the high-f_0 condition of Experiment 2 resulted in significant effects of formant amplitude. One possibility is that changes in formant amplitude may assume greater importance (relative to changes in formant frequency) when the separate contributions of two closely-spaced formants are not specified by distinct peaks in the spectrum envelope, as in vowels with a high f_0 (Beddor & Hawkins, 1990). Although two distinct peaks are not always present in the amplitude spectrum when F2 is close to F1 in frequency, other aspects of spectral shape, such as the amplitudes of the formants, overall spectral balance, the slope of the spectrum above F2, and the presence of a spectral shoulder corresponding to a poorly resolved formant peak may convey phonetic information. More work is needed to establish whether and how listeners combine spectral shape cues with the information provided by spectral peaks; it is unlikely that the mechanisms suggested by the FCOG hypothesis can provide an adequate characterization of this process.

REFERENCES

Ainsworth, W.A. & Millar, J.B. (1972). The effect of relative formant amplitude on the perceived identity of synthetic vowels. *Language and Speech*, *15*, 328–341.

Assmann, P.F. (1985). *The role of harmonics and formants in the perception of vowel quality*. Unpublished PhD dissertation, University of Alberta.

Assmann, P.F. & Nearey, T.M. (1987). The perception of front vowels: The role of harmonics in the first formant region. *Journal of the Acoustical Society of America*, *81*, 520–534.

Beddor, P.S. & Hawkins, S. (1990). The influence of spectral prominence on perceived vowel quality. *Journal of the Acoustical Society of America*, *87*, 2684–2704.

Bedrov, Y.A., Chistovich, L.A. & Sheikin, R.L. (1978). Frequency position of the "centre of gravity" of formants as a useful feature in vowel perception. *Soviet Physics-Acoustics*, *24*, 275–281.

Carlson, R., Fant, G., & Granström, B. (1975). Two-formant models pitch and vowel perception. In G. Fant & M.A. Tatham (Eds.), *Auditory analysis and perception of speech* (pp. 55–82). London: Academic Press.

Carlson, R., Granström, B., & Fant, G. (1970). Some studies concerning the perception of isolated vowels. *Speech Transmission Laboratory Quarterly Progress Status Report* (STL-QPSR 2/3): 19–35.

Chistovich, L.A. & Lublinskaya, V.V. (1979). The "centre of gravity effect" in vowel spectra and critical distance between the formants: Psychoacoustic study of the perception of vowel-like stimuli, *Hearing Research*, *1*, 185–195.

Chistovich, L.A. (1985). Central auditory processing of peripheral vowel spectra. *Journal of the Acoustical Society of America*, *77*, 789–805.

Darwin, C.J. (1984). Perceiving vowels in the presence of another sound: Constraints on vowel perception. *Journal of the Acoustical Society of America, 76*, 1636–1647.

Darwin, C.J. & Gardner, R.B. (1986). Which harmonics contribute to the estimation of first formant frequency? *Speech Communication, 4*, 231–235.

Delattre, P., Liberman, A.M., Cooper, F.S., & Gerstman, L. (1952). An experimental study of the acoustic determinants of vowel colour. *Word, 8*, 195–210.

Fant, G. (1956). On the predictability of formant levels and spectrum envelopes from formant frequencies. In M. Halle (Ed.), *For Roman Jakobson* (pp. 109–120). The Hague: Mouton.

Fant, G. (1960). *Acoustic theory of speech production*. The Hague: Mouton.

Flanagan, J.L. (1972). *Speech analysis, synthesis and perception* (2nd ed.). Berlin: Springer-Verlag.

Holmes, J.N. (1983). Formant synthesizers: Cascade or parallel? *Speech Communication, 2*, 251–273.

Karnickaya, E.G., Mushnikov, V.N., Slepokurova, N.A., & Zhukov, S. (1975). Auditory processing of steady-state vowels. In G. Fant & M.A.A. Tatham (Eds.), *Auditory analysis and perception of speech* (pp. 37–53). London: Academic Press.

Klatt, D.H. (1980). Software for a cascade/parallel formant synthesizer. *Journal of the Acoustical Society of America, 67*, 971–995.

Klatt, D.H. (1982a). Speech processing strategies based on auditory models. In R. Carlson & B. Granström (Eds), *The representation of speech in the peripheral auditory system* (pp. 181–196). New York: Elsevier.

Klatt, D.H. (1982b). Prediction of perceived phonetic distance from critical-band spectra: A first step. *Proc ICASSP, 82*, 1278–1281.

Klatt, D.H. (1985). A shift in formant frequencies is not the same as a shift in the centre of gravity of a multi-formant energy concentration. *Journal of the Acoustical Society of America, 77* (Supplement 1), S7(a).

Miller, R.L. (1953). Auditory tests with synthetic vowels. *Journal of the Acoustical Society of America, 25*, 114–121.

Moore, B.C.J. & Glasberg, B.R. (1983). Suggested formulae for calculating auditory-filter bandwidths and excitation patterns. *Journal of the Acoustical Society of America, 74*, 750–753.

Moore, B.C.J. & Glasberg, B.R. (1987). Formulae describing frequency selectivity as a function of frequency and level, and their use in calculating excitation patterns. *Hearing Research, 28*, 209–225.

Patterson, R.D. & Moore, B.C.J. (1986). Auditory filters and excitation patterns as representations of frequency resolution. In B.C.J. Moore (Ed.), *Frequency Selectivity in Hearing*, (pp. 123–177). London: Academic Press.

Peterson, G.E. & Barney, H. (1952). Control methods used in a study of vowels. *Journal of the Acoustical Society of America, 24*, 175–184.

Potter, R.K. & Steinberg, J. (1950). Towards the specification of speech. *Journal of the Acoustical Society of America, 22*, 807–820.

Schroeder, M.R. & Mehrgardt, S. (1982). Auditory masking phenomena in the perception of speech. *Journal of the Acoustical Society of America, 72* (Supplement 1a).

Schwartz, J.-L. & Escudier, P. (1989). A strong evidence for the existence of a large-scale integrated spectral representation in vowel perception. *Speech Communication, 8*, 235–259.

Zwicker, E. (1961). Subdivision of the audible frequency range in critical bands (Frequenzgruppen). *Journal of the Acoustical Society of America, 33*, 248.

Zwicker, E. & Terhardt, E. (1980). Analytic expressions for critical band rate and critical bandwidth as a function of frequency. *Journal of the Acoustical Society of America, 68*, 1523–1525.

Revised manuscript received 28 November 1990

THE QUARTERLY JOURNAL OF EXPERIMENTAL PSYCHOLOGY, 1991, *43A* (3) 449–458

Spectral Weights and the Profile Bowl

David M. Green and Bruce G. Berg
University of Florida, Gainesville, Florida, U.S.A.

In these experiments, listeners detected changes in the shape of a complex spectrum that varied in overall level. With multicomponent complexes, a typical finding is that the listeners were more sensitive to changes made in the middle components of the spectrum than to changes made at either edge. We used a technique developed by Berg (1989) to estimate the weight listeners attached to the different components of the spectrum in making these judgements. For reasons not understood, the pattern of spectral weights was nearly optimum for a change made in the middle component of the spectrum and much poorer when the change occurred at either edge.

In what we call a profile task, the listener is trying to detect a change in the amplitude spectrum of a complex sound. Often a multicomponent background composed of equal-amplitude components is used as the standard spectrum. The alteration in spectral shape, the signal, is produced by increasing the level of a single component. Typically, the frequencies of the complex range from 200 to 5000 Hz, and successive components are spaced at equal ratios (equal logarithmic spacing). We know that the listener is detecting a change in the shape of the spectrum, rather than a change in level of a single component, because the overall level of the sound is chosen randomly on each presentation. Thus, the absolute level of any component provides little relevant information about the spectral shape change. We also know that the temporal waveform is not a critical stimulus variable, because randomizing the phase of the components on each and every stimulus presentation does not affect the listener's ability to hear the spectral change. For a review of research on profile experiments, see Green (1987).

Requests for reprints should be sent to David M. Green, Psychoacoustics Laboratory, Department of Psychology, University of Florida, Gainesville, Florida 32611, U.S.A.

We wish to thank Dr Huanping Dai and Dr Jill Raney, who read an earlier draft of this paper. Drs D. R. J. Laming, Q. Summerfield, and an anonymous reviewer helped clarify a later draft of the manuscript. The research was supported by grants from the National Institutes of Health and from the Air Force Office of Scientific Research.

If 10 to 20 components are used in the standard, then a typical listener can detect a change of less than one decibel if the increment is added to a central component of the complex. Some listeners can detect this change in spectral shape better than they can detect the same increment added to the single component in isolation (Green & Mason, 1985). If the increment is added to non-central components, either higher or lower in frequency, then the listener's sensitivity to such a change is somewhat poorer. Plotting the threshold for detecting a change in level of a component as a function of the component frequency produces a bowl-shaped function, vaguely reminiscent of the absolute sensitivity of the ear (Green & Mason, 1985; Green, Onsan, & Forrest, 1987).

We know, however, that the bowl function is not related to absolute sensitivity, because the bowl shape remains the same when we make all the components of the standard equal in sensation level rather than equal in amplitude. In addition, the frequency associated with the minimum of the bowl function is clearly influenced by the locus of frequencies used in the complex. The minimum tends to stay near the mid-frequency components of the complex (Green & Mason, 1985; Green et al., 1987).

A new procedure developed by Berg (1989) allows us to estimate the weights given by the listener to the various components of the multitonal complex in arriving at a decision about the presence of a spectral change. We apply this technique to profile data collected with a spectral change at the low, middle, and high frequencies of the complex. The results suggest that the bowl shape arises because the spectral weights are near optimum for detecting a change in the middle components of the complex, but are distinctly non-optimum for detecting change at the extreme frequencies. This analysis provides an account for the bowl-like function, but it does not explain why the non-optimum assignment of weight occurs.

We begin the paper with a brief description of the methods used to collect the data. Next, we describe Berg's procedure. Finally, we present the results and discuss them.

Methods

A two-interval, forced-choice procedure was used to estimate the listener's ability to hear an increment in level of one tone of a multicomponent complex. The standard was an 11-tone complex, with all tones equal in amplitude. The tones ranged in frequency from 200 to 5000 Hz and were equally spaced on a logarithmic frequency scale. What we will call the signal is an increment, Δ_s, in one component of the complex produced by adding (in phase) a sinusoidal component to one component of the standard. In different conditions, the signal was 280, 1000, or 3620 Hz, corresponding to the 2nd, 6th, or 10th components of the 11-tone complex. We describe the signal threshold as the relative amplitude of the signal component re the component of the standard in decibels. Thus, if the signal to standard ratio were 0 dB, the signal would produce a 6-dB increment in the standard at that component frequency.

A 900-msec interval separated the standard or signal-plus-standard intervals, which were each 500 msec in duration. After the listener responded, feedback was presented on each trial. An adaptive procedure was used to estimate an initial threshold level. In the main experimental procedure, a mix of adaptive- and fixed-level presentations was used. Trials with a fixed-signal level were used to estimate spectral weights. The adaptive trials were used to monitor detection performance and to ensure that no change in sensitivity had occurred while the weights were being estimated. The listeners were undergraduates at the university. They observed two hours a day, five days a week, and had considerable practice in profile listening. For details of the experimental procedure, see Berg and Green (1990).

The level of the sounds presented on each trial requires some discussion. To construct a standard stimulus, we began by setting the level of each of the 11 components to 70 dB SPL. Next we added a small perturbation in level to each tone. This perturbation changed the level of each tone according to a Gaussian distribution with mean zero and standard deviation, denoted σ_X, equal to 1 dB. As will be explained, we will analyse how the probability of a choice in the forced-choice task is influenced by the size of these perturbations. In this way, we can infer the relative weight given to each of the components of the complex on the final decision. Finally, the overall level of the sound presented in any interval is a random variable. Specifically, we scaled the entire waveform by attenuating it according to a rectangular distribution ranging from 0 to 20 dB. We call the standard deviation of this distribution, σ_L equal to 5.7 dB. Thus, each component of the standard waveform had a median level of 60 dB and a $\pm$ 1 dB Gaussian perturbation about that level. All components of the resulting waveform were varied $\pm$ 10 dB in overall level. If a signal-plus-standard were desired, the signal component was added to the proper component of the standard. This procedure was followed for each and every stimulus presentation. We emphasize that independent samples were drawn for each presentation, even within the same trial. Thus, on a single forced-choice trial, the signal-plus-standard presentation might be at an average level of 53 dB and the standard presentation at 68 dB. In this example, to be correct, the listener has to choose the less intense sound.

Berg's Procedure

We now briefly outline how the spectral weights were estimated using Berg's procedure. For a more extended discussion, see Berg (1989) or Berg and Green (1990).

The basic rationale is to use the magnitude of each perturbation to assess the importance of each component in reaching a final decision. We call the perturbation in level of the *i*th component associated with the first interval of the forced-choice trial, x_{1i}. Suppose we tabulate a series of responses and find that the listener tended to select the first interval as x_{1i} increases in magnitude. We could then assert that the listener attached a positive weight to that component. To become more quantitativc in this assessment, let us assume a simple decision rule for selecting a particular interval in the forced-choice trial. Assume the listener will respond that *the signal is in interval one* whenever

$$\sum_{i=1}^{n} a_i(x_{1i}+L_1) > \sum_{i=1}^{n} a_i(x_{2i}+L_2) \tag{1}$$

where x_{1i} and L_1 are the perturbations and overall level on component *i* in the first interval, x_{2i} and L_2 are the perburbations and overall level on component *i* in the second interval, and a_i is the weight associated with the *i*th component. (Note that the overall level, *L*, is not double-subscripted because it is the same for all components.) We have omitted the fixed signal level, Δ_s, which is always presented in either the first or second interval. If the signal is presented in the first interval, then add Δ_s to the left-hand side of the inequality. If the signal is presented in the second interval, then add Δ_s to the right-hand side of the inequality.

In essence, the central idea of COSS (conditional-on-a-single-stimulus) analysis is to decompose the entire stimulus into separate parts and to examine the influence of each part on the final decision. To do this, we construct functions reminiscent of psychometric functions. Instead of plotting the probability of a certain response versus the magnitude of the stimulus, Δ_s, we plot response probability versus the magnitude of the perturbation difference in the two intervals, $(x_{1i}-x_{2i})$. The slope of the COSS function provides a measure of the influence of that component on the decision.

The application of this technique is illustrated in Figure 1, where we display five COSS functions constructed from another experiment in which there were only five components in the standard. Consider first the middle panel, which shows the analysis for the 1000-Hz component ($i=3$), the component to which the signal was added. The plot is the proportion of "interval one" responses as a function of the difference in level of the perturbations used in the first and second intervals. There are actually two separate data sets plotted: the upper set represents data where the signal was added to the first interval, and the lower set represents data where the signal was added to the second interval. The solid curves are theoretical fits to the data that we will discuss shortly. The two curves fall about $\pm\Delta_s$ from 0 dB,

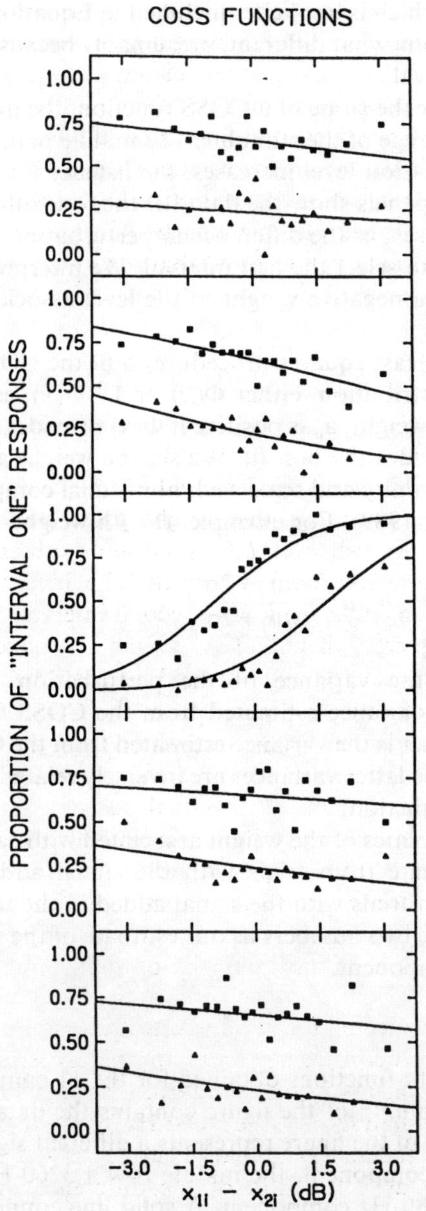

FIG. 1. Five COSS functions obtained from a five-component profile task. The abscissa is the difference in the perturbation level used in the first and second interval of the forced-choice task. The ordinate is the proportion of responses on which the listener chose the first interval.

which reflects the term which is implicitly included in Equation 1. The actual deviation from 0 dB is somewhat different, presumably because of a response bias favouring one interval.

Intuitively, the steeper the slope of a COSS function, the more the change in behaviour per unit change of the stimulus. The middle panel shows that as the difference in perturbation level increases, the listener tends to select the first interval. The other panels show the data for the four other (non-signal) components. In those cases, as the difference in perturbation level increases, the listener is less likely to select the first interval. We interpret this to mean that the listener applies a negative weight to the level associated with these components.

Specifically, we use a least-squares procedure to fit the COSS data with a cumulative Gaussian distribution, either $\Phi(x)$ or $1-\Phi(x)$, estimating both mean and variance. The weight, a_i, is positive if $\Phi(x)$ provides the best fit and negative if $1-\Phi(x)$ provides the best fit. We set the weight associated with the signal component to unity and scale each non-signal component relative to that weight (see Berg, 1989). For example, the *j*th weight, a_j, is given by

$$a_j^2 = \frac{\mathrm{var}_s + 2\sigma^2_x}{var_j + 2\sigma^2_x} \tag{2}$$

where σ_x^2 (=1 dB) is the variance of the perturbation on all of the components, var_s is the variance estimated from the COSS function of the signal component, and var_j is the variance estimated from the COSS function of the *j*th component. The latter variances are inversely related to the slope of their respective COSS function.

Two independent estimates of the weight associated with each component are obtained: one estimate from trials with the signal added in the first interval, the second from trials with the signal added in the second interval. We use the mean of these two numbers as our estimate of the spectral weight associated with that component.

Results

Figure 2 shows the weight functions obtained for the 11 components of the profile stimulus. Each column of the figure contains the data of one of the three listeners. Each row of the figure represents a different signal frequency: the top row a 1000-Hz component, the middle row a 3260-Hz component, and the bottom row a 280-Hz component. A solid line connects the weight estimates as a function of component number. The two small solid points that bracket (or fill) each open symbol represent the two independent estimates. In most cases, there is good agreement between the two estimates. The dotted line indicates a weight of zero.

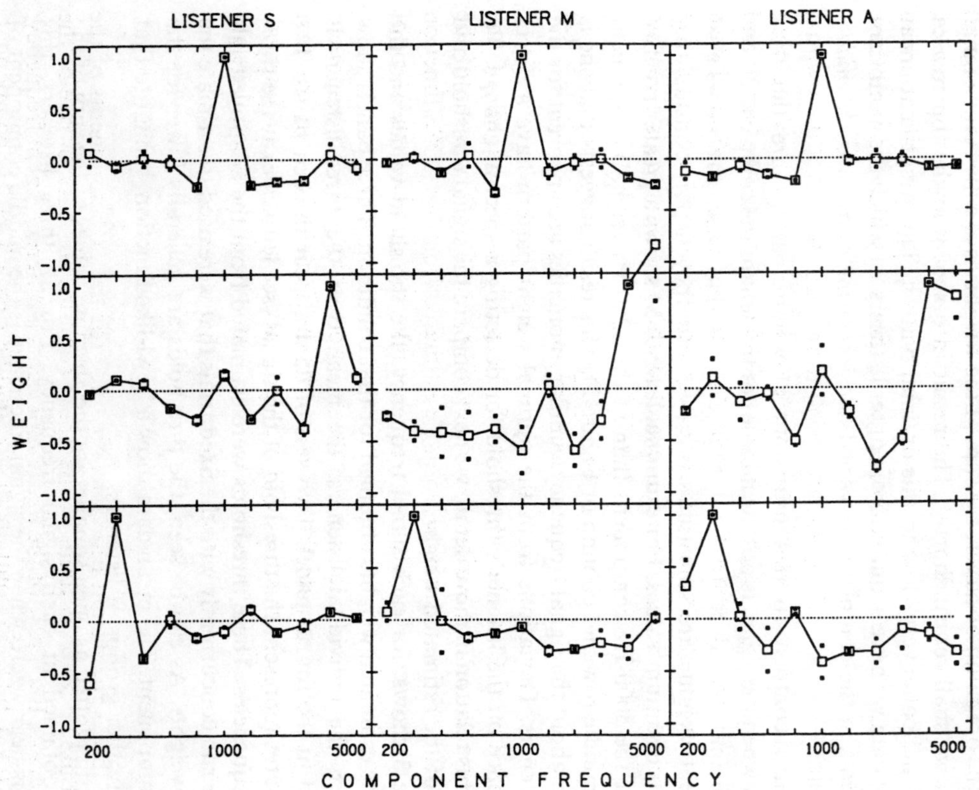

FIG. 2. Spectral weights obtained for each component of the profile stimulus. Data for the different listeners are shown in each column. The rows, top to bottom, show the data when the increment was added to a middle component (1000 Hz), a higher-frequency component (3260 Hz), or a lower-frequency component (280 Hz) of the complex. The arrow above the abscissa indicates the signal component.

A near-optimum (maximum likelihood ratio) strategy in the profile task is to compare the level at the signal component with the average level measured for the non-signal components (Berg & Green, 1990). If the signal component is given a weight of unity, then the weight of each non-signal component is $-1/(n-1)$, where n equals the total number of components. In our case, the optimum weight of each non-signal component is -0.1. Note that for the optimum observer, the sum of the weights is exactly zero, a point to which we shall return shortly. The results are shown in the top row of Figure 2 and come very close to this optimal pattern. This weight pattern is typical of data we have acquired from other listeners, in which the number of components in the complex was varied *and where the signal was the middle component*.

In sharp contrast to this near-optimal weight pattern are the data obtained when the signal is not the middle component of the complex, as seen in the second and third rows of Figure 2. In that case, the non-signal component weights are sometimes positive, and they depart considerably from their optimum values. For example, listener M shows a greater positive weight at the 5000-Hz component than at the 3280-Hz (signal) component (see the middle row and column of Figure 2). This result suggests that she is uncertain about the signal frequency. Similar anomalies are apparent for the other listeners. Deviations from the optimal weight pattern have a direct consequence on the listener's threshold for detecting a spectral change. To explore this relation in more detail, we next compare the signal threshold and the sum of the estimated weights.

Figure 3 shows, for each signal frequency, the threshold values and the sum of the estimated weights obtained for that condition. Three panels show data from the individual listeners; the mean over the three listeners is presented in the fourth panel. Two sets of data appear in each panel. The solid squares represent the threshold of the signal (see left scale) at the three signal frequencies. These thresholds were estimated from the adaptive trials that were run concurrently with the fixed trials that were used to estimate the spectral weights. As can be seen, the thresholds are generally lower for the middle component. The mean data show a bowl-like function, similar to that seen with other groups of listeners.

The data plotted as open squares are the absolute values of the sum of the weights obtained at each signal frequency. For all three listeners, this quantity is nearly zero when the signal frequency is the middle component of the complex, 1000 Hz. For the other frequencies, this quantity differs from zero, sometimes by a large amount. The mean data show an almost perfect covariation of the signal threshold and the absolute value of the sum of weights.

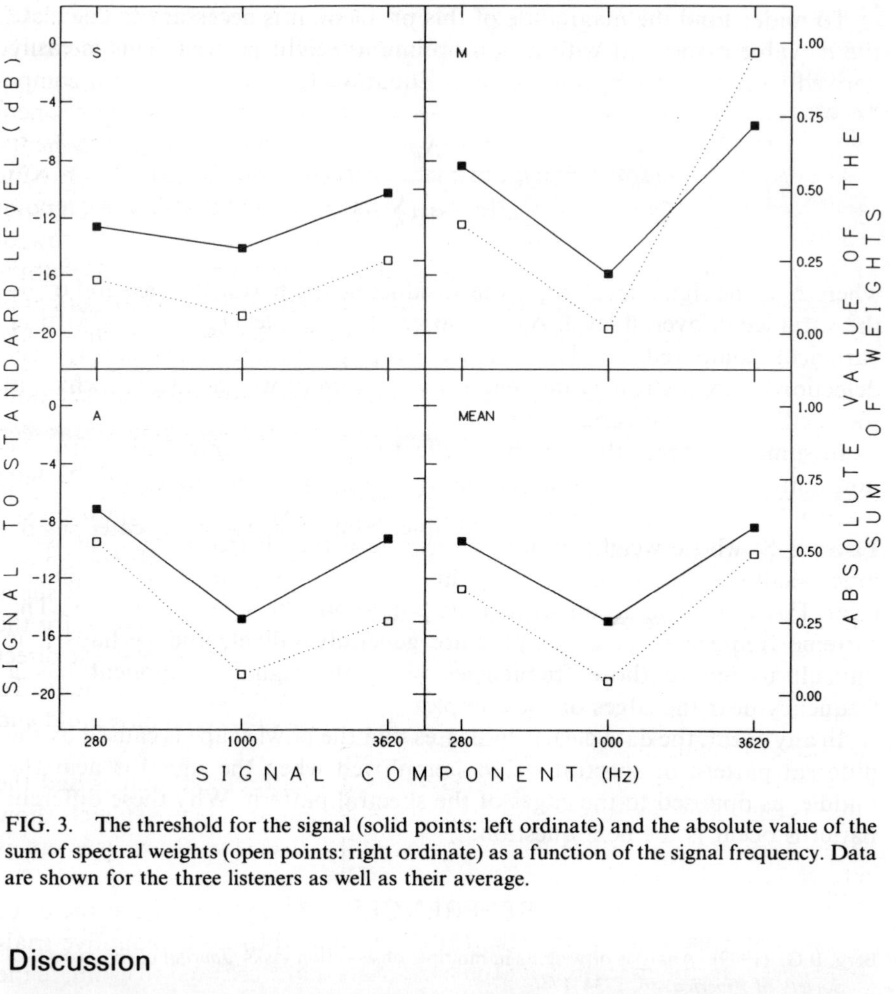

FIG. 3. The threshold for the signal (solid points: left ordinate) and the absolute value of the sum of spectral weights (open points: right ordinate) as a function of the signal frequency. Data are shown for the three listeners as well as their average.

Discussion

There are many aspects of optimum detection performance that can be compared with human observers' performance. In this discussion, we concentrate on a single feature because of its importance in this kind of detection task. For the optimum weight pattern, the sum of weights is exactly zero, as the signal component has a weight of one and the non-signal components have weights of $-1/(n-1)$. The reason for this constraint is that if the sum is non-zero, then the decision statistic will allow changes in overall stimulus level to influence the decision. Recall that overall level varied over a 20-dB range in this experiment. If one is trying to detect a small (1 dB) change in the level of the signal component, then it is clearly maladaptive to allow the changes in overall level to influence the decision rule, because these changes are unrelated to the occurrence of the signal.

To understand the magnitude of this problem, it is necessary to calculate the d' value associated with a non-optimum weight pattern. This is easily derived from the assumption made in Equation 1.

$$d' = \frac{\sqrt{2}\Delta_B}{\sqrt{\sum_{i=1}^{n} a_i^2\sigma_x^2 + \sigma_L^2(\sum_{i=1}^{n} a_i)^2}} \tag{3}$$

where Δ_s is the signal level, σ^2_x is the variance of the perturbations, and σ^2_L is the variance in overall level. As the range of overall level is 20 dB (33 dB in variance) compared to the variance of perturbation levels (1 dB), the detection index is strongly influenced by the sum of weights, $(\Sigma a_i)^2$, which is the coefficient of the variance in overall level.

In sum, it appears that the bowl effect in profile listening arises from a non-optimum use of weights in the decision rule. Note in Figure 3 that listener M, who has the largest sum of weights, displays the deepest bowl. Listener S, whose weight pattern is near zero for all frequencies, shows a much shallower bowl pattern. Why this should be the case is not completely clear. Possibly it has to do with confusion about the signal frequency. The extreme frequencies of a complex are generally salient, and perhaps it is difficult to ignore those frequencies when the signal component has a frequency near the edges of the complex.

In any event, the data clearly indicates that the bowl shape is caused by the different pattern of spectral weights employed when the signal is near the middle, as opposed to the edges of the spectral pattern. Why these different patterns occur is the next question.

REFERENCES

Berg, B.G. (1989). Analysis of weights in multiple observation tasks. *Journal of the Acoustical Society of America, 86*, 1734–1746.

Berg, B.G. & Green, D.M. (1990). Spectral weights in profile listening. *Journal of the Acoustical Society of America, 88*, 758–766.

Green, D.M. (1987). *Profile analysis: Auditory intensity discrimination.* New York/Oxford: Oxford University Press.

Green, D.M. & Mason, C.R. (1985). Auditory profile analysis: Frequency, phase, and Weber's law. *Journal of the Acoustical Society of America, 77*, 1155–1161.

Green, D.M., Onsan, Z.A., & Forrest, T.G. (1987). Frequency effects in profile analysis and detecting complex spectra changes. *Journal of the Acoustical Society of America, 81*, 692–699.

Revised manuscript received 5 July 1990

THE QUARTERLY JOURNAL OF EXPERIMENTAL PSYCHOLOGY, 1991, *43A* (3) 459–479

Perception of Spectral Changes in Multi-tone Complexes

Niek J. Versfeld and Adrianus J.M. Houtsma

Institute for Perception Research (IPO), Eindhoven, The Netherlands

Amplitude changes of the spectral components of a complex tone, relative to each other, are usually well perceived, even if the over-all intensity is kept fixed. Three experiments are reported: Experiment 1 dealt with the detectability of amplitude changes in two-tone complexes of fixed frequencies. Experiment 2 examined detection of slope changes in ramp-shaped spectral envelopes of two- and three-tone complexes as a function of spectral spacing. As a control experiment for some conditions a roving intensity level was used. Experiment 3 investigated the detectability of changes in the spectral slope of multi-tone complexes as a function of the number of components. The results of the experiments show that detection of spectral changes in a sound is strongly dependent on the frequency spacing of the components. It is concluded that the auditory system is capable of comparing the relative energy distributions over different critical bands. Within a critical band there exists an optimum frequency separation with respect to the detection of relative amplitude change.

This study deals with the ability of our auditory system to discriminate between multi-tone complexes of different spectral shapes. Knowing how and to what extent we can discriminate spectral shape is important for understanding speech communication and music perception. From a subjective viewpoint, one can see this as an investigation of primarily timbre discrimination, but it should be kept in mind that the subjective cues used to discriminate the various sounds may often also be pitch or loudness.

In most experiments dealing with this subject, an increment in amplitude in one of the components is to be detected. To prevent subjects from listening

---

Requests for reprints should be sent to Niek J. Versfeld, Institute for Perception Research (IPO), P.O. Box 513, 5600 MB Eindhoven, The Netherlands.

The authors thank C.J. Darwin and an anonymous reviewer for their very thoughtful comments on an earlier version of this manuscript.

This research was supported by the Netherlands Organization for the Advancement of Pure Research (N.W.O.) through the Psychon Foundation, Grant No. 560–262–034.

to pure intensity cues, a roving level is often used (Green, 1988), that is, the overall intensity is randomly varied between observation intervals. In our experiments stimuli have a constant overall intensity level, which means that overall intensity cannot be used as a cue for detection. This does not mean that local intensity cues are not used. Therefore a roving level paradigm for control has been applied in one experiment.

Because a spectrum can be varied in many other ways (time, frequency, amplitude, phase), some further specifications and restrictions are in order. Firstly, we will restrict ourselves to quasi-steady-state sounds and not become involved in perceptual effects of transients such as signal onset or offset, which are known to have significant consequences for both the effective spectrum as well as the percept of a sound (Berger, 1964; Smurzyński & Houtsma, 1989). Secondly, the focus of this study will be on sensitivity for amplitude changes of components with fixed frequency. Changes caused by frequency or phase shifts of components are not considered. Phase seems to have little influence on detection of spectral envelope changes in multi-tone signals (Green & Mason, 1985).

Spectral shape discrimination in the strict sense of the word applies to many discrimination experiments reported in the literature. On the one hand there are the many simple-tone intensity discrimination (Riesz, 1928; Rabinowitz, Lim, Braida, & Durlach, 1976; Jestaedt, Wier, & Green, 1977) and frequency discrimination (Shower & Biddulph, 1931; Wier, Jestaedt, & Green, 1977) experiments, which, in essence, do provide a measure of sensitivity for simple changes in spectral shape. On the other hand, discrimination measurements have been made for sounds with very complex broadband spectra such as speech-shaped noise (Farrar et al., 1987), peaked or notched broadband noise (Moore, Oldfield, & Dooley, 1989), and multi-tone complexes (Moore, Glasberg, & Shailer, 1984; Green, 1988). The multi-tone experiments of Moore and Green involved the selection of a specific spectral feature, for instance the centre frequency of a spectral peak or notch or the intensity of a single tone component, as the physical variable to be manipulated and discriminated. Finally, other experiments with band-limited tone and noise stimuli have been reported that could be viewed as spectral shape discrimination experiments. Buus (1983) investigated sensitivity for opposite frequency shifts of the components of a two-tone complex as a function of their frequency difference, whereas Feth and O'Malley (1977) did similar experiments for small intensity changes. Raney, Richards, Onsan, and Green (1989) have shown that tone-in-noise detection with signal uncertainty also can be considered as spectral shape discrimination.

Three experiments are reported in this paper. Experiment 1 deals entirely with the detection of incremental amplitude changes in one or two fixed-frequency tones, with and without the background of other non-varying tone components. Experiment 2 deals with detection of changes in the spectral slope of two- and three-tone complexes, as a function of frequency separation between components. Experiment 3 explores the detection of changes in the spectral slope of multi-tone complexes comprising between two and twelve components, as a function of spectral range. A computer implementation of Feth's EWAIF model (Feth, 1974; Feth & O'Malley, 1977; Feth, O'Malley, & Ramsey, 1982; Feth & Stover, 1987) was used to compare our results qualitatively with the model predictions. In a final section of the paper an attempt is made to identify some elements that should go into a model that can explain the most prominent features of discrimination behaviour observed in this study as well as in other studies from the literature.

EXPERIMENT 1

Experiment 1 dealt with the question of how well the human auditory system can discriminate signals that are comprised of fixed frequencies but differ in amplitude of one or more components. Detection threshold for an amplitude increase in one (or more) components was determined with an adaptive two-interval two-alternative forced-choice paradigm. Each sound contained discrete frequency components that remained fixed during the entire experiment. The number of components in the sounds varied from a single one (i.e. sounds were pure tones) to 20, although most sounds were two-tone complexes. The one- and two-tone experiments were done in three different frequency regions to study the frequency dependence of discrimination. The 20-tone experiment, in which the amplitudes of only two components were manipulated, was meant as a control experiment to assess the influence of the presence of other non-varying components on complex-sound discrimination (Green, Kidd, & Picardi, 1983; Green, Mason, & Kidd, 1984). In the profile analysis studies by Green and his co-workers the general approach was to measure detection of an amplitude increment of a single component of a tone complex. In the present study the focus is on the detection of some fixed increment of a single tone component being moved from one component to the next. The fact that we can track the placement of tones and tone voids in a sequence of complex tones has been shown in a recent pitch–motion study with random chord sequences (Allik, Dzhafarov, Houtsma, Ross, & Versfeld, 1989). In order to make sure that no loudness cues were used, Green and co-workers used a roving intensity level. In this experiment, discrimination of pure intensity differences and spectral shape differences are compared; thus the roving level paradigm was not used.

Method

Stimuli. Five types of stimuli were used, as illustrated in Figure 1, each stimulus containing two sound intervals:

1. two pure tones of frequency f_1, one with $L_p = L + \triangle L$, the other with $L_p = L$;
2. two two-tone complexes with tones at frequencies f_1 and f_2, one with tones at sound pressure levels of $L + \triangle L$ and L, the other with both tones at $L_p = L$;
3. two two-tone complexes with tones of frequencies f_1 and f_2, one with SPLs of $L + \triangle L$ and L, the other with SPLs of L and $L + \triangle L$;
4. two two-tone complexes with frequencies f_1 and f_2, one with both tones at $L_p = L + \triangle L$, the other with both tones at $L_p = L$;
5. two twenty-tone complexes with frequencies $f_n = 200 \cdot 20^{(n-1)/19}$ Hz ($1 \leqslant n \leqslant 20$), all at $L_p = L$ except the mth component in one interval and $(m+1)$th in the other interval, which had a sound pressure level of $L + \triangle L$.

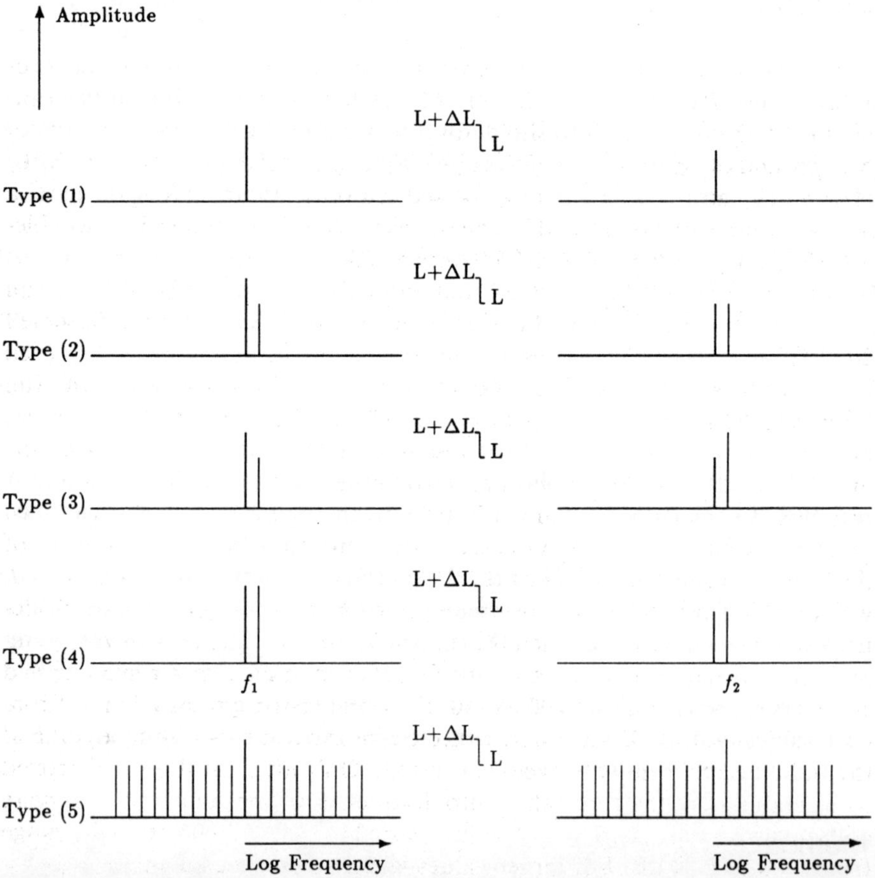

FIG. 1. Representation in the frequency-amplitude domain of the five stimuli types used in Experiment 1. Amplitudes are either L or $L + \Delta L$.

For stimulus types (2), (3), and (4), three different frequency pairs (f_1, f_2) were generated: a low pair (321.0, 375.8 Hz), a middle-range pair (826.6, 967.8 Hz), and a high pair (2128.9, 2494.5 Hz). They will be referred to as "l", "m", and "h". The 20-tone complex of stimulus type (5) consisted of equally-spaced components on a log-frequency scale, ranging from 200 to 4000 Hz, with a frequency ratio of 1.17 for successive components (about 2.7 semitones). Green, Mason, and Kidd (1984), Green, Onsan, and Forrest (1987) and Bernstein and Green (1987a) have shown that for this frequency separation the improvement of the threshold is maximized. The component pairs (4,5), (10,11), and (16,17) of this 20-tone complex correspond exactly to the three frequency pairs "l", "m", and "h" of stimulus types (2), (3), and (4). Each sound had a duration of 250 msec, including 20-msec on- and off-ramps. Sounds were separated by a 10-msec silent gap. Total stimulus duration was 510 msec.

Procedure. Stimuli were presented in an adaptive two-interval two-alternative forced-choice paradigm. All sessions started with the determination of the subject's threshold for the stimulus (with $\triangle L=0$), with a background of continuous white noise with a spectral density of 10 dB SPL/Hz (which, according to Hawkins and Stevens, 1950, corresponds to a sensation level of about 40 dB). The subject, who was seated in a double-walled (IAC) sound-insulated chamber, received the repeated stimulus binaurally through headphones and adjusted the sound level with an attenuator so that this stimulus was barely audible. Stimuli were presented 20 dB above this empirically established threshold. The white noise was used to mask unwanted distortion products of the ear (Plomp, 1965; Goldstein, 1967) and was continuously present throughout the experiment. There was no response time limit after the presentation of a stimulus during experimental runs, and feedback was provided immediately after each response. A response was given by pushing a button on the response-box. A two-down one-up adaptive procedure was used to establish the 70.7% correct point of the psychometric function (Levitt, 1971). Trials started with values for $\triangle L$ well above threshold. At the beginning of each run a simple one-down one-up procedure was used to reach the threshold quickly. The two-down one-up procedure was only adopted after the first four reversals. Each run contained 24 reversals, having about 100 to 150 trials, and lasted typically 4 min. From each subject at least 10 runs were collected for experiments with types (3) and (5) and at least 5 runs with types (1) and (2). Only after the threshold proved to be stable were the runs taken into account. For one subject, 5 runs were collected with type (4). The $\triangle L$ values varied in steps of 0.05 dB in the range from 0.00 to 2.00 dB. For larger values larger steps were taken.

All stimuli were calculated on a minicomputer system and were stored on disk. Stimuli were transformed into acoustical signals with a 12-bit D/A-converter at a sampling rate of 10 kHz, low-pass filtered at 4.3 kHz. The entire experiment was computer-controlled.

Subjects. Three subjects AH, JS, and NV, participated. They included both authors. All subjects had received musical training and had experience with psychoacoustic experiments.

Determination of thresholds

Thresholds were determined by fitting a normal probability function to the data with a least χ^2 fit, whereafter the 70.7% correct point was estimated. Signal detection theory provides an expression for the relation between Pc (the fraction correct responses) and the sensitivity d' in a two-interval two-alternative forced-choice paradigm (see Green & Swets, 1966):

$$\mathrm{Pc} = \Phi\left(\frac{d'}{\sqrt{2}}\right) \tag{1}$$

where $\Phi(z)$ is the normal probability function. The χ^2 statistics provide a goodness of fit criterion, and results will show that under all conditions and for all subjects a χ^2 fit is acceptable ($p > 0.01$) with a simple linear relationship between d' and ΔL, that is:

$$d' = \alpha \Delta L \tag{2}$$

Threshold is taken as that value for ΔL for which a 70.7% correct score is established. In this way, not only information from responses around threshold is used, but also information of trials that were well above or below threshold. Furthermore, a great experimental advantage compared to the conventional adaptive procedures, such as the two-down, one-up procedure (Levitt, 1971) is that now the stimulus step size can be chosen arbitrarily, as long as enough measurements are made for each stimulus value. A goodness of fit criterion is provided, and confidence intervals for the threshold can be given. It is also possible to perform ANOVA-like processing, for example, to decide whether averaging over subjects is allowed.

Results and Discussion

It became apparent from the beginning of the experiment that a variety of subjective cues played a role in the discrimination process of the signals of the different types. For types (1) and (4) it was only loudness cues, as expected, but for stimulus types (2), (3), and (5) subjects quite often reported using pitch jumps or timbre changes as discrimination cues. Pitch jumps, as reported by subjects in terms of musical intervals, appeared to correspond to the physical frequency components in which the change took place. No further attempt was made to investigate the subjective clues that were supposedly or actually used. The feedback that was given after every response simply enabled subjects to learn to use every possible cue in order to obtain a correct answer.

The results for stimulus types (1), (2), (3) and (5) are shown in Figure 2 for each individual subject, where the 70.7% correct thresholds ΔL (in dB) are plotted as a function of the stimulus type and frequency region. Filled symbols in Figure 2 indicate that inter-subject differences were not significant ($p > 0.01$), so that averaging over subjects was allowed. Six data points [AH and JS "h" for type (2) and (3); NV "l" and JS "h" for type (5)] differed significantly from the rest of the data. Omitting these 6 points, results showed that for each subject, results for stimulus type (1) differed significantly ($p < 0.001$) from the other types. Types (2) and (3) differed significantly, but no significant difference was found between types (2) and (5) or (3) and (5).

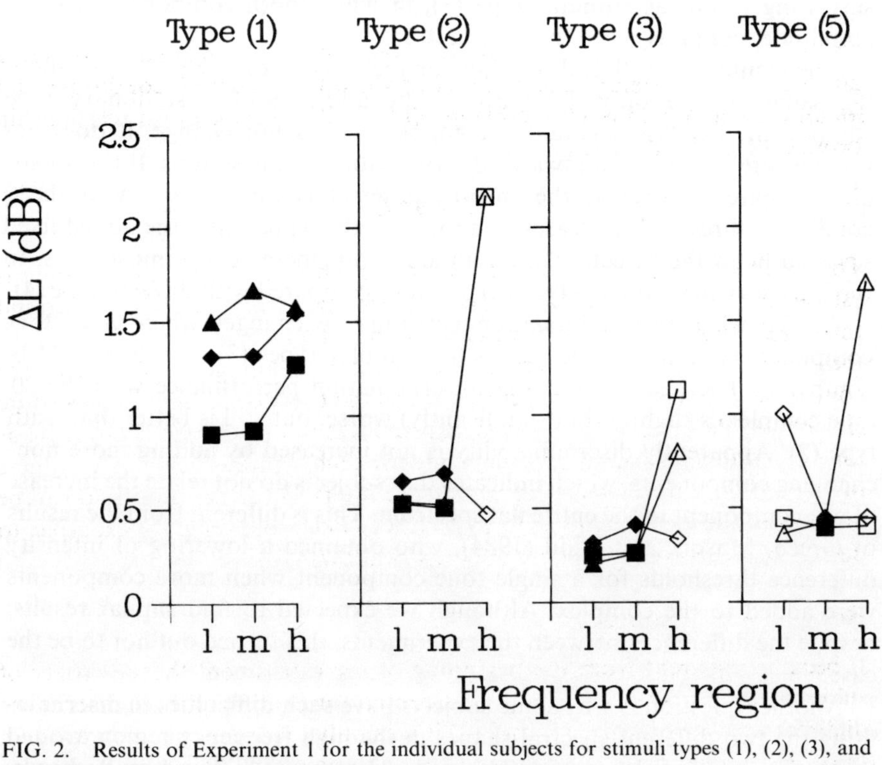

FIG. 2. Results of Experiment 1 for the individual subjects for stimuli types (1), (2), (3), and (5). Subjects AH (□), JS (△), NV (◇). The filled symbols indicate that averaging over subjects was allowed ($p > 0.01$). The three frequency regions are denoted with "l" (low), "m" (middle), and "h" (high). For type (4), middle region, threshold for NV was 1.04 dB.

Frequency region proved to be not significant if the six above-mentioned points are excluded, and averaging over both subjects and frequency region then was allowed for each type. For all subjects and all frequency regions, the four types differed significantly. The thresholds, averaged over subjects and frequency regions, are 1.22 dB for type (1); 0.57 dB for type (2); 0.33 dB for type (3); and 0.44 dB for type (5).

The results show that the pure-tone intensity discrimination thresholds for stimulus type (1) vary from 0.9 to 1.7 dB for all subjects and frequencies and are in good agreement with data from Florentine (1983) or Jesteadt et al. (1977) for sensation levels of 20 dB. As a control experiment only 5 runs were taken from subject NV for stimulus type (4) in the middle-frequency region. The threshold for this stimulus type was 1.04 dB, which is 0.3 dB lower than NV's threshold for pure tones. This result did not differ significantly from the other data of type (1), whereas it did for the other types. Results obtained with stimuli of types (2) and (3) show that for all conditions the thresholds for type (3) are about twice as small as for type (2). This in itself is not a very surprising result, as stimulus type (3), in which both components change amplitude, contains twice the information.

One would expect that thresholds for stimulus types (1) and (2) are about the same, as the only difference is the addition of a stationary tone component. Because this added component does not change, it does not provide any information towards discrimination of the sounds. If thresholds are compared, however, the surprising result is that in 7 out of the 9 conditions threshold decreases to about 0.5 dB. Apparently the added fixed sinusoid helps the detectability of an amplitude increment in most cases. In the same way the results of type (3) might be compared with those of type (4).

To see whether discrimination performance changes when more tone components are added, the results for stimulus types (3) and (5) should be compared. The results show that discrimination performance with the 20-tone complex is slightly (but significantly) worse, but still is better than with type (2). Apparently discriminability is not increased by adding more non-changing components, which indicates that subjects do not relate the increase of one component to the entire flat spectrum. This is different from the results of Green, Mason, and Kidd (1984), who obtained a lowering of intensity difference thresholds for a single tone component when more components were added to the complex. Although we expected to find similar results, despite the differences between the experiments, this turned out not to be the case.

Another question is why some subjects have such difficulties in discriminating the two different spectral shapes in the high frequency region around 2 kHz. Experiments by Green, Onsan, and Forrest (1987) and by Richards, Onsan, and Green (1989) showed that subjects perform best near 1 kHz. Spiegel and Green (1982) noticed a break point in frequency beyond which detection of a tone increment became more difficult. These effects, however, are too small to account for our results. We believe that, just as Kidd, Mason, and Green (1986), we are dealing here with a learning effect. It can be seen that for two out of the six outlying data-points, four are close to pure-tone threshold values. The other two are smaller. We think that even after 10 to 20 runs some subjects were still unable to use fully the special cue, and that additional training should have helped.

Perhaps the most interesting results of this experiment are the very low threshold values, which, for some conditions, were as low as 0.2 dB. When the spectral shape of a signal changes, as happened in stimulus types (2), (3), and (5), thresholds are lower than when only magnitude changes, as in stimulus types (1) and (4). It seems that the change of spectral shape in itself provides a powerful discrimination cue to the auditory system, and probably reflects the same behaviour that Green (1988) has referred to as *profile analysis*. However, no roving level for intensity has been used in the present experiment; thus one might expect that intensity cues still may have played a role. The very small intensity difference thresholds on the one hand, and the subjects' report of using different cues (pitch jumps) on the other hand, do suggest that for these types no overall loudness cues have been used, as for types (3) and (5) overall intensity remained constant for the two stimulus intervals.

Feth and Stover (1987) reported computations on complex signals using the envelope weighted average instantaneous frequency (EWAIF) as a means of discriminating complex tones (Feth, 1974). The model is based on the assumption that a change in the amplitude of a component in a complex signal introduces a change in pitch, on the basis of which discrimination takes place. It can be shown that an arbitrary time signal $A(t)$ can be written as

$$A(t) = E(t) \cos [p_i(t)], \tag{3}$$

where $E(t)$ is the envelope function and $p_i(t)$ the instantaneous phase angle. The instantaneous frequency is now defined as the time-derivative of $p_i(t)$

$$f_i(t) = \frac{1}{2\pi} \frac{\partial p_i(t)}{\partial t} \tag{4}$$

One now can determine the EWAIF of a sound of a period T by computing

$$\text{EWAIF} = \frac{\int_0^T E(t) f_i(t) dt}{\int_0^T E(t) dt} \tag{5}$$

Threshold of discrimination is said to be reached if the EWAIF-difference between two signals has a certain value. Applying this model to our stimuli, we see that the model does predict a factor of two difference in the thresholds found with types (2) and (3). The model, however, also predicts that discrimination improves with increasing frequency separation between two tones, or with an increasing number of (non-changing) components of fixed separation. If one keeps in mind that with our stimuli, the frequency separation increases from the lower- to the higher-frequency region (namely from 55 to 366 Hz), such an improvement in threshold is not found. This is due to the fact that the EWAIF model operates on linear frequency, whereas the ear's resolving power is logarithmic for the frequency range in question. Also, there is no improvement for type (5) compared to type (3), as the model predicts, but quite the contrary.

By manipulating the frequency ratio of successive partials one might reach an optimum value for which discriminability is best. To find out what the optimum frequency ratio is and how much the already rather low threshold values for type (3) might improve, Experiment 2 was performed.

EXPERIMENT 2

This experiment is designed to study threshold behaviour for spectrally symmetric amplitude changes in two- and three-tone complexes. The two-tone complexes are identical to type (3) of the previous experiment, but with varying inter-tone frequency ratio. The three-tone complexes are identical to the two-tone complexes, except for a non-changing component put in the geometric centre. Thus, if a two-tone complex has an intertone spacing of N semitones, then the corresponding three-tone complex has an inter-tone spacing of $N/2$ semitones, whereas for both complexes the outer-most components are N semitones apart.

The general idea of this experiment is to investigate whether and how discrimination improvements, observed in Experiment 1 under some conditions, change when the total range and/or the inter-tone frequency ratio are changed. As a control experiment, it was investigated to what extent a roving intensity level would affect discrimination performance for two-tone complexes.

Method

Stimuli Two types of stimuli were used, each containing two sound intervals:

1. two two-tone complexes with tones of frequencies f_1 and f_2, centred geometrically around 1000 Hz, one complex with sound pressure levels of $L+\Delta L$ and L respectively, the other with SPLs of L and $L+\Delta L$.

This stimulus is in essence similar to the one used by Feth and O'Malley (1977);
2. two three-tone complexes, derived from the two-tone complexes described above, but with a fixed frequency component of 1000 Hz and a fixed sound pressure level of $L+\Delta L/2$ added.

The temporal structure of the stimuli was the same as in Experiment 1, i.e. sounds had a duration of 250 msec and were separated by a 10-msec silent period. When a roving level for intensity was used, the intensity was varied randomly from interval to interval uniformly between 10 and 30 dB above the empirically established threshold in white noise.

Procedure. The procedure was the same as the one described in Experiment 1. From each subject at least 10 runs (containing 24 reversals) were collected for each condition if the threshold proved to be stable. For stimulus type (1) there were 13 different frequency–ratio values, ranging from 0.25 to 11 semitones. For stimulus type (2) six different range ratios, that is, ratios of the highest and lowest frequency, were investigated. They ranged from 1 to 10 semitones. Thresholds were determined by the same method as was described in the previous section by fitting a normal probability function to the data, after which the 70.7% correct point was estimated.

Subjects. With the two-tone complexes 5 subjects participated for ratios of 0.25, 0.5, 1, 3, 5, 7, 9, and 11 semitones. One of those and two other subjects participated for ratios of 1, 2, 4, 6, 8, and 10 semitones for both two- and three-tone complexes. For the experiment with two-tone complexes, having roving levels for intensity, two subjects (both authors) participated for ratios of 1, 5, and 11 semitones. All subjects had some experience with psychoacoustic experiments. Their degree of musical experience varied greatly.

Results and Discussion

Results obtained with the two-tone stimuli are plotted for all individual subjects in Figure 3. The figure shows the threshold intensity difference between sound components, ΔL, as a function of the range f_2/f_1 expressed in semitones. Each adaptive run represents on the average more than 100 discrimination trials, so that each symbol corresponds to at least 1000 trials. Also, the results of Experiment 1 for the type (3) middle-frequency region are plotted (2.7 semitones). The results of both experiments are in good agreement with each other.

Feth and O'Malley (1977) performed a comparable experiment in which they used stimuli similar to ours, but with a fixed intensity difference of 1 dB

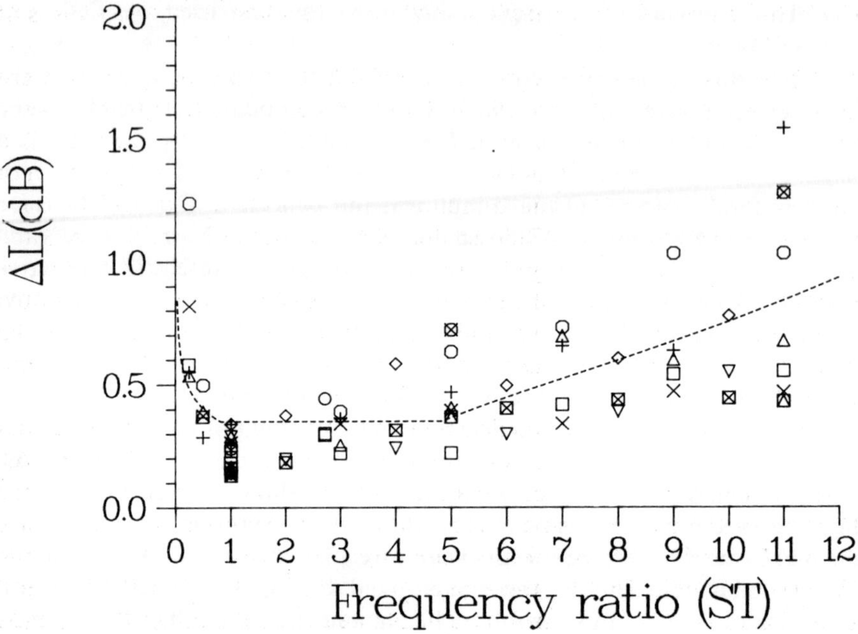

FIG. 3. Results of Experiment 2. Threshold values ΔL of two-tone complexes are plotted as a function of the frequency ratio in semitones. Each symbol denotes a different subject. A fit to Feth and O'Malley's data (1977) for 1000 Hz is plotted as a dashed curve.

between tone components, and measured percent-correct discrimination scores. From the three-line fit they made to their data taken around 1000 Hz, we calculated the equivalent 70.7% correct threshold, on the assumption that their data contained no large response bias and that sensitivity d' is proportional to the intensity difference (in dB) between the tone components. The result of this calculation, which is represented by the dashed function in Figure 3, appears to be quite consistent with our results.

To explain Feth and O'Malley's data, Feth and Stover (1987) invoked the earlier-mentioned EWAIF model. This model was shown to account, at least qualitatively, for their data and, by inference, also for our present data. When $f_2=f_1$, the two-tone complexes to be distinguished will be physically identical, as long as the phase angle between the two identical frequencies remains constant, and will therefore be indistinguishable. This corresponds with an infinite ΔL. When f_2/f_1 increases, the envelope-weighted instantaneous frequency will become increasingly more different between the two complexes; discrimination will therefore improve, and ΔL will decrease. If, however, f_2/f_1 reaches the point where the two frequency components of the complex tone become aurally resolved, the EWAIF mechanism breaks down, discrimination deteriorates, and ΔL will increase again. Ultimately it is expected to level off at the intensity difference limen for single pure tones of 1–1.5 dB.

Although the EWAIF account of Feth and O'Malley's and our present data is qualitatively plausible, there are some quantitative aspects that the model does not explain very well. One is the observed fact that there is a plateau in the original Feth and O'Malley data—or, equivalently, a region of constant low ΔL between 1 and 5 semitones for the manner in which we have plotted the data. The EWAIF model does not describe what keeps ΔL limited to about 0.3 dB in that region. Another problem is that a conservative estimate of the bandwidth of the filters that separate the tones, represented by the breakpoint of the curve at about 5 semitones, is very wide compared with the conventional estimates of the critical bandwidth (about 3 semitones).

For our present data one could argue that a plateau is not so evident and that they are best fit by an asymmetric U-shaped curve with a minimum ΔL for a frequency ratio of 1 or 2 semitones. This would largely resolve the dilemma of the plateau and the location of the breakpoint. The difference limen ΔL simply decreases with increasing f_2/f_1 because of the increasing EWAIF difference between the signals, until the trend is reversed by aural resolution of the tone components. The plateau in Feth and O'Malley's data can easily be accounted for by their paradigm of using a constant component intensity difference of 1 dB, which caused performance saturation of 100% correct responses.

In order to see whether our experimental task should be viewed as spectral shape discrimination and not as intensity discrimination, a control experiment with a roving intensity level was performed. The experiment was identical in all respects, except that the overall intensity was varied randomly over a range of 20 dB for each sound; 70.7% thresholds for the two individual subjects are given in Table 1.

The results show that despite the roving level, subjects are still able to discriminate in a correct sense, which indicates that they use across-channel information. Furthermore, the similar trend of the thresholds for the roving

TABLE 1
Results from Experiment 2 for Two-Tone Complexes, With and Without a Roving Intensity Level, for Frequency Separations of 1, 5, and 11 Semitones

	1 ST		*5 ST*		*11 ST*	
	fixed	*roving*	*fixed*	*roving*	*fixed*	*roving*
AH	0.14	0.28	0.72	1.04	1.40	2.29
NV	0.18	0.28	0.37	0.50	0.43	1.13

and non-roving paradigm strongly suggests that a roving level simply adds noise at some central level (Durlach, Braida, & Ito, 1986). This enables us to think of the discrimination process with fixed intensities as being based on the perception of changes in the spectral shape.

Figure 4 shows the results of the second part of the experiment for three subjects. Solid data points represent results for the three-tone complexes, open data points for two-tone complexes. 70.7% correct thresholds are plotted as a function of the bandwidth of the signal, expressed in semitones. Each symbol represents about 1000 trials.

One can see that generally thresholds decrease when partials come closer in frequency, just as was observed with two-tone complexes. In general thresholds for three-tone complexes resemble those of the two-tone ones. For small inter-tone values (1–2 semitones), three-tone complexes have a larger threshold. The EWAIF model predicts this correctly. Although no smaller inter-tone distances were tried, ΔL is expected to increase again when the range is reduced. The data show that thresholds for three-tone complexes are not as low as those for the two-tone complexes. For 8 and 10 semitones, discrimination thresholds for three-tone complexes are lower than those found for two-tone stimuli. The reason for this is not obvious, because the

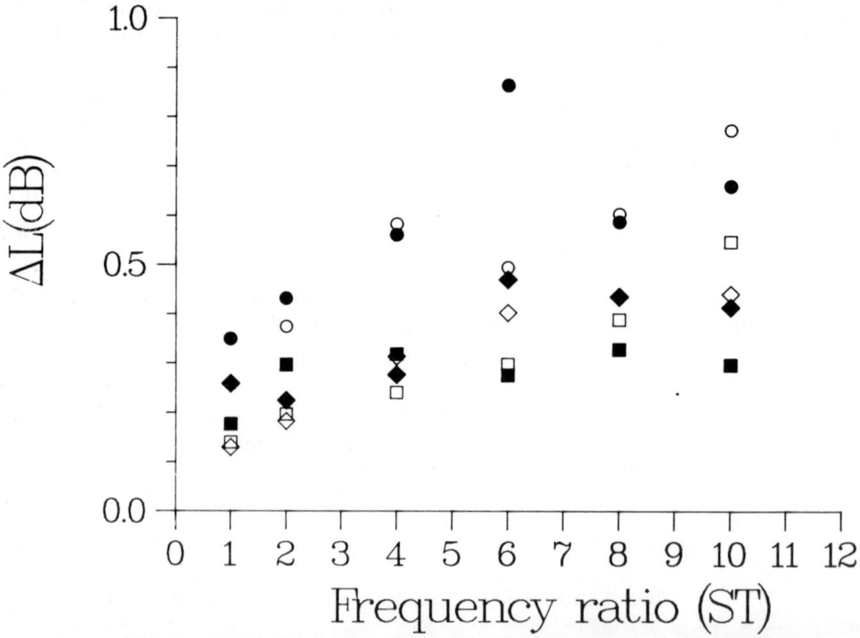

FIG. 4. Results of Experiment 2. Threshold values ΔL of two- (open symbols) and three-tone complexes (filled symbols) are plotted as a function of the frequency ratio of the outer components in semitones. Each different symbol denotes a subject.

added third tone did not change amplitude. It is our belief that when the added third tone is also resolved, cross-comparison is easier, because it enables the subject to use one extra point to estimate the spectral shape. Bernstein and Green (1987a) provide an analoguous explanation.

EXPERIMENT 3

Experiment 3 deals with the perception of changes in the spectral slope of multi-tone complexes. It is designed to investigate how discrimination improves when the total frequency range is changed, and the inter-tone spacing remains constant.

Method

Stimuli. The stimulus used contained two sound intervals, as illustrated in Figure 5 for a two-, four-, and a twelve-tone complex. Each sound interval contained a multi-tone complex with tones geometrically centred around 1000 Hz, all tones being separated by one semitone, and with a ramp-shaped spectral envelope on a log-frequency scale. One complex had a positive spectral ramp—that is, its lowest-frequency partial at sound pressure level L and its highest partial at $L+\Delta L$—the other complex a similar negative spectral ramp.

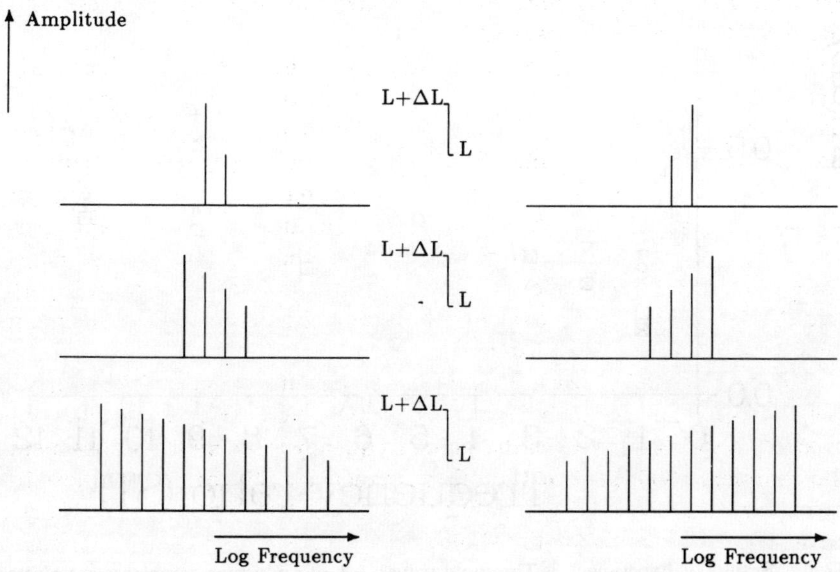

FIG. 5. Representation in the frequency-amplitude domain of the stimulus type used in Experiment 3. Stimuli with 2, 4, and 12 components are plotted. Amplitudes varied between L and $L+\Delta L$. Inter-tone spacing always was 1 semitone.

The temporal structure of the stimuli was the same as in Experiment 1—that is, sounds had a duration of 250 msec and were separated by a 10 msec silent period.

Procedure. The procedure was the same as the one described in Experiment 1. From each subject at least 10 runs (containing 24 reversals) were collected for each condition if threshold proved to be stable. Thc number of components in the complex was either 2, 4, 6, 8, 10, or 12, resulting in a spectral bandwidth of 1, 3, 5, 7, 9, or 11 semitones. 70.7% correct thresholds were determined by the same method as was described in Experiment 1.

Subjects. Four subjects participated, including one of the authors (NV). All had some experience with psychoacoustic experiments. Their degree of musical experience varied greatly.

Results and Discussion

Figure 6 shows the results, where threshold is plotted as a function of the bandwidth of the multi-tone complex, expressed in semitones. Again one

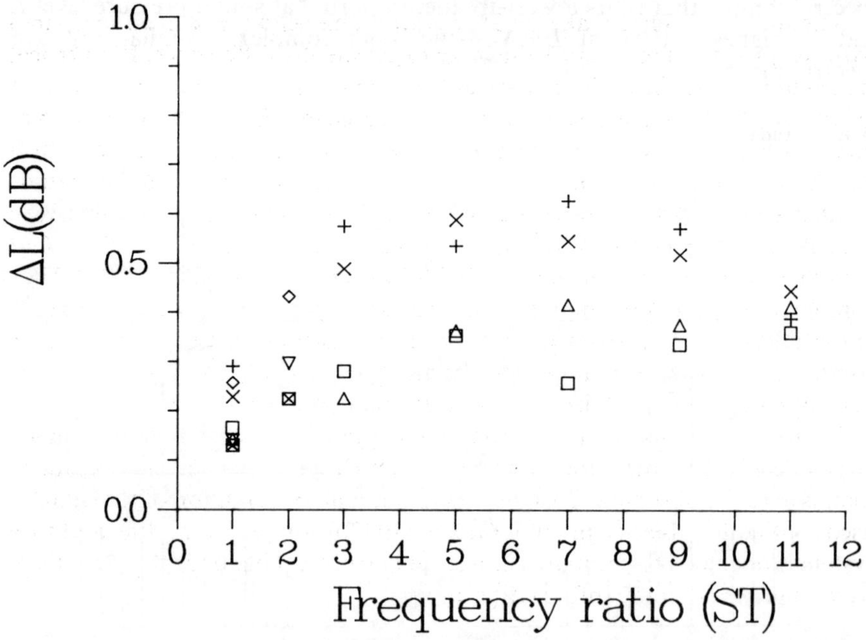

FIG. 6. Results of Experiment 3. Threshold values ΔL of multi-tone complexes are plotted versus the frequency ratio of the outer components (in semitones) for four subjects. For comparison also some results of Experiment 2 are plotted. Each different symbol represents a different subject.

symbol represents on the average 1000 trials. For comparison, also the data of Experiment 2 for two- and three-tone complexes with a separation of 1 semitone are plotted. The results of both experiments are in excellent agreement. The figure as a whole shows that, starting from the two-tone condition as a reference, addition of tone components make discrimination threshold increase until about 4 or 5 components are present (3 to 4 semitones). Addition of more tone components does not increase the threshold level any further but, on the contrary, seems to cause a slight but statistically significant decrease. The subjective cue, as reported by the subjects, appeared to be a change in "sharpness" of the timbre, which was also reported by Bismarck (1974a, 1974b).

The left part of Figure 6, showing an upward trend, is not consistent with the prediction of the EWAIF model. This model predicts a downward trend for ΔL, when tone components of one-semitone spacing are added. Beyond a total complex tone range of 3 or 4 semitones one might expect a decline in performance—that is, an increase in ΔL, because our auditory filter will begin to separate the tone complex into different spectral parts. The data, on the other hand, show a plateau for ΔL up to about 7 semitones, and beyond that a slight decrease.

The study by Green et al. (1983) provides some data that can be compared with the present ones, despite the large experimental differences. If a vertical cross-cut is made through the data displayed in Figure 4 of Green's study, at an abscissa value of 5 units, which is comparable to our stimulus condition of one semitone separation, a function of four data points is obtained, which has the same general shape as our function in Figure 6. Absolute magnitude comparisons cannot be made because of the fundamental difference between the roving-level paradigm that Green used and our fixed-level paradigm. Our stimuli also resemble those used by Bernstein and Green (1987b). They compared a 21-component flat spectrum with a spectrum having a ramp on a amplitude–log frequency scale. Because they used only one complex-tone condition, results cannot be compared. They showed, however, that the percept could be catagorized as spectral shape discrimination.

Vector summation of d' for each changing component predicts a much larger decrease in threshold when more and more components are added than is actually observed. This implies that not all information of the signal is used optimally. Bernstein and Green (1987b) suggest that the auditory system is only able to compare changes in two critical bands at the same time, which may leave some information unused.

Learning Effects

Figure 7 shows subject RC's threshold ΔL as a function of run number for three different frequency ratios employed in the first part of Experiment 2.

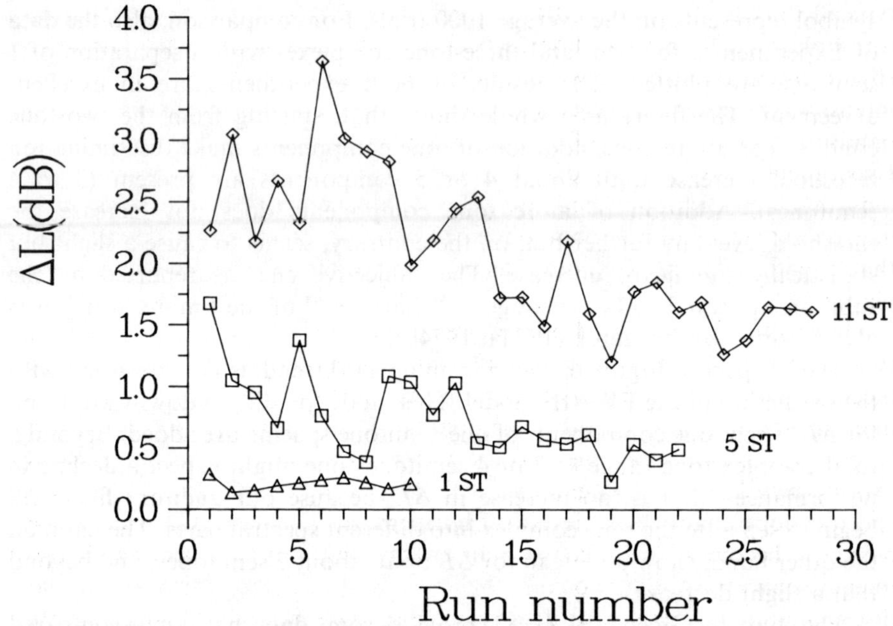

FIG. 7. Results from Experiment 2 for subject RC. Threshold values ΔL are plotted for frequency ratios of 1, 5, and 11 semitones as a function of the run number.

Especially for frequency separations larger than three semitones, subjects took time (sometimes even up to 2500 practice trials) to reach a relatively stable threshold. Large learning effects were also reported by Kidd, Mason, and Green (1986), who reported similar numbers of practice trials needed before threshold was stable. It is believed that strong learning effects exist because subjects have to learn to compare sounds that are not in the same critical band.

Apart from learning effects, robustness of the threshold—that is, variation of the threshold between the consecutive runs—varies for different frequency ratios. This robustness appears to depend on threshold value in the sense that the variance increases with increasing threshold. This may be partly due to the experimental set-up, where, in a two-down one-up adaptive procedure, a linear relationship between d' and ΔL (which determines the shape of the psychometric function) causes an increasing variance with increasing threshold.

GENERAL DISCUSSION

The most striking feature of this study is the apparent fact that discrimination thresholds for intensity changes, which under most conditions are typically in the order of 1 dB for signals of 20 or 30 dB above hearing threshold, can become as low as 0.2 dB. The control experiments with a roving intensity level show that discrimination is not based on simple intensity cues and that subjects are able to make comparison across critical bands. The facts that even for large frequency separations (a) thresholds in Experiment 2 stay near 0.5 dB, (b) three-tone complexes have lower thresholds than the corresponding two-tone complexes, and (c) discrimination improves with added tone components in Experiment 3 also strongly indicate that a pattern or profile comparison across different channels must take place.

Originally we interpreted our data as if the auditory system is limited by two different mechanisms when detecting spectral shape changes. One mechanism operates on the conventional measure of relative energy changes in critical-band filters, the other on global or local changes of spectral slope. If this idea is applied to the two-tone data shown in Figure 3, one would expect them to fit a straight line that goes through the origin (constant spectral slope change) and levels off horizontally (constant ΔL) when slope detection becomes less effective than energy detection. At very small frequency separations, the two components were thought to interact such that discrimination worsens. Our data seem to fit such a curve (Versfeld, 1989). The data of Experiment 3, however, show that the concept of simple spectral slope discrimination by the auditory system for more complex changes is untenable. If spectral slope discrimination were the mechansism, for Experiment 3 one would expect an ever-increasing threshold as a function of the bandwidth.

The EWAIF model of Feth (1974) can, at least qualitatively, account for some of the data presented in this study, but not for all. The model does roughly predict the observed shape of the ΔL function of Experiment 2 shown in Figure 3, but it predicts just about the opposite trends for the data of Experiment 1 shown in Figure 2 [type (3)] or the results of Experiment 3 shown in Figure 6.

Another approach to interpreting our data might be to consider the beat interference pattern of signals as a possible basis for discrimination. The lowest ΔL value found in Experiment 2 was for a tone separation of one semitone, as seen in Figure 3. This is about the same spacing for which Plomp and Levelt (1965) and Plomp and Steeneken (1968) found a maximum of subjective roughness or dissonance in two-tone complexes. Inside the critical band, the relatively low thresholds may be caused by the detection of a change in regularity of an interference pattern from incompletely resolved partials. Especially if there are only two partials, a symmetrical amplitude change as happened in stimulus type (3) of Experiment 1 will cause a shift in the carrier phase with respect to the signal envelope, which may constitute a detection cue. With three partials in the stimulus, the signal envelope will be much less regular, because the tones are spaced equally on a log-frequency scale and are usually not harmonically related. A change of carrier phase with respect to an irregular envelope may be much more difficult to detect, explaining the rise of threshold. With four partials present, the advantage of the interference pattern cue has just about disappeared. Presumably, if stimulus partials had been chosen harmonically, as is the case in most musical and voiced-speech sounds, the curves of Figure 4 and Figure 5 would have shown a quite different shape. It is left to future research to find out whether this is true.

REFERENCES

Allik, J., Dzhafarov, E.N., Houtsma, A.J.M., Ross, J., & Versfeld, N.J. (1989). Pitch motion with random chord sequences. *Perception & Psychophysics, 46*, 513–527.

Berger, K.W. (1964). Some factors in the recognition of timbre. *Journal of Acoustical Society of America, 36*, 1888–1891.

Bernstein, L.R. & Green, D.M. (1987a). The profile analysis bandwidth. *Journal of the Acoustical Society of America, 81*, 1888–1895.

Bernstein, L.R. & Green, D.M. (1987b). Detection of simple and complex changes of spectral shape. *Journal of the Acoustical Society of America, 82*, 1587–1592.

Bismarck, G. von (1974a). Timbre of steady sounds: A factorial investigation of its verbal attributes. *Acustica, 30*, 146–159.

Bismarck, G. von (1974b). Sharpness as an attribute of the timbre of steady sounds. *Acustica, 30*, 159–172.

Buus, S. (1983). Discrimination of envelope frequency. *Journal of the Acoustical Society of America, 74*, 1709–1715.

Durlach, N.I., Braida, L.D., & Ito, Y. (1986). Towards a model for discrimination of broadband signals. *Journal of the Acoustical Society of America, 80*, 63–72.

Farrar, C.L., Reed, C.M., Ito, Y., Durlach, N.I., Delhorne, L.A., Zurek, P.M., & Braida, L.D. (1987). Spectral shape discrimination. I. Results from normal-hearing listeners for stationary broadband noises. *Journal of the Acoustical Society of America, 81*, 1085–1092.

Feth, L.L. (1974). Frequency discrimination of complex periodic tones. *Perception & Psychophysics, 15*, 375–378.

Feth, L.L. & O'Malley, H. (1977). Two-tone auditory spectral resolution. *Journal of the Acoustical Society of America, 62*, 940–947.

Feth, L.L., O'Malley, H., & Ramsey Jr., J.W. (1982). Pitch of unresolved, two-component complex tones. *Journal of the Acoustical Society of America, 72*, 1403–1412.

Feth, L.L. & Stover, L.J. (1987). Demodulation processes in auditory perception. In: W.A. Yost and C.S. Watson (Eds.), *Auditory processing of complex sounds* (pp. 76–86). Hillsdale, NJ: Lawrence Erlbaum Associates, Inc.

Florentine, M. (1983). Intensity discrimination as a function of level and frequency and its relation to high-frequency hearing. *Journal of the Acoustical Society of America, 74*, 1375–1379.

Goldstein, J.L. (1967). Auditory nonlinearity, *Journal of the Acoustical Society of America, 41*, 676–689.

Green, D.M. (1988). *Profile analysis: Auditory intensity discrimination*. Oxford: Oxford University Press.

Green, D.M., Kidd Jr., G., & Picardi, M.C. (1983). Successive versus simultaneous comparison in auditory intensity discrimination. *Journal of the Acoustical Society of America, 73*, 639–643.

Green, D.M. & Mason, C.R. (1985). Auditory profile analysis: Frequency, phase and Weber's Law. *Journal of the Acoustical Society of America, 77*, 1155–1161.

Green, D.M., Mason, C.R., & Kidd Jr., G. (1984). Profile analysis: Critical bands and duration. *Journal of the Acoustical Society of America, 75*, 1163–1167.

Green, D.M., Onsan, Z.A., & Forrest, T.G. (1987). Frequency effects in profile analysis and detecting complex spectral changes. *Journal of the Acoustical Society of America, 81*, 692–699.

Green, D.M. & Swets, J.A. (1966). *Signal detection theory and psychophysics*. New York: Krieger.

Hawkins, J.E. & Stevens, S.S. (1950). The masking of pure tones and of speech by white noise. *Journal of the Acoustical Society of America, 22*, 6–13.

Jesteadt, W., Wier, C.C., & Green, D.M. (1977). Intensity discrimination as a function of frequency and sensation level. *Journal of the Acoustical Society of America, 61*, 169–177.

Kidd Jr., G., Mason, C.R., & Green, D.M. (1986). Auditory profile analysis of irregular sound spectra. *Journal of the Acoustical Society of America, 79*, 1045–1053.

Levitt, H. (1971). Transformed up-down methods in psychoacoustics. *Journal of the Acoustical Society of America, 49*, 467–477.

Moore, B.C.J., Glasberg, B.R., & Shailer, M.J. (1984). Frequency and intensity difference limens for harmonics within complex tones. *Journal of the Acoustical Society of America, 75*, 550–561.

Moore, B.C.J., Oldfield, S.R., & Dooley, G.J. (1989). Detection and discrimination of spectral peaks and notches at 1 and 8 kHz. *Journal of the Acoustical Society of America, 85*, 820–836.

Plomp, R. (1965). Detectability threshold for combination tones. *Journal of the Acoustical Society of America, 37*, 1110–1123.

Plomp R. & Levelt, W.J.M. (1965). Tonal consonance and critical bandwidth. *Journal of the Acoustical Society of America, 38*, 548–560.

Plomp R. & Steeneken, H.J.M. (1968). Interference between two simple tones. *Journal of the Acoustical Society of America, 43*, 883–884.

Rabinowitz, W.M., Lim, J.S., Braida, L.D., & Durlach, N.I. (1976). Intensity perception. VI. Summary of recent data on deviation from Weber's law for 1000-Hz tone pulses. *Journal of the Acoustical Society of America, 59*, 1506–1509.

Raney, J.J., Richards, V.M., Onsan, Z.A., & Green, D.M. (1989). Signal uncertainty and psychometric functions in profile analysis. *Journal of the Acoustical Society of America, 86*, 954–960.

Richards, V.M., Onsan, Z.A., & Green, D.M. (1989). Auditory profile analysis: Potential pitch cues. *Hearing Research, 39*, 27–36.

Riesz, R.R. (1928). Differential intensity sensitivity of the ear. *Physics Review, 31*, 867–875.

Shower, E.G. & Biddulph, R. (1931). Differential pitch sensitivity of the ear. *Journal of the Acoustical Society of America, 3*, 275–287.

Smurzyński, J. & Houtsma, A.J.M. (1989). Auditory discrimination of tone-pulse onsets. *Perception & Psychophysics, 45*, 2–9.

Spiegel, M.F. & Green, D.M. (1982). Signal and masker uncertainty with noise maskers of varying duration, bandwidth and center frequency. *Journal of the Acoustical Society of America, 71*, 1204–1210.

Versfeld, N.J. (1989). Intensity perception in two-tone complexes. *Proc. 28th Acoustic Conference on Physiological Acoustics, Psychoacoustics, Acoustics of Music and Speech*, Štrbské Pleso, Czechoslovakia, pp. 167–170.

Wier, C.C., Jestaedt, W., & Green, D.M. (1977). Frequency discrimination as a function of frequency and sensation levels. *Journal of the Acoustical Society of America, 61*, 178–184.

Revised manuscript received 19 October 1990

THE QUARTERLY JOURNAL OF EXPERIMENTAL PSYCHOLOGY, 1991, *43A* (3) 481–501

The Detection of a Tone Added to a Narrow Band of Noise: The Energy Model Revisited

Virginia M. Richards and Laurie M. Heller
University of Pennsylvania, Philadelphia, Pennsylvania, U.S.A.

David M. Green
University of Florida, Gainesville, Florida, U.S.A.

In an effort to determine whether cues related to changes in energy contribute to the detection of a tone added to a narrow band of noise, we examined the effect of level variation on detection thresholds. In the first experiment, the level of each waveform was randomly varied on each presentation. Level variation had only marginal effects on performance. In addition, detection thresholds were obtained using bands of noise with equal energy across intervals. Neither increasing nor decreasing the variance of the noise-alone and tone-plus-noise energy difference distributions altered the detectability of a tone added to noise. Thus, the changes in energy that are concomitant with the addition of the tone are not the sole cue for the detection of the tone. In a second experiment, three psychometric functions were measured. One function was determined using no level variation, one was measured in the presence of level variation, and one was measured in the context of level variation, but for trials without level variation. The context of level variation slightly reduced detectability. In a third experiment, we compared detectability in three conditions: no level variation, across-trial level variation, and across-interval level variation. The thresholds obtained in the absence of level variation were superior to those measured in the presence of level variation, regardless of the manner in which the level variation was incorporated.

The detectability of a tone added to noise has received a great deal of attention in the history of the hearing sciences, primarily as a measure of frequency resolution. One class of descriptive models asserts that the ability

---

Requests for reprints should be sent to Virginia M. Richards, Department of Psychology, University of Pennsylvania, 3815 Walnut Street, Philadelphia, PA, U.S.A.

This research was supported in part by a grant from NIH, in part by a grant from the Air Force Office of Scientific Research, and in part by a grant from the University of Pennsylvania Research Foundation. We thank Drs Bruce G. Berg, Laurel H. Carney, Brian C.J. Moore, Jacob Nachmias, and an anonymous reviewer for their help in the preparation of this paper.

to detect the added tone depends on the change in the power, or the energy, that is concomitant with the addition of the tone (Fletcher, 1940; Schafer, Gales, Shewmaker, & Thompson, 1950; Swets, Green, & Tanner, 1962). For example, the energy model of Green and Swets (1966) posits that the observer compares the energy in the noise-alone and the tone-plus-noise waveforms, and the tone is judged to be present in the stimulus with the larger energy value. The energy model is familiar to many psychologists in part because of its success in describing basic auditory data, and in part because of its formulation in terms of the theory of signal detection. The energy model is frequently the model of comparison as it is specific both about the relevant stimulus parameters and the decision statistic.

The energy model has not always been completely successful in describing the detection of a tone added to noise, however (Ahumada & Lovell, 1971; Ahumada, Marken, & Sandusky, 1975; Moore, 1975; Pfafflin & Mathews, 1966). In recent years, particularly strong evidence against the energy model has emerged (Gilkey, 1987; Kidd, Mason, Brantley, & Owen, 1989). In these experiments, the energy levels of the noise-alone and the tone-plus-noise waveforms were independently and randomly chosen on each stimulus presentation. Thus, the stimulus energy was no longer coupled with the presence or the absence of the tonal signal. The energy model predicts that the threshold level of the tone must increase in order to overcome the external changes in level. Instead, only marginal effects of level variation were obtained. For example, Gilkey (1987) found that for 50-Hz wide bands of noise centred at 500 Hz, the introduction of a 40-dB level variation yielded only a 4.4-dB elevation in threshold relative to conditions for which no level variation was present. More recently, Kidd et al. (1989) examined the effect of level variation as a function of masker bandwidth for bands of noise centred at 900 Hz. When a bandwidth of 10 Hz was employed, the effect of a 32-dB level variation was to increase thresholds an average of 5 dB. For bandwidths greater than or equal to 50 Hz, the effect of level variation was negligible. From these data it is apparent that variability associated with the difference between the energy in the tone-plus-noise and in the noise-alone intervals has little effect on the detectability of a tone added to noise.

Alternatives to the energy model include models of detection that rely on the temporal or dynamic aspects of the stimuli (Moore, 1988). The envelopes of the noise-alone and the tone-plus-noise waveforms differ significantly (Jeffress, 1964). For example, the tone-plus-noise waveform tends to have a flatter envelope. It is also the case that adding a tone to a narrow band of noise forces the fine structure towards a more periodic, less random function (Rice, 1954). Whereas the energy model captures the difference in mean envelope values, it does not reflect all of the changes produced by the added tone. Unfortunately, recent work has yet to reveal what aspect of those differences are critical (cf. Schooneveldt & Moore, 1989), but it is apparent that changes in the envelope (Hartmann & Pumplin, 1988) and changes in the fine structure (Moore, 1975) can, in some instances, alter the detectability of a tone added to noise.

The series of experiments described below represents an initial effort to determine the relative contribution of energy-related and non-energy-related cues for the detection of a tone added to noise. These experiments address only one half of the problem, asking whether energy-based cues do in fact contribute to the detection of a tone added to a narrow band of noise. In addition, we attempted to determine whether a single decision strategy was employed both when level variation was present and when it was absent. The complementary experiments that examine the other, non-energy-based comparisons require a different experimental approach, and are currently under study.

The first experiment described below extends the results described by Gilkey (1987) and Kidd et al. (1989). A two-interval, forced-choice (2IFC) paradigm was employed. Observers indicated which of two 100-Hz-wide bands of noise centred at 2000 Hz contained the added 2000-Hz tone. On each and every stimulus presentation, the level of the stimulus, either noise-alone or tone-plus-noise, was randomly varied. The ranges of external level variation were 0 (no external variation), 30, and 60 dB. We will refer to these conditions as the 0-dB, 30-dB, and 60-dB conditions.

Consistent with Gilkey and Kidd et al., the data indicated an effect of level variation far smaller than predicted by the energy model. Thus, the energy model is not accurate for the case in which large ranges of variation are present, but it may still be valid for the condition that historically led to its adoption—namely, the 0-dB condition. For example, it might be the case that energy-based comparisons are employed when no external level variation is present, and that some other mechanism(s) emerges only when the energy-based cues become unreliable. For that reason, we completed a condition in which the variation in the distribution of energy differences (noise-alone vs. tone-plus-noise waveforms) was decreased rather than increased. If an energy-based strategy is employed for the 0-dB condition, then reducing the across-interval variability in energy should yield improved performance levels. An improvement was not observed.

Two additional experiments were completed in an effort to determine the mechanism by which level variation slightly alters detectability. In the second experiment, we examined the possibility that listeners employ different decision strategies, depending on the presence or absence of level variation. Psychometric functions were obtained for conditions in which ranges of level variation of either 0 or 40 dB were present. Embedded in the 40-dB condition were occasional trials for which there was no level variation. Three psychometric functions resulted; one for the 0-dB condition, one for the 40-dB condition, and one for trials that had no level variation but were presented in the context of level variation. The data indicate that the context of level variation is sufficient to increase detection thresholds.

In the third experiment, the effects of level variation were more fully explored. Using a 2IFC paradigm, detection thresholds were measured for three different conditions: no level variation (fixed-level condition), level variation that was present across trials but not across intervals (roving-standard condition), and level variation that was present both across intervals and across trials (random-level condition). The range of level variation, when present, was 40 dB. For both the fixed-level and the roving-standard conditions the predictions of the energy model are the same. The energy model predicts that performance should deteriorate only when across-interval variability is present. However, if performance is reduced by simply increasing the range of levels to which the observer is exposed, then thresholds measured using a roving standard would be poorer than thresholds obtained in the fixed-level condition. That result was obtained.

EXPERIMENT 1

Effects of Changes in the Variability of Energy

In a 2IFC paradigm, observers were asked to indicate which of two intervals contained the tone-plus-noise stimulus rather than the noise-alone stimulus. The level of the signal needed for 71% correct discrimination was measured. The bands of noise were 100-Hz wide and were centred at 2000 Hz. The signal to be detected was a 2000-Hz tone. In addition to the changes in level due to the choice of random noise tokens, external level variation with a range of 0, 30, or 60 dB was present. For example, when a range of 30 dB was employed, the waveform to be presented was attenuated by a value chosen from a uniform distribution of attenuation values that varied over a 30-dB range. In a fourth condition, the bands of noise that were presented in the two intervals had the same energy. Thus, for the four conditions considered, the variance associated with the distribution of energy differences (tone-plus-noise minus noise-alone) varied from nearly zero variance (equal-energy across intervals) to a value typically associated with the tone in noise task for the parameters employed here (approximately 25 dB), to a distribution having an additional variance of 600 dB (based on the difference distribution expected when a 60-dB variation in level is present).

Methods

Stimuli

The narrow bands of noise were digitally generated by summing tones that were separated by 5 Hz in the range from 1950 to 2050 Hz. The amplitudes of the tones were Rayleigh distributed, and the phases were uniformly distributed from 0 to 2π (see Richards, 1987, for further details). The average amplitude of the tones was chosen so that the largest value across all stimuli utilized the full 16-bit resolution allowed by the digital-to-analog converter (D/A).

Thirty-six such bands were generated. Generating bands of noise by summing tones separated by 5 Hz yields 200 msec of independent noise. For this experiment, 300-msec waveforms were generated, so that the last 100 msec of each waveform duplicated the first 100 msec. Thus, several 200-msec stimuli could be obtained from each waveform by varying the starting point from within the first 100 msec of the waveform. Prior to each experimental session, 12 waveforms were read into computer memory. On each stimulus presentation, one of those 12 waveforms was randomly chosen, a starting place was randomly drawn from the first 80 msec of the waveform, and a 210-msec token of the waveform was presented. For one group of listeners the 2000-Hz tone was also computer generated. For a second group of listeners, an oscillator (Hewlett Packard 200 AB) was employed.

The narrow bands of noise were presented via a 16 bit D/A at a presentation rate of 25,000 samples/sec. When a computer-generated signal was used, the tone was presented via the second channel of the D/A. The computer-generated stimuli were lowpass filtered at 10 kHz (Kemo VBF/8, attenuation rate approximately 85 dB/oct) and then passed through a programmable attenuator. The noise and tone were added and gated synchronously using a 5-msec cosine-squared onset/offset ramp. For each stimulus presentation, the steady-state duration was 200 msec, and the duration of the stimulus was 210 msec. The noise had an average spectrum level of 40 dB SPL.

Equal-Energy Bands of Noise. Although increasing level variation increases variability in the tone-plus-noise minus the noise-alone distribution, it is important to recognize that even in the absence of level variation, the tone-plus-noise and noise-alone energy distributions do not have zero variance. One source of variability that affects only the tone-plus-noise distribution is due to the fact that the phase of the tone, relative to the phase of the noise, is not fixed. A second, and larger, source of variance is due to the fact that different noise tokens, which have different energy values, are chosen for the two intervals.

One way to reduce the variance of the noise-alone and the tone-plus-noise difference distributions is to present the same noise waveform on each interval of a trial.[1] However, we wished to generate a stimulus that had the

[1] The use of such "frozen noise" has been employed in the past (Pfafflin & Mathews, 1966; Spiegel & Green, 1982). However, if some non-energy-based cue mediates, or contributes to, the detection of a tone added to noise, the use of frozen noise would in all likelihood reduce the variability of that unknown cue as well.

same energy value across the two intervals of each trial but had envelope patterns that differed across the two intervals.

The equal-energy bands of noise were generated in pairs. First, tones ranging from 1950 to 2050 Hz and spaced at 5-Hz separations were summed. The amplitudes of the tones were chosen from a Rayleigh distribution, and the phases were chosen from a uniform distribution that ranged from 0 to 2π. The resulting waveform is a narrow band of Gaussian noise. The second band of each pair, however, was not independently generated. The paired band was also a sum of tones, and again the frequencies ranged from 1950 to 2050 Hz. The amplitudes of the tones were identical to those used to generate the initial band, with one important exception: the order of the amplitudes was randomly re-assigned. For each of the paired bands, the phases were independently chosen from a uniform distribution ranging from 0 to 2π.

Waveforms generated using summed tones with the same amplitudes, but amplitudes that are ordered differently, have equal power. However, in order for short-duration stimuli to have equal energy, the noise bands must be presented for an integral number of cycles. Because the tones that were used to generate the stimuli were separated by 5 Hz, the bands of noise will repeat every 200 msec. As a consequence, any 200-msec token chosen from either band will have the same energy value as any other 200-msec token.

When the bands of noise are shaped by onset and offset ramps, they do not have exactly equal energy. We used a 5-msec cosine-squared ramp that allowed for a steady-state portion of 195 msec, or a total duration of 205 msec. Numerical computations indicated that, for stimuli so generated and ramped, the error in the equal-energy requirement is small. On average, the paired bands had zero differences in energy, and the standard deviation of the differences was less than 1% of the total energy. Furthermore, the goal of generating stimuli that had different patterns across intervals was reasonably met. Although the paired bands had equal-energy values, the paired waveforms were not correlated (average across 100 random sample pairs, $r = 0.01$, SEM $= 0.015$). In addition, analytic signals were generated in order to determine the envelopes of the paired bands, and the envelopes were found to be uncorrelated ($r = 0.013$, SEM $= 0.02$).

It should be noted that for these stimuli, the equal-energy claim relies on the existence of a wide-band analysing system. It is essential that the tones within the 100-Hz band are given equal weight by any processing filter. If the components of the noise were differentially attenuated, then the amplitudes would no longer be elements of the same set. Although the auditory system is not a wide-band system, the 100-Hz wide bands of noise are narrow relative to the putative critical bandwidth in the region of 2000 Hz. Thus, we are treating the auditory system as wide-band relative to the stimuli. The results of Hartmann and Pumplin (1988) support this assumption.

A total of 36 pairs of equal-energy bands was generated, each pair being based on a band of independent Gaussian noise. As before, each waveform had a 300-msec duration, allowing several beginning points for D/A conversion. An analog oscillator was used to generate the tone.

Procedure

A two-down one-up 2IFC adaptive procedure (Levitt, 1971) was used to estimate the level of the tone needed for 71% correct judgements. The step size was initially 4 dB, and was reduced to 2 dB following three reversals. The procedure was terminated after 50 trials, and the last even number of reversals, excluding at least the first three, were averaged in order to obtain a threshold. The initial signal level was approximately 15 dB above threshold.

Six college students with normal hearing were hired to participate in the experiments, three of whom completed the equal-energy condition. Observers were seated in a sound-attenuated room. They listened to the stimuli over either Sennheiser HD-414 or Sennheiser HD-410 earphones driven in-phase at the two ears. The two intervals were accompanied with a visual warning, and visual feedback was presented after each response. The two intervals of each trial were separated by 400 msec of quiet.

None of the observers had prior experience in psychophysical tasks. A minimum of 6 blocks of 50 trials was completed for each condition before data collection began. Each threshold is based on a minimum of 18 blocks of 50 trials, or 18 threshold estimates. Because these data were completed as a control for an unrelated experiment, it was not uncommon that a week or more would pass between periods of data collection. The order of the level variation conditions was random. The equal-energy condition was completed after the level variation conditions were completed.

Computer Simulations. In order to generate the predictions of the energy model described by Green and Swets (1966), their formulation of the energy model was programmed on a microcomputer. The computer simulations employed the same stimuli and the same stimulus presentation program that was used in the psychophysical experiment, with the exception that rather than human responses, the computer "listened" to each waveform, computed the energy, and assigned the response "signal present" to the waveform with the larger energy value.

The sequence of events was as follows: On each "trial", a stimulus waveform was chosen and was translated into real numbers; when appropriate, a tonal signal was added. The waveform was then attenuated in accordance with a value randomly chosen from a uniform distribution (multiplication rather than analog attenuation was employed), and onset/offset ramps were applied. The resultant waveform was subjected to a point-by-point squaring and then summed. The model's decision rule was that the stimulus with the larger energy value would be chosen as the stimulus with the added tone. Simulations were completed for ranges of level variation of 0, 10, 20, 30, 45, and 60 dB, and for the equal-energy bands. An adaptive procedure was used to estimate the "threshold".

Results and Discussion

Figure 1 presents the results of both the human experiment and the computer simulations. Signal threshold, presented as the ratio of the signal energy to the noise spectrum level (E/N_0) in dB, is plotted as a function of the range of level variation, either 0, 30, or 60 dB. The left-most point indicates the data for the equal-energy condition. The dotted lines indicate the human data; there is one line for each of the six observers. Note that only three of the observers completed the equal-energy condition. The standard error of the mean was computed for each subject, and for each condition, based on either 18 or 24 threshold estimates. Standard errors of the mean ranged from 0.3 to 1.3 dB.

The open squares indicate the predictions of the energy model. In order to appreciate the energy-model predictions as a function of the range of level variation, simulations were completed for several ranges of level variation. The predictions are based on an average of three sets of 20 threshold estimates, and the standard errors of the mean across the three sets are indicated as error bars. The filled symbols are described later.

Increasing the external level variation from 0 to 60 dB led to an average

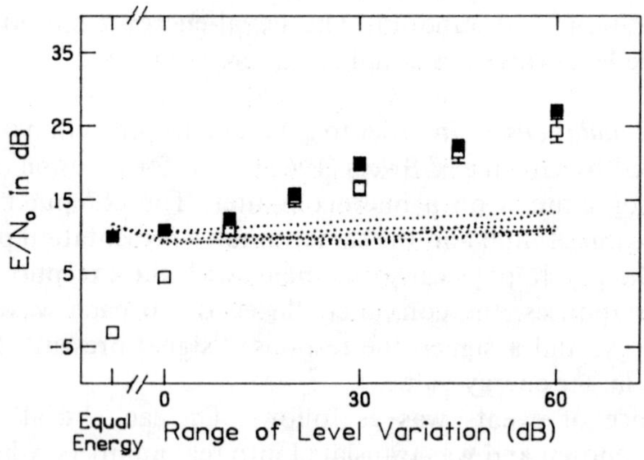

FIG. 1. Estimated threshold signal energy *re* noise spectrum level (E/N_0) in dB is plotted as a function of the range of level variation and for equal-energy bands of noise. The results for the human observers are indicated as dotted lines. The results of the energy model simulations are indicated as open squares. Predictions based on the energy model plus internal noise are indicated as filled squares. Error bars indicate standard errors of the mean across three simulation replicates.

increase in the human listeners' threshold of 1.9 dB. Across all listeners, the difference in thresholds range between a 0.3-dB advantage in the 60-dB condition relative to the 0-dB condition, to a 2.9-dB advantage in the 0-dB condition relative to the 60-dB condition. In contrast, the simulations indicate a 20-dB advantage in the 0-dB condition relative to the 60-dB condition.

The psychophysical thresholds measured in the equal-energy condition are similar to those obtained in the other conditions. In contrast, the energy model predicts a reduction in threshold of 7.5 dB relative to that obtained using independent noise tokens (equal-energy vs. 0 dB). It might be surprising that when equal-energy bands of noise are used, the energy model does not predict perfect detection (i.e. thresholds arbitrarily close to negative infinity). This less-than-perfect performance may be attributed to the fact that (1) the tone-plus-noise stimulus sometimes had less energy than the noise-alone stimulus (the phase of the tone was random relative to the phase of the band of noise), and (2) the decision "tone present" was assigned to the interval with the largest energy value.

Based on these results, it would appear that energy cues are not critical for the detection of a tone added to noise. Neither increasing nor decreasing the variability in the noise-alone and the tone-plus-noise difference distribution alters detectability to the extent predicted by the energy model. Next we will show that if a large "internal noise" is postulated, the energy model predicts that the equal-energy and the 0-dB conditions should yield similar thresholds.

Internal Noise

The data presented above suggest that non-energy-based comparisons dominate the detection of a tone added to a narrow band of noise. Here, we consider the role that "internal noise" might play in the interpretation of the results described above. As is clear in Figure 1, for the 0-dB condition the energy model predicts detection thresholds that are lower than those obtained psychophysically. Before rejecting the energy model, it is important to address that difference, and then to reconsider the effects of level variation.

There are at least two sources of variability that might contribute to the relatively poor levels of performance exhibited by our observers (relative to the predictions of the energy model). First, it is reasonable to assume that the sound waveform is not transduced by the auditory apparatus in a way that is error-free. Such errors might go under the heading of "neural jitter" and would add variability to the estimate of the stimulus energy. Additionally, variability at the level of the decision processes must exist. In the computer simulations described below, we determined the amount of combined "internal" variance that must exist in order to yield the human results obtained in the 0-dB condition. Then, using that estimate of internal noise, we repeated the energy model simulations. The equal-energy bands of noise were used for the equal-energy condition only. For the 0-dB, the 30-dB, and the 60-dB conditions, independent noise tokens were used. The variance associated with the internal noise was fixed, regardless of the range of level variation—that is, increases in level were not mirrored in the variance of the internal noise, even though such changes in the internal noise have been reported in psychophysical tasks (Green, 1964). As a result, the simulations represent a conservative estimate of the effects of internal noise when external level variation is present.

The computer program was the same as the one described above, except that in order to introduce internal noise, an independent zero-mean normal deviate was added to each energy estimate. By adjusting the variance of the added deviate, the predicted performance levels were roughly matched to those obtained experimentally. The resulting threshold predictions are indicated as filled squares in Figure 1. For the stimulus levels employed, and for the 0-dB condition, over 90% of the total variance (the sum of the external and internal) was due to internal noise.

When the range of external variation is large, internal noise has little effect on predicted thresholds. For example, for a 75-dB range of external level variation (not shown), threshold estimates obtained using added internal noise were as likely to be smaller than the estimates for the energy model as they were to be larger than the estimates for the energy model. This relatively small effect of internal noise is obtained because the internal variability is small compared to the external variability. Because the sum of independent random variables has variances that add, the same amount of internal noise will contribute a relatively smaller portion of the total variance for large ranges of external variation. In contrast, when the range of external variation is small, internal variability dominates the total variance.

The simulations indicate that the internal noise may be sufficiently large to overcome the reduction in variance gained by the use of equal-energy bands. Thus, the observation that the equal-energy bands and the bands of Gaussian noise yielded similar thresholds in the 0-dB condition does not rule out an energy model that includes a large internal noise. However, when the range of level variation is equal to or greater than 30 dB, the energy model cannot predict the data, even when the role of internal noise is considered.

EXPERIMENT 2

Effects of Context

In this experiment, we attempted to determine whether the mechanisms and/or decision processes responsible for the detection of a tone added to a narrow band of noise were the same in the presence and in the absence of level variation. Using a 2IFC paradigm, psychometric functions were measured. The bands were 100-Hz wide, centred at 2000 Hz, and presented for 105 msec including 5-msec onset/offset ramps. Equal-energy bands of noise were employed.

Either no external level variation was present, or a 40-dB range was used. When level variation was present, 15% of the trials had no across-interval level variation. Those 0-dB trials occurred randomly. If the introduction of level variation yields a change in strategy, then the context in which the 0-dB trials occur would be expected to have an effect.

Of the four observers tested, two were aware of the experimental manipulation (the first two authors served as subjects). Neither reported awareness of those trials for which the level variation was fixed to zero. The manipulation of level variation was obvious to all observers.

Methods

The experimental methods were similar to those described above. Sixty pairs of noise waveforms with equal energy were generated, each pair being based on an independent band of Gaussian noise. The tones summed to generate the bands were separated by 10 Hz and ranged from 1950 to 2050 Hz, inclusive. Each generated waveform represented 200 msec of noise, or two periods of the 10-Hz fundamental. The signal was a computer-generated 2000-Hz tone and was gated on and off with the masker. The starting points of the two bands were independently chosen from the initial 80 msec of each waveform. The 5-msec onset/offset ramps were digitally generated such that the stimuli presented to the observers had a total duration of 105 msec, or a 95-msec steady-state portion. The median noise spectrum level was 50 dB SPL.

Percent correct was measured as a function of either four or five different signal levels. For most listeners and most conditions, energy to spectrum level ratios ranged uniformly from 5 to 14 dB, in 3-dB steps. Occasionally, measurements at 2 or 17 dB were required due to individual differences in sensitivity. The signal level was fixed within 70-trial blocks. Each of the four levels was completed in random order. Then a new order was chosen, and the set of blocks was repeated. In the 0-dB condition, four repetitions were completed, yielding a total of 280 judgements at each signal level. For the 40-dB condition, a total of seven replicates were completed, yielding 490 judgements at each signal level. The data obtained in the 40-dB condition were then separated into two groups: those trials with and those trials without level variation. The average number of trials per signal level was 412 and 78 trials, respectively. For the 0-dB trials embedded in the 40-dB condition, the true range of trials per signal level was 65 to 92 trials.

Four normal-hearing observers ranging in age from 23 to 33 years of age participated in the experiment. Three of the four observers had extensive experience in psychoacoustic tasks. Each observer completed a minimum of 150 trials in the 0-dB condition prior to the collection of data in the 0-dB condition. Three of the observers completed a minimum of 250 trials in the 40-dB condition prior to collection of data in the 40-dB condition. For Observer 4, only 70 trials were completed prior to data collection in the 40-dB condition. Observers 1 and 2 completed the 40-dB condition first; the other two observers completed the 0-dB condition first.

Results and Discussion

Figure 2 plots the percent correct judgements as a function of the signal energy *re* the noise spectrum level, E/N_0, in dB. The open squares indicate data collected in the 0-dB condition, filled squares indicate performance levels obtained for the 0-dB trials embedded in the 40-dB condition, and filled circles indicate performance in the 40-dB condition. Each panel presents the data for a single subject, and the error bars represent the standard errors of the mean.

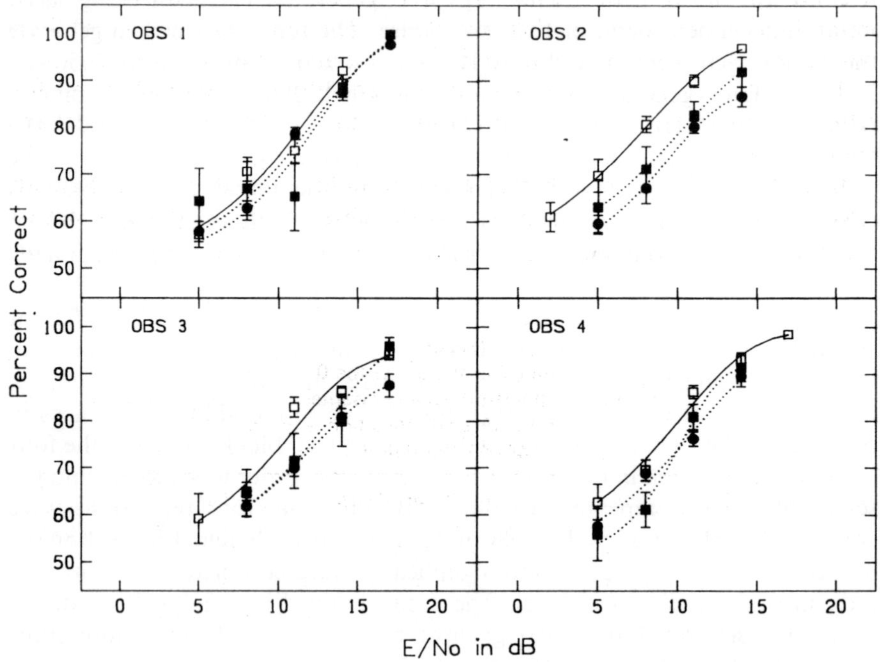

FIG. 2. Percentage of correct judgements is presented as a function of E/N_0, in dB. Each panel presents the data of a single observer. Open squares present data collected in the absence of level variation; filled circles represent data collected in the 40-dB condition; filled squares represent data collected in the 40-dB condition, but for those trials for which no level variation was present; solid and dotted lines indicate fits to the 0- and 40-dB conditions, respectively.

For each observer, percent correct scores were fitted to a psychometric function using a cumulative Weibull distribution and three free parameters (Watson, 1979; Nachmias, 1981).[2] The three estimated parameters correspond roughly to the position of the curve along the abscissa, the steepness of the curve, and the upper asymptote of the curve. The functions were forced to achieve a lower asymptote of 50% correct (chance level for 2IFC). The functions were fitted to the data using weights proportional to the number of observations and the percent correct value—that is, weights appropriate for Bernoulli trials were used. For all but two of the data sets, the fitted function accounted for more than 95% of the total variance in the data. For the 0-dB trials that were extracted from the 40-dB condition, only 58% (Observer 1) and 87% (Observer 3) of the total variance was accounted for by the fitted functions. The fitted functions are shown in Figure 2. The solid curve represents the fits to the 0-dB condition, and the dotted curves present the fits to the data obtained in the 40-dB condition.

As in Experiment 1, the effect of level variation was small. For Observer 2, the psychometric functions are orderly, showing relatively consistent effects of context. For Observers 3 and 4, the 0-dB condition produces the best performance levels, and the other conditions are not strongly delineated. For Observer 1, the psychometric functions do not appear to be orderly.

Thresholds, defined as the signal level needed for 76% correct ($d' = 1$ for 2IFC), were estimated from the fitted functions. The resulting estimates are presented in Table 1.

In order to determine whether the thresholds differed significantly, an ANOVA was completed which treated the observers and the experimental

TABLE 1
Estimated Thresholds for the 0-dB Condition, the 0-dB Trials Presented in the Context of 40-dB Level Variation, and the 40-dB Condition

Obs.	*0-dB*	*0-dB/from 40-dB*	*40-dB*
1	10.5	11.5	11.0
2	6.9	9.3	10.0
3	10.5	12.3	12.6
4	9.1	10.4	10.6

[2] The data were also fitted using a linear, least-squares fit of d' vs. signal level. The data were better fit by the psychometric function described in the text (which has one more parameter), and the statistical analysis and conclusions obtained using a linear least-squares fit were consistent with those obtained using the 3-parameter fit described in the text.

condition as random and fixed factors, respectively. The effect of experimental condition was found to be significant, $F(2, 6) = 12.9$, $p < 0.01$. Scheffé comparisons indicated that the thresholds obtained in the 0-dB and the 40-dB conditions differed significantly, $F(1, 3) = 11.0$, $p < 0.05$, and that the thresholds in the 0-dB condition and the 0-dB trials presented in the context of level variation were significantly different, $F(1, 3) = 26.8$, $p < 0.05$. The difference between the thresholds obtained for the 40-dB condition and the 0-dB trials presented in the context of level variation was not significant [$F(1, 3) = 0.73$].

Although the effect was small (see Figure 2), thresholds measured for 0-dB trials that were presented in the presence of level variation were larger than thresholds obtained in the absence of level variation. Stimuli for those two conditions were selected from the same set, and so the effect of level variation reflects an effect of context.

Two possible models of the data seem appropriate. First, the obtained context effect might reflect a change in the decision strategy employed by the listener. For this model, an energy-based strategy might be employed in the absence of level variation, and the increased threshold obtained in the presence of level variation would reflect a change from an energy-based strategy to some other, non-energy-based strategy.

Alternatively, a single non-energy-based comparison may be responsible for detection both in the presence and in the absence of level variation. For such a model, the slight reduction in detectability with level variation would reflect what is often called a "range effect" (for example, Parducci, 1965), and the reduction in performance might be attributed to a change in internal noise (cf. Durlach & Braida, 1969). Ways in which the internal noise might be increased include uncertainty as to the optimal location of the decision criterion, an increase in the "neural jitter", or an increase in the variability of a number of processes that contribute to the detection judgement. In this setting, the effect of context observed in Experiment 2 would be due to a net change in internal noise, not a change in the decision-making process.

EXPERIMENT 3

Comparing Fixed-level, Roving-Standard and Random-level Conditions[3]

In the previous experiments, the reliability of energy-based cues and the presence of level variation covaried. In Experiment 3, level variation was not necessarily associated with a reduction in the reliability of energy-based cues.

[3] The conditions completed in Experiment 3 and the resulting analyses were suggested by Dr Jacob Nachmias. We gratefully acknowledge his suggestions.

Three experimental conditions were completed, each with an increased amount of uncertainty concerning the energy level of the stimuli. In one condition, the random-level condition, the energy level of each stimulus was randomly chosen from a 40-dB range on an interval-by-interval basis (40-dB condition above). In the second, roving-standard condition, the levels of the stimuli were varied across trials, but not across the intervals within a trial. In the third, fixed-level condition no level variation was present (0-dB condition above). Comparing the fixed-level and the roving-standard conditions allows an assessment of the effects of level variation between two conditions for which an across-interval comparison of energy remains an effective detection scheme.

The simulations presented in Figure 1 compare the predictions of the energy model with the human data, and it is clear that the listeners' decision "signal present" is not based solely on the difference in energy associated with the addition of the signal. Although it was obvious to all observers that overall loudness did not correlate with the presence of the tonal signal, we wished to determine whether the listeners' responses were at all dependent on the relative intensity of the stimuli. Here, the listeners' responses were partitioned in order to determine whether, in the random-level condition, the listeners' detection decision depended on the energy values associated with the stimuli presented in the two intervals.

In examining the observers' responses conditional on stimulus level, we may determine whether the observers' decisions are based, even in part, on changes in energy. If energy-based cues are employed, there would be a tendency to respond "signal present" for the interval with the most intense stimulus. In order to examine that possibility, the observers' response bias was measured. For all trials for which the spectrum level of two maskers differed by more than 5 dB, the proportion of the times that the listener responded "signal present" to the interval with the more intense stimulus was determined. The 5-dB window was necessary in order to ensure that the addition of the tone did not yield a "tone-plus-noise" stimulus with a larger (smaller) energy value even though the noise spectrum level was smaller (larger).

A second prediction for an energy-based decision is that when the tone-plus-noise stimulus is more intense than the noise-alone stimulus, thresholds should be superior to those obtained when the tone-plus-noise stimulus is less intense than the noise-alone stimulus. In order to determine whether the observers exhibited such a pattern of thresholds, the observers' responses were partitioned according to the following three stimulus conditions: (1) the tone-plus-noise stimulus was more intense than the noise-alone stimulus; (2) the noise-alone and the tone-plus-noise stimuli were within 20 dB of one another; and (3) the tone-plus-noise stimulus was less intense than the noise-alone stimulus. Should the listeners incorporate energy-related changes into their responses, then these three conditions would respectively yield increasingly poor detection thresholds.

Methods

The experimental methods were similar to those described in Experiment 2. For most conditions, psychometric functions were derived using signal energy *re* spectrum level ratios (E/N_0) ranging uniformly from 3 to 15 dB, in 3-dB steps. Occasionally, measurements at 0 or 18 dB were required due to individual differences in sensitivity. The signal level was fixed within 50-trial blocks. Each of the five levels was completed in random order. Then a new order was chosen, and the set of blocks was repeated. For each of the conditions tested, five repetitions were completed, yielding a total of 250 judgements at each signal level, and typically yielding 1250 decisions per psychometric function.

When the random-level condition was employed, the observers' responses were analysed in order to determine the proportion of all trials for which the observer responded "signal present" to the interval with the more intense stimulus. As described above, only those stimuli with spectrum level differences of at least 5 dB were included in the measurement of bias. Additionally, a total of four psychometric functions were derived from the random-level trials; one based on all of the data, one based only on those trials for which the tone-plus-noise interval had an attenuation value 20 dB greater than the noise-alone interval, one based on those trials for which the tone-plus-noise and the noise-alone interval had attenuation values that differed by less than 20 dB, and one based on those trials for which the noise-alone interval had attenuation values 20 dB greater than the tone-plus-noise interval. The psychometric functions based on trials with intensity differences in excess of 20 dB were formed using an average of 160 judgements, and the psychometric functions based on trials with intensity differences less than 20 dB were formed using an average of 940 judgements.

Three normal-hearing listeners ranging in age from 19 to 33 years participated in the experiment. One of the listeners had participated in Experiment 2 (Observer 2) and completed this experiment after completing Experiment 2. The two remaining observers were highly trained in tone-in-noise experiments. Two observers (2 and 5) achieved stable levels of performance with only 4 hours of practice; the third (Observer 6) required 10 hours before stable performance levels were obtained. Each observer completed the three conditions in random order, with the provision that no two observers completed the three conditions in the same order. Each participant completed at least 250 practice trials before data were collected in a new condition.

Results and Discussion

Table 2 presents the estimated detection thresholds (76 percent correct) for the fixed-level, roving-standard, and random-level conditions. As described above, percent correct scores were fitted to a psychometric function using a cumulative Weibull distribution and three free parameters. Of the functions fitted to the data, the poorest fit accounted for over 80% of the variance present in the data. All other fits accounted for over 90% of the variance present in the data. In order to estimate the variability of the estimated thresholds, each replicate psychometric function was fitted, and the standard error of the mean across the threshold estimates was computed. The resulting standard errors of the mean are indicated in parentheses.

In this experiment, the average difference in threshold between the random- and fixed-level conditions was 3.9 dB. Although the effect of level variation was small, it was larger than the 1.9-dB difference obtained in Experiment 1 and the 1.8-dB difference obtained in Experiment 2. Part of that difference was due to the extreme sensitivity demonstrated by Observer 5 in the fixed-level condition. The other two listeners' data are more consistent with values obtained in Experiments 1 and 2.

Table 2 shows that detection thresholds increase as level uncertainty increases. An analysis of variance that treated the replicates as a random factor and the observers and experimental factors as fixed, indicated that the effect of level uncertainty was significant, $F(2, 8) = 21.7$, $p < 0.005$. The difference between the fixed-level and the roving-standard conditions was significant, $F(1, 4) = 34.4$, $p < 0.01$, as was the difference between the roving-standard and the random-level, $F(1, 4) = 15.1$, $p < 0.02$.[4]

TABLE 2
Estimated Thresholds, E/N_0 in dB, for the Fixed-Level, the Roving-Standard, and the Random-Level Conditions

Obs.	*Fixed level*	*Roving standard*	*Random level*
2	7.5 (0.4)	9.3 (0.6)	9.7 (0.7)
5	3.9 (0.5)	7.7 (0.5)	9.6 (0.4)
6	7.2 (0.3)	8.0 (0.4)	11.0 (0.8)

Note: The standard errors of the mean for the estimated thresholds are indicated in parentheses.

[4] It should be noted that in treating the observers as a fixed factor we accept that standard psychophysical procedures are tests of individual highly trained observers. The between-subject differences were significant, but our interest was whether the data were lawful for each observer. In Experiment 2, the number of trials in each condition was restricted, and so replications were not available for analysis.

As detection thresholds obtained in the roving-standard condition are poorer than those obtained in the fixed-level condition, it is reasonable to conclude that the presence of level variation, in and of itself, leads to decreased sensitivity. Thus, these data are consistent with the hypothesis that introducing level variation acts to increase internal noise. It seems unlikely that the reduced detection thresholds obtained in the roving-level condition are due to changes in sensitivity at the extremes of the range of stimulus levels. In that regard, the data in the literature generally support the energy model's prediction that E/N_0 is constant over a wide range of overall levels (Green & Swets, 1966; Moore, 1975). The observation that the thresholds obtained in the roving-standard condition and the random-level were reliably different suggests little: not only were energy-related cues rendered unreliable, but there was increased uncertainty concerning the level of the stimuli.

Table 3 presents the data obtained in the random-level condition partitioned in accordance with changes in stimulus level. The first three columns of Table 3 present thresholds for trials for which the difference in spectrum level between the tone-plus-noise and the noise-alone stimuli was (1) at least 20 dB, (2) was between +20 and −20 dB, and (3) at most −20 dB. The standard errors of the mean were estimated for each listener and each condition and are indicated in parentheses. The individual psychometric functions for (1) and (3) above were based on relatively few points, and on some occasions the resulting psychometric functions were sufficiently non-monotonic that meaningful threshold estimates could not be obtained. For those occasions, the standard errors of the mean presented in Table 3 are based on only four replicates and are indicated with an asterisk.

For only one of the observers, 6, is there a consistent effect of across-interval level difference. For Observer 6, when the signal is present in the more intense interval, thresholds are best. When the signal is present in the

TABLE 3

Estimated Thresholds, E/N_0 in dB, as a Function of the Difference in the Spectrum Level of the Tone-plus-Noise and the Noise-Alone Stimuli

Obs.	*D* > *20 dB*	− *20 dB* < *D* < *20 dB*	− *20 dB* < *D*	*Bias*
2	9.1 (0.7*)	9.7 (1.0)	9.3 (0.3*)	0.48
5	8.7 (0.9*)	9.4 (1.3)	8.8 (2.1)	0.47
6	6.1 (1.2)	10.5 (0.6)	14.8 (0.4)	0.57

Note: The difference, D, takes on values of: (a) $D > 20$ dB, (b) $-20\text{ dB} < D < 20$ dB, and (c) $D < -20$ dB. The final column indicates the proportion of times that the observer indicated that the signal was in interval with the largest energy value. The standard error of the mean for the estimated threshold is indicated in parentheses, and an asterisk (*) indicates that the standard error of the mean is based on four rather than five threshold estimates.

least intense interval, thresholds are poorest. Thus, it appears that Observer 6 incorporated energy-based cues even though level variation had rendered those cues inappropriate.

The final column of Table 3 indicates response bias, or the proportion of times that the observer chose the more intense interval as the one containing the signal. Treating each judgement as an independent Bernoulli trial, proportions in excess of 0.54 and less than 0.46 would exceed the 95% confidence interval surrounding random responses. Only Observer 6 exceeded those tertiary limits. Thus, Observer 6 exhibits both a response bias and a pattern of thresholds that suggest that he used a response strategy that included energy-based cues. In contrast, Observers 2 and 5 do not demonstrate a simple energy-related pattern of response.

In short, the results of Experiment 3 suggest two conclusions: (1) It is apparent that introducing level variation disrupts performance, even when energy-based cues are not degraded and (2) when energy-based cues are unreliable, at least one listener based his detection judgements on energy-related changes. For the other two listeners, we were unable to demonstrate any effect of an energy-based decision process.

GENERAL DISCUSSION

The first experiment expanded on observations presented in the past (Gilkey, 1987; Kidd et al., 1989). Neither increasing nor decreasing the variability of the energy present in the tone-plus-noise and the noise-alone difference distribution has a large effect on the detectability of a tone added to a narrow band of noise. In the presence of level variation, energy cues are not the determinant of detection. In the second experiment, we found that the context of level variation acts to increase detection thresholds for the equal-energy bands of noise. The third experiment demonstrated that (1) in the presence of level variation, even when energy-based cues were reliable, thresholds increased, and (2) when across-interval level variation was present, at least one listener responded as though his detection scheme relied in part on energy differences.

As a whole, the data presented here are consistent with two hypotheses: (1) The detection of a tone added to noise may rely on a single, non-energy-based decision stategy. For that model, the effect of level variation would amount to an increase in the internal noise associated with the decision processes. The observation that across-trial level variation led to poorer thresholds relative to those obtained in the absence of level variation supports this hypothesis. (2) Two or more cues may be combined in order to detect a tone added to noise. For such a model, we cannot reject the possibility that energy-based comparisons contribute to detection when level variation is absent. If several cues are combined, then the introduction of an across-interval level variation would render energy-based cues unreliable, and so the observer would alter his/her decision strategy in order to restrict reliance on energy-based cues. The resulting change in threshold would depend on the weight of the energy-based cue relative to the weight of other cues (cf. Green & Swets, 1966; Richards, 1986) and on whether all cues are combined optimally. We note that Observer 6 provides an example of someone who appears to have adopted such a combination strategy but failed to act optimally in the sense that he incorporated energy-based cues even when energy-based cues were unrelated to the presence of the tonal signal.

When comparing these alternative models, it should be noted that in adopting a model that posits a change in the way that different cues are combined, the possibility that level variation increases internal noise remains valid. Indeed, for an optimal combination of information, increases in internal noise necessarily produce changes in the weighting of the contributing cues.

As was indicated in the introduction, it is becoming evident that non-energy-related properties of the stimuli contribute to the detectability of a tone added to noise, and in all probability such cues contributed to the detection strategies employed by our observers. For example, the phenomenological reports of our observers and reports described by Kidd et al. (1989) suggest that observers make their decision based on the "loudness", "clarity", "roughness", and "goodness" of the sounds. If changes in the dynamic properties of the envelope and the fine-structure of the stimuli contribute to detection, then phenomenal changes in the "roughness" or "clarity" of the sounds would be a reasonable consequence.

REFERENCES

Ahumada, A. Jr. & Lovell, J. (1971). Stimulus features in signal detection. *Journal of the Acoustical Society of America*, *49*, 1751–1756.

Ahumada, A. Jr., Marken, R., & Sandusky, R. (1975). Time and frequency analyses of auditory signal detection. *Journal of the Acoustical Society of America*, *57*, 385–390.

Durlach, N.I. & Braida, L.D. (1969). Intensity perception I. Preliminary theory of intensity resolution. *Journal of the Acoustical Society of America*, *46*, 372–383.

Fletcher, H. (1940). Auditory patterns. *Review of Modern Physics*, *12*, 47–65.

Gilkey, R.H. (1987). Spectral and temporal comparisons in auditory masking. In W.A. Yost & C.S. Watson (Eds.), *Auditory processing of complex sounds*. Hillsdale, NJ: Lawrence Erlbaum Associates, Inc.

Green, D.M. (1964). Consistency of auditory detection judgements. *Psychological Review*, *71*, 392–407.

Green, D.M. & Swets, J.A. (1966). *Signal Detection Theory and Psychophysics*, New York: Robert E. Krieger Publishing.

Hartmann, W.M. & Pumplin, J. (1988). Noise power fluctuations and the making of sine signals. *Journal of the Acoustical Society of America*, *83*, 2277–2289.

Jeffress, L.R. (1964). A stimulus-oriented approach to detection. *Journal of the Acoustical Society of America, 36*, 766–774.

Kidd, G., Mason, C.R., Brantley, M.A., & Owen, G.A. (1989). Roving-level tone-in-noise detection. *Journal of the Acoustical Society of America, 86*, 1310–1317.

Levitt, H. (1971). Transformed up-down methods in psychoacoustics. *Journal of the Acoustical Society of America, 49*, 467–477.

Moore, B.C.J. (1975). Mechanisms of masking. *Journal of the Acoustical Society of America, 57*, 391–399.

Moore, B.C.J. (1988). Dynamic aspects of auditory masking. In G.M. Edelman, W.E.Gall, W.M. Cowan (Eds.), *Auditory function: Neurological bases of hearing*. New York: John Wiley.

Nachmias, J. (1981). On the psychometric function for contrast detection. *Vision Research, 21*, 215–223.

Parducci, A. (1965). Categorical judgement: A range frequency model. *Psychological Review, 72*, 407–418.

Pfafflin, S.M. & Mathews, M.V. (1966). Detection of auditory signals in reproducible noise. *Journal of the Acoustical Society of America, 39*, 340–345.

Rice, S.O. (1954). Mathematical analysis of random noise. In N. Wax (Ed.), *Selected Papers on Noise and Stochastic Processes*. New York: Dover Publications.

Richards, V.M. (1986). *The effect of bandwidth on frequency discrimination*. Unpublished doctoral dissertation, University of California, Berkeley.

Richards, V.M. (1987). Monaural envelope correlation perception. *Journal of the Acoustical Society of America, 82*, 1621–1630.

Schafer, T.H., Gales, R.S., Shewmaker, C.A., & Thompson, P.O. (1950). The frequency selectivity of the ear as determined by masking experiments. *Journal of the Acoustical Society of America, 19*, 609–619.

Schooneveldt, G.P. & Moore, B.C.J. (1989). Comodulation masking release (CMR) as a function of masker bandwidth, modulation bandwidth, and signal duration. *Journal of the Acoustical Society of America, 85*, 273–281.

Spiegel, M.F. & Green, D.M. (1982). Signal and masker uncertainty with noise maskers of varying duration, bandwidth, and center frequency. *Journal of the Acoustical Society of America, 71*, 1204–1210.

Swets, J.A., Green, D.M., & Tanner, W.P. (1962). On the width of critical bands. *Journal of the Acoustical Society of America, 34*, 108–113.

Watson, A.B. (1979). Probability summation over time. *Vision Research, 19*, 512–522.

Revised manuscript received 19 October 1990

THE QUARTERLY JOURNAL OF EXPERIMENTAL PSYCHOLOGY, 1991, *43A* (3) 503–516

Lateralization of Very-short-duration Tone Pulses of Low and High Frequencies

Trevor M. Shackleton and John M. Bowsher
University of Surrey, Guildford, Surrey, U.K.

Ray Meddis
University of Technology, Loughborough, Leicestershire, U.K.

The position and image-width of the simultaneous images produced by very short tone pulses were measured as a function of interaural time difference (ITD) at both low- (250 and 800 Hz) and high- (2500 and 8000 Hz) frequencies using a direct-estimation technique.

Primary images are lateralized towards the ear receiving the leading stimulus. At low frequencies image position is proportional to interaural phase-difference (IPD) below 90° and remains at the lead-ear for larger values. At high frequencies image position is proportional to ITD up to 500–1000 µsec. Secondary images are reported on the opposite side of the head for IPDs greater than 180° at low frequencies, and at ITDs greater than 500 µsec at high frequencies. Image width is approximately constant for all ITDs and both images at a given frequency, but becomes more compact as frequency increases.

The data are discussed in terms of onset cues and stimulus fine-structure cues. The best explanation is in terms of an onset mechanism, but one that is calibrated in terms of IPD at low frequencies. The existence of double images is explained in terms of a breakdown in the mechanism determining fusion.

Lateralization is the name given to the perception of a sound-image inside the head when a binaural stimulus is presented over headphones. This perception arises from an analysis of the differences between the waveforms

---

Requests for reprints should be sent to Trevor M. Shackleton, Speech and Hearing Laboratory, Department of Human Sciences, University of Technology, Loughborough, Leicestershire, LE11 3TU, U.K.

This research was supported by an SERC CASE studentship awarded to Trevor Shackleton at the University of Surrey. The authors wish to thank the University of Technology, Loughborough, for making the facilities available for writing up this experiment, and the two anonymous reviewers for their helpful comments.

presented to each ear. These differences are of two forms: (1) interaural level differences (ILDs), and (2) interaural time differences (ITDs). In this paper we shall be exclusively concerned with the role of ITDs.

In a natural environment, ITDs arise because the sound from a source away from the medial-saggital plane arrives at one ear before the other. This results in an ITD that is a function of azimuth and is almost constant as a function of stimulus frequency (Kuhn, 1977). We might reasonably expect that the lateralization of a stimulus will increase with ITD, and that for a constant ITD it will be almost independent of stimulus frequency. The validity of these expectations will be discussed in the following paragraphs.

An alternative method of expressing ITDs is as interaural phase differences (IPDs). The IPD is proportional to the ITD multiplied by the frequency. We have argued that naturally occurring objects in the same position produce similar ITDs. So we would expect stimuli of the same IPD but different frequencies (and hence different ITDs) to be perceived in different positions. However, experiments using pure tones have shown that the extent of lateralization for a constant IPD is almost constant across frequency (Yost, 1981; Sayers, 1964). In addition, the just-noticeable difference (jnd) for ITD using pure-tone stimuli is almost constant when expressed in terms of IPD for frequencies below 800 Hz (Bloom & Jones, 1978; Klump & Eady, 1956; Zwislocki & Feldman, 1956; Yost, 1974, 1976).

These results appear to suggest that IPD is the determinant of the extent of lateralization. This raises problems for the lateralization of interaurally delayed broad-band stimuli. All the frequency components of an interaurally delayed stimulus have the same ITD, and therefore different IPDs. If IPD is the determinant of lateral position, then the lateralization of broad-band stimuli ought to broaden as bandwidth increases, and perhaps become ambiguous. In fact, clicks (which are very broad-band stimuli) have a compact image, which is easily lateralized (e.g. Babkoff & Sutton, 1966; Guttman, 1962; Sayers & Toole, 1964; Teas, 1962; Toole & Sayers, 1965).

The paradoxical results for narrow-band and broad-band stimuli represent a fundamental challenge for theories of lateralization. The most fully worked-out theories involve the cross-correlation of the critical-band filtered waveforms from each ear (e.g. Blauert & Cobben, 1978; Jeffress, 1948; Lindemann, 1986a, 1986b; Stern & Colburn, 1978; Stern, Zeiberg & Trahiotis, 1988). These are explicitly ITD-based models, which predict different positions for pure tones with the same IPD as their frequency is altered.

We therefore have the problem of how to resolve the paradox of the results of experiments using pure tones and clicks. We notice that clicks and pure tones are extreme stimuli. Clicks are of very short duration, are broad-band, and have rapid onsets and offsets. Pure tones, on the other hand, are of relatively long duration, are very narrow-band, and generally have slow onsets and offsets (to ensure that energy is not spread into adjacent frequency bands). It is therefore very possible that clicks and pure tones engage different aspects of the lateralization mechanism and may even reveal two separate mechanisms, which are usually complementary. Therefore it is desirable to examine the lateralization of stimuli that have a different mix of properties from either pure tones or clicks. We have chosen to use very-short-tone pulses which are formed from narrow-bandpass-filtered clicks. These stimuli are narrow-band, are short, and have rapid onsets and offsets. They therefore have a mix of the properties of pure tones and clicks, which should help to elucidate the lateralization mechanism(s).

In this experiment we also seek to answer three further questions. The first of these is, "are there any similarities between ITD processing at low and high frequencies?" It has been known since the days of Rayleigh (1907) that it is not possible to lateralize high-frequency pure tones. However, it is possible to discriminate between amplitude-modulated high-frequency stimuli based on differences in the ITD of the envelope of a low-frequency modulator (e.g. Henning 1974a, 1974b, 1980a, 1980b). In this experiment we address the problem of whether a single cycle of amplitude modulation is enough to allow lateralization. The band-pass stimuli we use can be regarded as a single cycle of modulation and are similar in structure at both high- and low-frequency stimuli.

The second question is, "do multiple images arise simultaneously?" Some studies have already indicated that for a given ITD two images can arise in completely different positions (Sayers, 1964; Yost, 1981; Hafter & Jeffress, 1968; Babkoff & Sutton, 1966; Guttman, 1962; Teas, 1962). However, many lateralization experiments only allow the subjects to report a single image position. This may produce anomalous results, as subjects could be inconsistent about which images they use, or average across images. In this experiment we allow and encourage subjects to report the positions of multiple simultaneous images.

The third question is, "does image width vary with frequency, ITD, or image number?" Very few experiments have sought information about image width in a systematic manner. The discussion above has illustrated the theoretical importance of image width, so it is vital that methods are developed for reporting image width in addition to image position.

Method

In this experiment we ask subjects to report the perceived lateral position and image widths for all the images perceived as the stimulus ITD and frequency were varied. The stimuli consist of tone pulses derived by band-pass filtering clicks at one of four centre frequencies. The position estimation procedure is based upon the methods of Yost (1981) and Sayers (1964).

Stimuli. The tone pulses were generated by passing a 60-μsec duration click through one of a set of narrow-bandpass filters with centre frequencies of 250, 800, 2500, and 8000 Hz. The bandwidths of the filters were chosen to be just narrower than the critical bandwidth (e.g. Zwicker, Flottorp & Stevens, 1957). The bandwidth was 75 Hz at a centre-frequency of 250 Hz, and 10% of the centre-frequency for the other frequencies.

Unfortunately these stimuli confound the parameters of frequency, duration, and onset rate; however, the authors believe that this is unimportant in this experiment. The intention was not to examine the interplay of the above parameters, but to present stimuli that represent a compromise between pure tones and impulses. This compromise has two aspects: (1) All stimuli are contained within a single critical band, and so are like pure tones in terms of their spread of excitation following peripheral filtering. (2) They are of the shortest duration consonant with their bandwidth, and so are like impulses temporally.

The signal levels were set at a sensation level of 50–60 dB SL. Levels were maintained to within 0.5 dB over the period of the experiment by measuring the output of each earphone with a microphone placed touching the grille over the earphone diaphragm. This method was found both to be very quick and the most precise of several tried.

Procedure. A lateralization-pointing technique similar to one developed by Yost (1981) was used. A reference stimulus of 0 ITD corresponding to the mid-point of the visual scale was presented three times. Following a gap of 1 sec, the test stimulus was then repeated four times. The gap between stimuli was 0.5 sec.

The subjects were then required to indicate the position of the sound by placing a pointer somewhere along a line of length approximating to the head width on a computer screen upon which were marked the positions of the ears and the centre of the head. Subjects could take as long as they wished over this and signalled that they had reached a decision by pressing a push switch. Subjects were then requested to indicate the perceived width of the stimulus on a scale varying from "very compact" to "filled head".

Following this, the subjects were asked whether they had heard other sound images in different positions. If they had, the whole response sequence was repeated until they reported no other images. The sounds were not repeated. Once the subject was satisfied that all the image positions had been reported, the next stimulus sequence was started.

Apparatus. A single microcomputer, the Acorn BBC B (based upon a 2-MHz 6502 8-bit processor), was used to control this experiment and collect subject responses. The computer generated a logic pulse of varying duration (1 μsec to 65,000 μsec), corresponding to the ITD required. This pulse was fed through a computer-controlled invert/non-invert switch. The rising edge of the pulse was used to trigger a monostable multivibrator in the left channel of the apparatus to produce a 60-μsec-long click. Similarly, the trailing edge of the pulse was used to produce a click in the right channel of the apparatus. Thus clicks separated by an ITD accurate to 1 μsec could be produced, with either the click in the left or right channel leading. These impulses were then amplified and fed in parallel through a carefully matched pair of filter banks comprising four bandpass filters each (at 250, 800, 2500, and 8000 Hz centre frequencies). In each channel the filter output required was selected using computer-controlled switches and attenuated by Marconi TF2162 manual attenuators (so the level could be set correctly). The outputs of the attenuators were then amplified and presented to the subject through Beyer DT48 headphones with circumaural cushions. Apart from the named equipment, all the electronics were designed and constructed by the first author. Subject responses were collected using an Acorn joystick connected to the computer analogue input.

Subjects. Five male undergraduates (aged 20–22) took part in the experiment. They were unpaid and received no prior training, except for a familiarization exercise at the beginning of the first experimental session. None of the subjects had previously taken part in any psychophysical experiment. None reported any hearing problems. They all reported that they found the lateralization task easy. The method chosen thus appears to impose few difficulties upon the subject in reporting their perceptions.

Design. All subjects participated in two sessions, which were separated by less than a week. The sessions lasted between 40 min and 1 h, depending upon the response rate of the subject. The sessions were split into four blocks, with a rest of at least 1 min between each block. The four different frequencies were split between the four blocks in a session, with only a single frequency presented per block. The order of frequencies in the session was decided for each subject and session by using a fresh selection from a table of random permutations (of fourth order). In every block all of the 13 ITDs were repeated three times each (non-consecutively), in a randomized order.

A practice session designed to familiarize the subjects with the response procedure preceded the first data collection session. In this session, which lasted about a quarter of an hour, every ITD at each frequency was presented once. In other words, all 52 conditions were presented covering the entire range of lateralizations.

Results

Subjects were encouraged to report as many, or as few, images as they wanted. In fact they all reported either one or two images. The proportion of reports of double images summed across all subjects as a function of ITD is shown in Figure 1. There were very few double images at 250 and 800 Hz when the IPD was less than 180°; however, almost all subjects reported double images when the IPD was greater than this. Almost all subjects reported double images at the extreme ITDs for frequencies of 2500 and 8000 Hz. Most of the double images reported at 2500 and 8000 Hz for ITDs less than 750 μsec were reported by a single subject.

The reported image width was not found to vary greatly with either ITD or image number; however, as frequency was increased, the sounds tended to be more compact (Table 1).

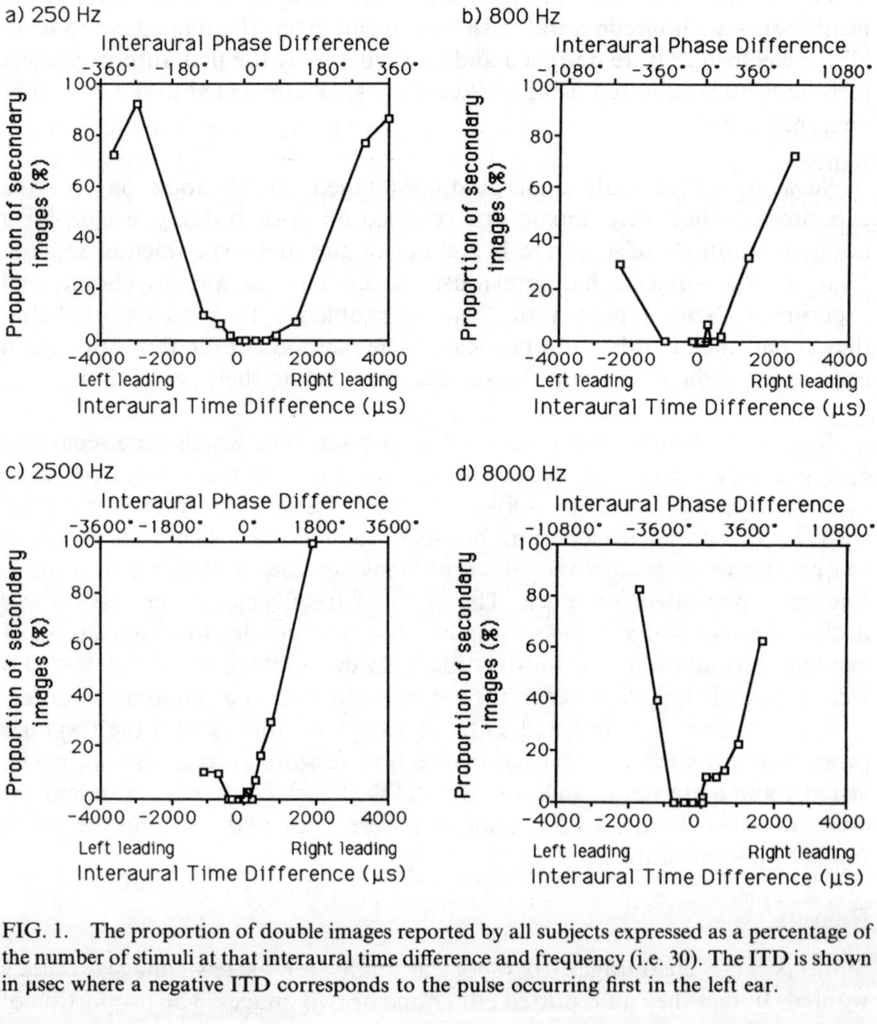

FIG. 1. The proportion of double images reported by all subjects expressed as a percentage of the number of stimuli at that interaural time difference and frequency (i.e. 30). The ITD is shown in μsec where a negative ITD corresponds to the pulse occurring first in the left ear.

TABLE 1
Mean Width of Auditory Images Averaged Across All ITDs for Primary and Secondary Images

	Primary Image		*Secondary Image*	
Frequency (Hz)	*Width*	*S.E.*	*Width*	*S.E.*
250	53.7	1.1	48.4	3.5
800	49.6	0.7	49.1	2.5
2500	39.0	0.6	26.5	3.8
8000	25.0	0.8	21.6	1.9

Note: A width of 100 corresponds to subjects' judgement of "filled head". A width of 0 corresponds to subjects' judgement of "very compact". The standard error of the estimates of mean width are shown in columns three and five.

The lateralization reports averaged across all five subjects are shown in Figure 2. All subjects exhibited very similar patterns and magnitudes of lateralization responses, so it was felt that no information would be lost, and presentational difficulties minimized, by presenting the mean of all subjects' responses. There were few outliers in the response data, which were also symmetrical, so the mean and median give very similar results.

At 250 and 800 Hz the lateralization function for the primary image follows the pattern expected from earlier work (e.g. Yost, 1981; Sayers, 1964), up to a 180° phase shift. Although the slopes of the 250 and 800 Hz functions around 0 ITD are very different when expressed in terms of ITD, they are more similar when expressed in terms of IPD (Table 2). Above an IPD of 180°, the primary images are lateralized near the leading ear (rather

TABLE 2
Slope of the Straight Portion of the Lateralization Function for Each Frequency Calculated by Linear Regression

Frequency (Hz)	*Slope (%/μsec)*	*S.E. (%/μsec)*	*Slope (%/deg)*	*S.E. (%/deg)*	*Range (μsec)*
250	0.086	0.005	0.953	0.056	± 1000
800	0.211	0.006	0.732	0.019	± 300
2500	0.138	0.003	0.154	0.003	± 400
8000	0.096	0.008	0.033	0.003	± 600

Note: The slopes are given as a percentage of the headwidth (± 100% is the position of the ears as marked on the judgement scale), divided by either the interaural time difference (%/μsec) or the interaural phase difference (%/deg). The standard errors of the estimated slopes are given in the third and fifth columns. The range of ITD over which the calculation was performed is shown in the final column; in all cases this constitutes three points on either side of zero ITD.

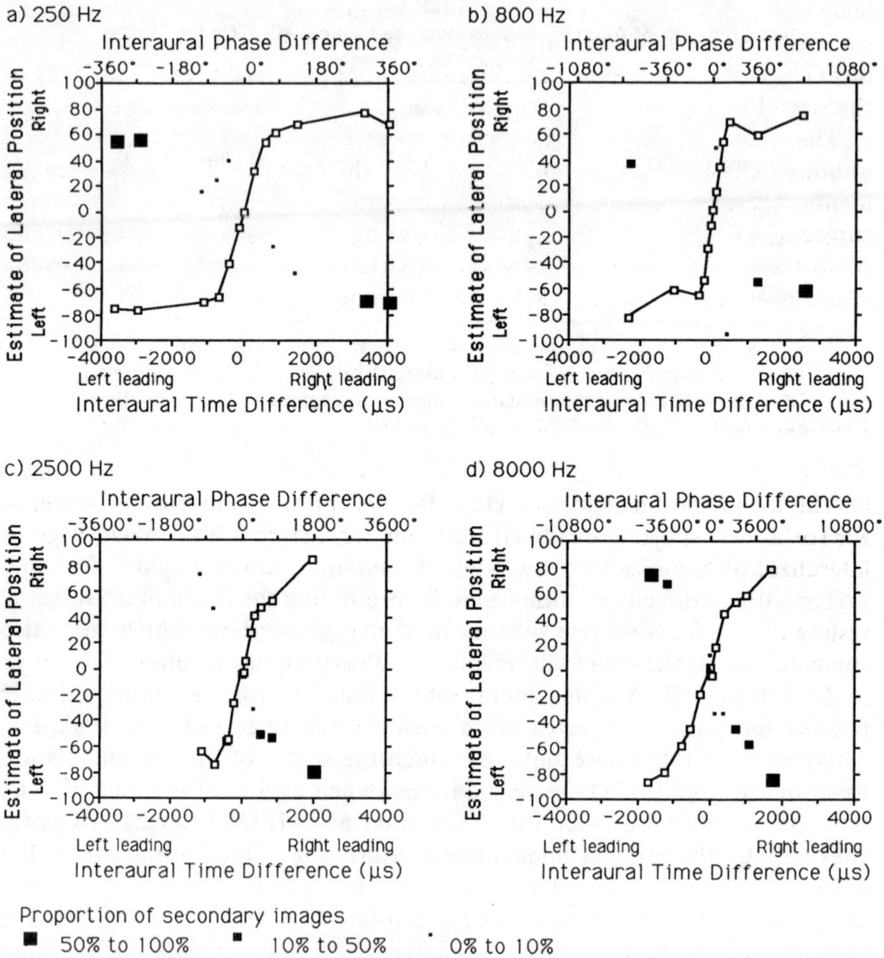

FIG. 2. The mean lateral position of primary and secondary images. Primary images were reported on 100% of occasions and are shown by open symbols joined by lines. Secondary images were only reported on some trials and are shown by filled symbols; the size of the symbol represents the proportion of secondary images reported as a percentage of the total number of stimuli at that interaural time difference and frequency (i.e. 30). The subjective lateral position is indicated on a scale of ± 100, where − 100 corresponds to the position on the screen of the left ear and + 100 to that of the right. The ITD is shown in μsec where a negative ITD corresponds to the pulse occurring first in the left ear.

than following the cyclic pattern reported by Sayer, 1964). There are very few secondary images below 180°, but above 180° they appear on the opposite side of the head to the primary images (i.e. the lagging side) and are closer to the centre for smaller ITDs.

Interestingly, the primary images at the higher frequencies of 2500 and

8000 Hz also exhibit a sigmoidal curve. Around 0 ITD these functions have similar slopes as each other and the 250-Hz function when expressed in terms of ITD (Table 2). Lateralization does not appear to be linked to the IPD of the stimulus.

The first author also took part in these experiments as a subject, and although his results are not included in this paper, they were virtually identical. This is important, as the author was more highly trained than the subjects (having served as a listener during numerous pilot studies) and performed more repeats during the experiment. In other words, learning effects appear to be negligible in this experiment.

DISCUSSION

Primary Images at 250 Hz and 800 Hz

The results at the lower two frequencies show that for these stimuli lateralization is a function of IPD; that is, up to $\pm 180°$ lateralization is approximately proportional to IPD, but for larger IPDs the image is lateralized at the leading ear.

The "phase-calibration"-like nature of our results is consistent with the results of several others, who found that the jnd for IPD is approximately constant for frequencies below 800 Hz (Bloom & Jones, 1978; Klump & Eady, 1956; Zwislocki & Feldman, 1956; Yost, 1974, 1976). However, these jnd measurements only tell us about the accuracy of lateralization, which is determined by both the slope of the lateralization function and the intrinsic noise in the lateralization mechanism. As increasing the number of chances of observing a lateralization cue will decrease the effective noise, careful consideration of the confounding effects of frequency, duration, and number of cycles is necessary in these experiments. Furthermore, these experiments only provide information about lateralization near the midline. The results presented in this paper thus complement the jnd measurements, providing information about lateralization function slope over a wide range of IPDs and removing the need to worry about the confounding effects.

In addition, these results demonstrate that phase calibration occurs with very short stimuli that have rapid rise-times (within the constraint of their spectrum being contained within a critical band). It appears that irrespective of the duration or rise-time of the signal, phase calibration occurs if the stimulus is sufficiently narrow-band. Comparing our results with those of Sayers (1964) and Yost (1981) shows that duration does not greatly affect the slope of the lateralization function up to 180°.

The factor that does appear to be influenced by duration and rise-time is whether the lateralization function cycles around for IPDs greater than 180°. Using longer stimuli and longer rise-times, Sayers (1964) found that lateralization switched from the lead ear to the lagging ear when the IPD exceeded

180° and got closer to the centre as IPD was increased towards 360°. The function repeated for multiples of 360°. We find, using short stimuli with rapid rise-times, that lateralization remains at the lead ear for IPDs greater than 180°. The difference could be due to either rise-time or duration. Abel and Kunov (1983) and Kunov and Abel(1981) found that rapid rise-times led to pure tones being lateralized at the lead ear for all IPDs and that durations between 25 and 200 μsec gave similar results. This suggests that it is rise-time that is the determinant of the shape of the lateralization function for IPDs greater than 180°. However, duration does have some effect upon lateralization, as is demonstrated by the experiment of Tobias and Schubert (1959). They used a broad-band noise signal and could vary the ITD of the envelope and the fine structure of the noise separately. They looked for the combinations of envelope and fine-structure ITDs that combined to give a centred image. They found that the envelope ITD was more salient for shorter stimuli.

Two mechanisms are suggested by these data. The first mechanism, called the ongoing mechanism, uses the ongoing, fine structural difference between the waveforms at each ear to determine the lateral position of the stimulus. An example of such a process is the use of the time-difference between a peak in the waveform at one ear and the next peak at the other, to indicate lateral position. A related example is the popular cross-correlation model (e.g. Blauert & Cobben, 1978; Jeffress, 1948; Lindemann, 1986a, 1986b; Stern & Colburn, 1978; Stern et al., 1988). Such a model would predict that the lateral position of a periodic stimulus should cycle around as the ITD is increased and that maximum lateralization should occur at odd multiples of 180°.

The second mechanism, called the onset mechanism, only uses the time difference between the onsets of the waveforms at each ear to determine lateral position or, equivalently, temporal differences in the envelope of the waveform. This mechanism would predict that the position of tone pulses should remain at the lead ear for values of ITD greater than 1/2 period of the fine-structure of the waveform.

We can see that both an onset and ongoing mechanism are necessary from Tobias and Schubert's (1959) data, and that the onset mechanism dominates in stimuli with short rise-times and short duration. Tobias and Schubert (1959) provide no data about how the onset mechanism is calibrated, as they use broad-band stimuli; our results suggest that it is calibrated in terms of IPD, like the ongoing mechanism.

Primary Images at 2500 Hz and 8000 Hz

The fact that lateralization is possible at high frequencies using our stimuli is perhaps not surprising given the jnds can be found and time-intensity-trades carried out for high-pass filtered clicks (e.g. David, Guttman, & van Bergeijk,

1959), and that jnds have been found for amplitude-modulated high-frequency carriers (e.g. Henning 1974a, 1974b, 1980a, 1980b). However, we have demonstrated that lateralization at high frequencies is still possible using a single cycle of modulation and band-limited stimuli. In other words, the only reason that high-frequency pure tones cannot be lateralized is because they have no resolved structure, the fine structure having been removed by the decline in phase locking of the auditory nerve (e.g. Rose, Brugge, Anderson, & Hind, 1967).

Secondary Images

Perhaps the most interesting result in this experiment is the form of the secondary images. Double images are most numerous at extreme ITDs, being reported on approaching 100% of all trials at the largest ITDs. It is difficult to see how secondary images could arise from an onset mechanism. An ongoing mechanism would produce ambiguous information regarding sidedness at odd multiples of 180°, possibly leading to multiple images (cf. Sayers, 1964, Figure 2). However, secondary images are produced at IPDs other than 180°, so the ongoing mechanism does not appear to explain their generation either.

Secondary images might appear because there is more than one lateralization mechanism. Such mechanisms would normally act cooperatively to produce a single image, but with abnormal stimuli the concurrence between the mechanisms may break down. We have already suggested that primary images occur through onset-cue processing. Can secondary images occur due to ongoing-cue processing? This seems unlikely for high-frequency stimuli, because, as discussed above, there is little fine-structure information available in the high-frequency stimuli. It also seems unlikely for low-frequency stimuli, because the secondary images do not follow the appropriate pattern. The ongoing model predicts that at 250 Hz there will be a central image for an ITD of 4000 μsec (360°); plus one half-way to the left at 3289 μsec (−60°); and others half-way, and most of the way to the right at −3667 and −3000 μsec, respectively (30° and 90°). At 800 Hz the secondary images ought to be in the centre for ITDs of 1250 and 2500 μsec (360° and 720°) and half-way to the right at −2345 and −1100 μsec (both 45°). The observed secondary images do not follow this trend. We therefore must reject the possibility that secondary images are produced by an ongoing mechanism.

We are therefore forced to fall back on the argument that the binaural mechanism is failing to fuse the stimuli at each ear into a single image. In other words, the binaural mechanism receives cues that are too extreme to allow it to reconcile them with a single acoustical event. This breakdown in fusion would appear to suggest that each component of double images should be extremely lateralized. Figure 2 shows that this is not the case.

Primary and secondary image positions appear to mirror one another. We would suggest that although the fusion mechanism has broken down, this does not mean that the waveforms from each ear do not influence one another.

In summary, it seems likely that the pattern of secondary images is best discussed in terms of a breakdown of the fusion process, coupled with an interference of the waveforms at each ear with each other, resulting in both images being pulled towards the centre.

CONCLUSIONS

Low-frequency transients have ITD lateralization functions that are very similar in slope when plotted in terms of IPD. However, the image does not cycle round like the image of long, low frequency tones, but remains lateralized at the lead ear. A secondary image does not normally appear until ITDs exceed 180°. These secondary images do not follow a pattern dictated by IPD; they tend to indicate that the binaural mechanism can no longer fuse the stimulus.

The results confirm and extend our knowledge of the processing of low-frequency tones. Like low-frequency tones with slow onsets, the lateralization response appears to be dictated by IPDs, but the sidedness is dependent only upon the onset. Here we have new information about an onset cue, one that appears to be calibrated in terms of IPD. The results are unlike those previously reported for low-frequency transients (which were relatively broad-band), as low-pass filtered pulses are processed in terms of time differences. We may conclude that the phase-like calibration of ITD response is dependent upon using narrow-band signals, and that the time-like response to low-pass pulses is due to the signal being processed in many critical bands.

The results obtained from high-frequency transients are new. Here we have ITD lateralization functions that are very similar to the 250-Hz function in terms of the slope as a function of time difference.

In summary, this experiment has verified that the processing of low-frequency, band-limited transients is in some ways similar to that of long-duration tones. It has also shown that use of an ITD cue is possible at high frequencies when there is only a single cycle of envelope modulation. Secondary images occur when the ITD is too long for fusion to take place.

REFERENCES

Abel, S.M. & Kunov, H. (1983). Lateralization based on interaural phase differences: Effects of frequency, amplitude, duration, and shape of rise/decay. *Journal of the Acoustical Society of America, 73*, 955–960.

Babkoff, H. & Sutton, S. (1966). End point of lateralization for dichotic clicks. *Journal of the Acoustical Society of America, 39*, 87–102.

Blauert, J. & Cobben, W. (1978). Some consideration of binaural cross correlation analysis. *Acustica, 39*, 96–104.

Bloom, P.J. & Jones, P.J. (1978). Lateralization thresholds based on interaural time differences for middle and high frequency three tone harmonic complexes. *Acustica, 39*, 283–291.

David, E.E., Guttman, N., & van Bergeijk, W.A. (1959). Binaural interaction of High-Frequency complex stimuli. *Journal of the Acoustical Society of America, 31*, 774–782.

Guttman, N. (1962). A mapping of binaural click lateralizations. *Journal of the Acoustical Society of America, 34*, 87–92.

Hafter, E.R. & Jeffress, L.A. (1968). Two-image lateralization of tones and clicks. *Journal of the Acoustical Society of America, 44*, 563–569.

Henning, G.B. (1974a). Detectability of interaural delay in high-frequency complex waveforms. *Journal of the Acoustical Society of America, 55*, 84–90.

Henning, G.B. (1974b). Lateralization and the binaural masking level difference. *Journal of the Acoustical Society of America, 55*, 1259–1262.

Henning, G.B. (1980a). Some observations on the lateralization of complex waveforms. *Journal of the Acoustical Society of America, 68*, 446–454.

Henning, G.G. (1980b). Lateralization of complex waveforms. In G. van den Brink & F.A. Bilsen (Eds.), *Psychophysical, physiological and behavioral studies in hearing. Proceedings of the fifth International Symposium on Hearing* (pp. 387–392). Delft, Netherlands: Delft University Press.

Jeffress, L. A. (1948). A place theory of sound localization. *Journal of Comparative and Physiological Psychology, 41*, 35–39.

Klump, R.G. & Eady, H.R. (1956). Some measurements of interaural time difference thresholds. *Journal of the Acoustical Society of America, 28*, 859–860.

Kuhn, G.F. (1977). Model for the interaural time difference in the azimuthal plane. *Journal of the Acoustical Society of America, 62*, 157–167.

Kunov, H. & Abel, S.M. (1981). Effects of the rise/decay time on the lateralization of interaurally delayed 1 kHz tones. *Journal of the Acoustical Society of America, 69*, 769–773.

Lindemann, W. (1986a). Extension of a binaural cross-correlation model by contralateral inhibition. I. Simulation of lateralization for stationary signals. *Journal of the Acoustical Society of America, 80*, 1608–1622.

Lindemann, W. (1986b). Extension of a binaural cross-correlation model by contralateral inhibition. II. The law of the first wavefront. *Journal of the Acoustical Society of America, 80*, 1623–1630.

Rayleigh, Lord, J.W.S. (1907). On our perception of sound direction. *Philosophical Magazine, 13* (6th Series), 214–232.

Rose, J.E., Brugge, J.F., Anderson, D.J., & Hind, J.E. (1967). Phase-locking response to low frequency tones in single auditory nerve fibres of the squirrel monkey. *Journal of Neurophysiology, 30*, 769–793.

Sayers, B.McA. (1964). Acoustic-image lateralization judgments with binaural tones. *Journal of the Acoustical Society of America, 36*, 923–926.

Sayers, B.McA. & Toole, F.E. (1964). Acoustic image lateralization judgments with binaural transients. *Journal of the Acoustical Society of America, 36*, 1199–1205.

Stern, R.M. & Colburn, H.S. (1978). Theory of binaural interaction based on auditory-nerve data. IV. A model for subjective lateral position. *Journal of the Acoustical Society of America, 64*, 127–140.

Stern, R.M., Zeiberg, A.S., & Trahiotis, C. (1988). Lateralization of complex binaural stimuli: A weighted-image model. *Journal of the Acoustical Society of America, 84*, 156–165.

Teas, D.C. (1962). Lateralization of acoustic transients. *Journal of the Acoustical Society of America, 34*, 1460–1465.

Tobias, J.V. & Schubert, E.D. (1959). Effective onset duration of auditory stimuli. *Journal of the Acoustical Society of America, 31*, 1595–1605.

Toole, F.E. & Sayers, B.McA. (1965). Lateralization judgments and the nature of binaural acoustic images. *Journal of the Acoustical Society of America, 37*, 319–324.

Yost, W.A. (1974). Discriminations of interaural phase-differences. *Journal of the Acoustical Society of America, 55*, 1299–1303.

Yost, W.A. (1976). Lateralization of repeated filtered transients. *Journal of the Acoustical Society of America, 60*, 178–181.

Yost, W.A. (1981). Lateral position of sinusoids presented with interaural intensive and temporal differences. *Journal of the Acoustical Society of America, 70*, 397–409.

Zwicker, E., Flottorp, G., & Stevens, S.S. (1957). Critical band width in loudness summation. *Journal of the Acoustical Society of America, 29*, 548–557.

Zwislocki, J. & Feldman, R.S. (1956). Just noticeable differences in dichotic phase. *Journal of the Acoustical Society of America, 28*, 860–864.

Revised manuscript received 23 October 1990

THE QUARTERLY JOURNAL OF EXPERIMENTAL PSYCHOLOGY, 1991, *43A* (3) 517–541

A Computer Model of Auditory Stream Segregation

Michael W. Beauvois and Ray Meddis
University of Technology, Loughborough, U.K.

A computer model is described which simulates some aspects of auditory stream segregation. The model emphasizes the explanatory power of simple physiological principles operating at a peripheral rather than a central level. The model consists of a multi-channel bandpass-filter bank with a "noisy" output and an attentional mechanism that responds selectively to the channel with the greatest activity. A "leaky integration" principle allows channel excitation to accumulate and dissipate over time. The model produces similar results to two experimental demonstrations of streaming phenomena, which are presented in detail. These results are discussed in terms of the "emergent properties" of a system governed by simple physiological principles. As such the model is contrasted with higher-level Gestalt explanations of the same phenomena while accepting that they may constitute complementary kinds of explanation.

The area of auditory stream segregation has been investigated extensively for almost 20 years since an initial study by Bregman and Campbell (1971). However, in this time there has been only one attempt (Williams, 1989) to use a computer model to simulate or reproduce the phenomena found in an extensive literature. In this paper we present a new computer model, which simulates some aspects of auditory stream segregation for successive pure-tone stimuli. We also present the results of an empirical study, which are compared directly with the performance of the model.

Auditory stream formation theory concerns itself with how the auditory system assigns acoustic events to different sound sources—a sound source being defined as a sequence of acoustic events emanating from one location or object. A "stream" is a psychological organization that represents such a

---

Requests for reprints should be sent to Michael W. Beauvois, Speech and Hearing Laboratory, Department of Human Sciences, University of Technology, Loughborough LE11 3TU, U.K.

This research was supported by a grant from the Science and Engineering Research Council of Great Britain. We would like to thank Trevor Shackleton and Michael Hewitt for technical help and Chris Darwin and Al Bregman for their comments on an earlier version of this paper.

sequence and displays a continuity that allows that sequence to be interpreted as a "whole" and contrasted with other auditory objects. The term "temporal coherence" is used to describe the subjective impression that a sequence of tones forms a connected series. The phenomenon has much in common with the visual separation of scenes into "figure" and "ground".

In auditory terms, figure-ground effects can be reproduced by using an alternating tone sequence composed of two tones at different frequencies (A and B), which is repeated continuously (i.e. A B A B, etc.). At long tone-repetition times (the time interval between the onset of consecutive tones in the sequence) the observer will hear one tone changing in frequency with a rhythm equal to the tone-repetition time (temporal coherence). At short tone-repetition times two alternating tones will be heard, but the observer's attention will be focused on only one of the tones. The stimulus will appear to have a longer periodicity equal to twice the tone-repetition time (streaming). The length of the silences between the tones does not affect this phenomenon, so long as the time interval between the tone onsets is held constant (Dannenbring & Bregman, 1976a).

The perception of auditory streams in sequences of alternating tones is influenced by several factors—for example, frequency difference between tones, rate of occurrence of events (tone-repetition time), and relative intensity of tones and timbre (see McAdams & Bregman, 1979). For the purpose of the present investigation, however, we can say that empirical studies have clearly shown that temporal coherence is more likely to occur when there is a small frequency difference between tones A and B and when there is a long tone-repetition time (McAdams & Bregman, 1979).

Existing auditory stream formation theories use Gestalt perceptual principles to explain streaming phenomena. The Gestalt approach taken by Bregman's (1984, 1990) theory of auditory scene-analysis postulates that the auditory system decomposes a sound mixture by assigning the resolvable frequency components of the mixture to the separate perceptual structures that are used to represent individual sound sources. These grouping mechanisms are claimed to operate according to Gestalt perceptual principles. For example, the principle of *good continuation* is demonstrated by connecting the tones of an alternating-tone sequence by glides. This reduces the tendency to hear the A and B tones as separate streams (Bregman & Dannenbring, 1973). Likewise, the principle of *similarity* is demonstrated by the tendency of tones to form streams when they are in the same frequency region and there is a small frequency difference between them (Van Noorden, 1975).

Stream segregation is thought to occur as a consequence of a "scene-analysis" process, whereby the system attempts to group auditory components into streams, each of which represents a separate sound source (Bregman, 1984, 1990). A computational auditory scene-analysis approach taken by Williams (1989) uses Gestalt perceptual principles to define the properties of the components of auditory scenes and groups them together on the basis of the Gestalt relationships between the components. These relationships are then displayed as frequency/time graphs.

An alternative approach, and one that we will utilize in this paper, is to consider the action of the lower levels of the auditory nervous system. It is possible that the physiology of the peripheral auditory system, rather than higher-level mechanisms, is responsible for the effects of some Gestalt perceptual principles. These perceptual principles could prove to be the "emergent properties" of a simple low-level processing system. In this paper we propose a model of the auditory system that uses physiological principles rather than Gestalt perceptual principles to account for some examples of auditory streaming. Our model is based upon simple circuits analogous to electronic or physiological systems. We shall demonstrate that this model exhibits similar behaviour to that of human listeners for certain simple stimuli. Although we have contrasted the two approaches for the purposes of introduction, we see our approach as quite possibly complementary to the Gestalt approach, but at a different level of explanation.

A novel feature of the model is the introduction of a random process that introduces "noise" into the system. A previous study (Anstis & Saida, 1985) has shown that auditory perception is indeed subject to noise. In this study it was found that when subjects were played an alternating A B A B tone sequence (fA = 800 and fB = 1200 Hz) that had a length of 30 sec, the percept fluctuated unpredictably from temporal coherence to streaming and back again over time, even though the signal was invariant. In addition to this, the probability of a streaming percept increased over the length of the sequence, suggesting an accumulation of the effects of this noise. These results suggested the inclusion of a "random-walk" mechanism in the model where small changes accrue over time, eventually leading to a large overall change. In the current model this is achieved by generating small random fluctuations in the output from each filter and then accumulating these fluctuations over time, with a separate random walk for each channel.

This article reports the results of testing the model using two simple but robust examples of auditory stream segregation. They illustrate how the model can explain the dependence of auditory streaming phenomena on tone-frequency separation, tone-repetition rate, and the overall duration of the stimulus.

MODEL DESCRIPTION

The model presented here uses a number of basic ideas drawn from auditory science in general and from the streaming literature in particular. These are: (1) a peripheral frequency analysis feeding "channels" characterized by a bandpass frequency response to stimuli; (2) an assumption that the system is inherently "noisy"; (3) a "leaky integration" principle, which allows excitation to build up in the channels and to dissipate slowly over time; and (4) an attentional mechanism that responds selectively to the channel with the greatest activity. A diagram showing the construction of the model is given in Figure 1.

Filter Bank

The stimulus input to the filter bank is a sequence of two alternating pure tones each computed as

$$s_t = \cos(2\pi f_j t) \qquad 1$$

where s_t is the instantaneous amplitude level of the tone, t is the time, and f_j is the frequency of the tone. In this implementation only one stimulus level was used. A tone sequence consists of tones of only two frequencies (fA and fB) and intervening silences. In what follows fA is always equal to 1000 Hz.

The first stage of the model is a multi-channel bandpass filter bank, which, in principle, has a large number of filters. However, when the stimulus is composed of tones of only two frequencies, the only relevant channels for our purposes are those with centre frequencies (CF) equal to the frequency of the two stimulus tones and one channel midway between the two (harmonic mean frequency).

The filter bank imitates the arrangement of the basilar membrane where any tone stimulating a filter will also stimulate adjacent filters. This stage of the model calculates the power attenuation (W_{ij}) of the signal output from the ith filter using formulae suggested by Glasberg and Moore (1990)—see also Patterson and Moore (1986), for a detailed discussion of this topic. The formula used was

$$W_{ij} = [1 + (p_i g_i)] \exp(-p_i g_i) \qquad 2$$

where W_{ij} is the power attenuation in the ith channel to the frequency f_j (fA or fB), and

$$p_i = 4f_j / \mathrm{ERB}(\mathrm{CF}_i) \qquad 3$$

and

$$g_i = (\mathrm{CF}_i - f_j)/\mathrm{CF}_i \qquad 4$$

where CF_i is the centre frequency of the ith filter in Hz. The ERB (equivalent rectangular bandwidth) of the filter was calculated by using the formula given by Glasberg and Moore (1990):

$$\mathrm{ERB}(\mathrm{CF}_i) = 107.939(\mathrm{CF}_i/1000) + 24.7 \qquad 5$$

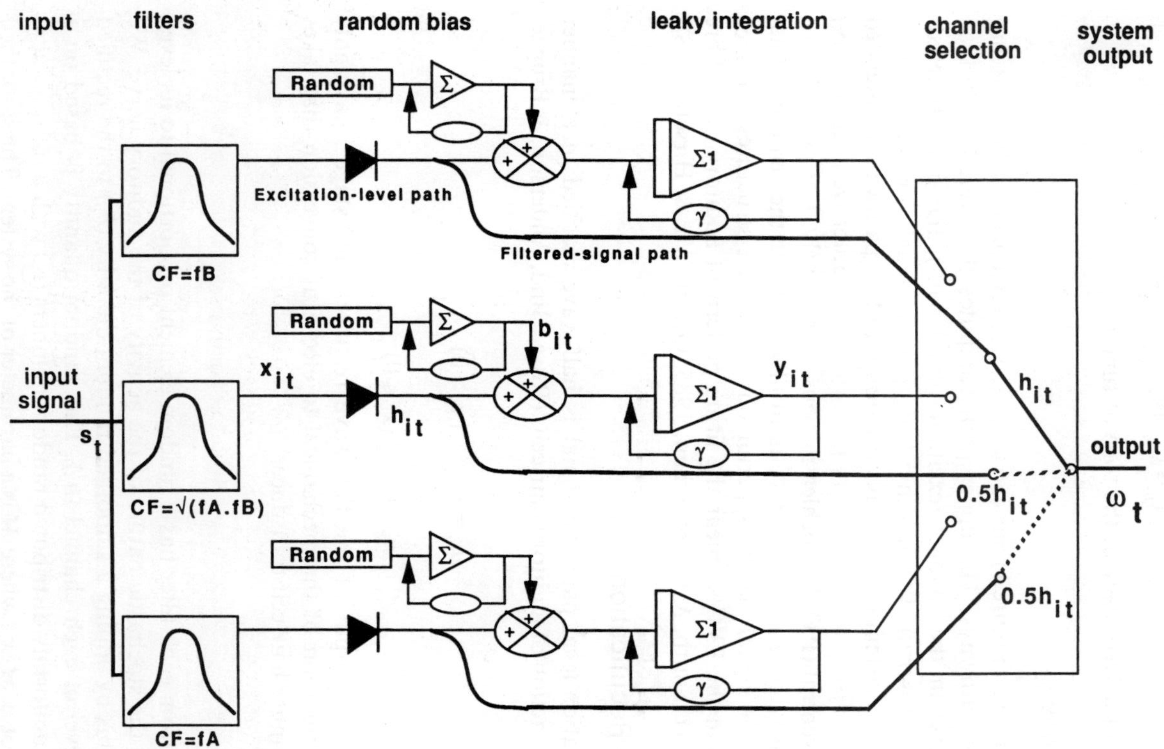

FIG. 1. The structure of the computer model. The output from the filters divides into two lines, an excitation-level path (thin line) and a filtered-signal path (thick line). The output from the model is taken from the filtered-signal branch of the channel that shows the greatest instantaneous excitation level. In this diagram the channel with a CF corresponding to *f*B is the dominant channel.

—see Figure 2. The output from each filter (x_{it}) is the input signal attenuated by the filter function,

$$x_{it} = s_t\sqrt{W_{ij}} \qquad 6$$

Note that j is the frequency of the tone at time t.

Dual Pathway

From the diagram (Figure 1) one can see that each channel is in fact split into two separate pathways. The upper path computes the overall, smoothed excitation level in the channel (excitation-level path); the other (filtered-signal path) preserves the unsmoothed filtered signal for later use in determining the system output. This division into two pathways is intended to reflect the division of the auditory pathway at the anteroventral (AVCN) and posteroventral (PVCN) cochlea nucleus, respectively. For example, the spherical bushy cells in the AVCN faithfully transmit the temporal fine-structure of the signal via the superior olive to higher structures, whereas stellate cells in the PVCN smear the firing pattern of auditory nerve fibre inputs (Frisina, Smith, & Chamberlain, 1985; Oertel, Wu, & Hirsch, 1988).

Half-wave Rectification

In the excitation-level path the signal is half-wave rectified in a manner similar to the action of auditory hair-cells (Rose, Hind, Anderson, & Brugge, 1971):

$$h_{it} = x_{it} \qquad (x_{it} > 0) \qquad 7$$

and

$$h_{it} = 0 \qquad (x_{it} \leqslant 0) \qquad 8$$

where h_{it} is the output of the half-wave rectifier. This stage is a highly simplified simulation of the mechanical to electrical conversion that takes place at the inner hair-cell transducer.

Random Bias

The output from each filter has a random element proportional to its level. This reflects the stochastic nature of the activity of the auditory nerve. We implement this by adding a smoothed random quantity (b_{it}) to the rectified excitation level of each channel (h_{it}). This random quantity is based on a sequence of uniformly distributed random numbers (r_{it}) with a mean of zero and a range of $\pm M \cdot x_{it}$, where M is a parameter of the system. The smoothed bias applied to the ith channel is computed as shown in Figure 1 by the following feedback loop:

$$b_{it} = b_{i(t-1)} + r_{it} \qquad 9$$

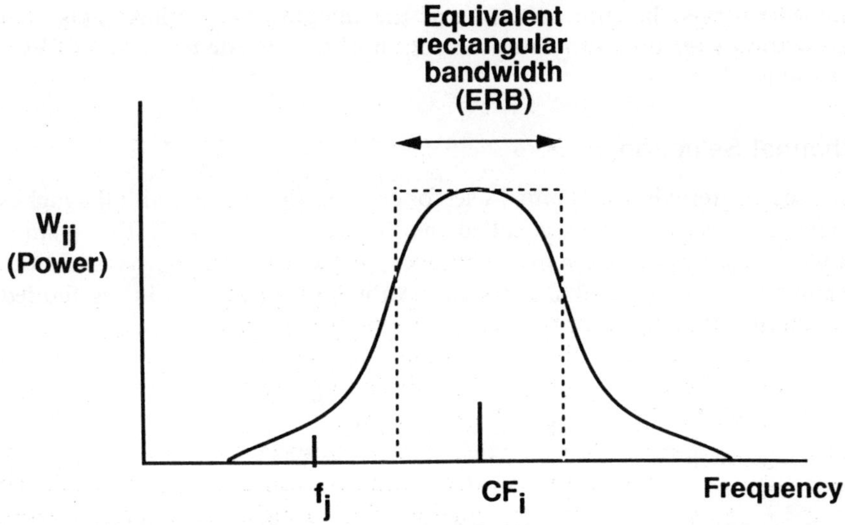

FIG. 2. Schematic representation of an auditory filter showing the equivalent rectangular bandwidth (ERB).

This procedure is used to generate a different random walk for each channel. The moderator value (M) of the random bias was found by optimizing model performance using data from Anstis and Saida (1985, Figure 2)—see further on.

As the random bias is proportional to the level of the stimulus, the onset of a tone that follows a period of silence is preceded by a history of little bias. However, the effect of the bias will accumulate over the first few presentations of the tone. As a consequence, the first few seconds of the stimulus are always characterized by temporal coherence, irrespective of the stimulus parameters, and streaming is more likely to occur after a few seconds.

Excitation Integration

The combined signal of each channel ($h_{it}+b_{it}$) then passes through a cumulative exponential accumulation and decay function (a leaky integrator). This is designed to give a slow build-up in excitation when a tone is playing and a slow decline in excitation once the tone has ended. This provides temporal integration of the filter output. A variable (γ) controls the time constant of the integrator. The output of the excitation-level pathway (y_{it}) is computed using the formula

$$y_{it} = \mu y_{i(t-1)} + [h_{it} + b_{it}] \qquad 10$$

where

$$\mu = \exp(-dt/\gamma) \qquad 11$$

and where γ is the time constant of the integrator in milliseconds. This summation over time simulates the action of the stellate cells in the PVCN (Oertel et al., 1988).

Channel Selection

At 1-msec intervals, the channel selector chooses the channel with the highest excitation level (y_{it}). This is called the "dominant channel". This channel experiences no attenuation in its filtered-signal path output, whereas all other channels experience a 50% reduction in the level of activity in the filtered-signal path; that is,

$$q_i = h_{it} \qquad 12$$

when i is the dominant channel, and

$$q_i = 0.5h_{it} \qquad 13$$

when i is not the dominant channel.

The system output is found by adding together the resulting levels of all the filtered-signal channels:

$$\omega_t = \sum q_i \qquad 14$$

In Figure 1 we have assumed, for the purposes of illustration, that the channel with a CF corresponding to fB is the dominant channel.

The process used in this section of the model is speculative. However, a multi-channel analogue of this possible mechanism has been explored by Meddis and Hewitt (submitted).

Streaming/Temporal Coherence Decision

Streaming occurs when the system output fluctuates in level giving a high output for one tone and a low output for the other tone. Temporal coherence occurs when the system output is approximately equal in response to the two tones. To evaluate this, we find the average level in response to tone A (ω_A) and compare it with the average level in response to tone B (ω_B) over a 1-sec period:

$$Z = \omega_A / \omega_B \qquad 15$$

When Z, or $1/Z$, exceeds a critical value, Z_{crit}, the system output is judged to be streaming. This judgement is made at the end of each second from the beginning to the end of the stimulus.

Z_{crit} is a parameter of the model. In the demonstrations described below, a Z value of 5.0 was used because, when $\gamma = 300$ msec and $M = 0.004$, this criterion yielded a satisfactory range of values for the percentage of coherent responses.

EXAMPLE STIMULI

We can illustrate the working of the model with an alternating A B A B tone sequence stimulus (similar to Figure 8) to show how frequency proximity and tone-repetition time affect the model output. In these examples the CF of Channel 1 corresponds to the frequency of tone A (fA), the CF of Channel 3 corresponds to the frequency of tone B (fB), and the CF of Channel 2 is placed midway between the two at $\sqrt{(fA\,fB)}$. The tone duration in all the examples is 40 msec. When reading the figures, it is important to note that the excitation in a channel builds up when a tone is played at its centre frequency and declines at other times. This gives the excitation curves their characteristic oscillatory appearance (Figure 3).

In most cases the filter whose CF corresponds to the tone frequency will contain the highest excitation level. This means that the output from that filter will dominate the system output because the output from the other filters will be attenuated. However, in some cases the most excited channel

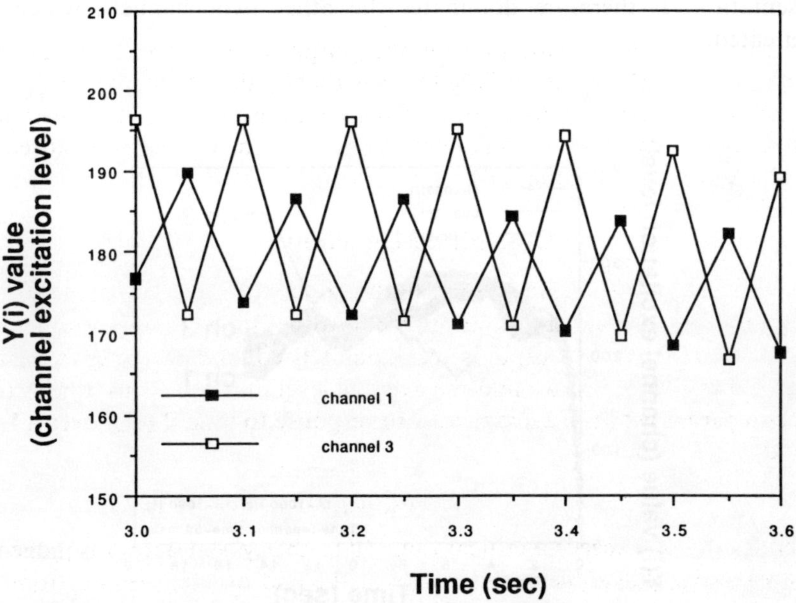

FIG. 3. Excitation levels for Channel 1 (CF=fA) and Channel 3 (CF=fB) showing the overlapping vertical excursions of the excitation levels. This figure is a blown-up segment of Figure 6.

will not correspond to the one being maximally stimulated, and this will reduce the system output in response to that tone because that channel has an attenuated contribution. This may arise when two frequency channels are close together and an intermediate channel can accumulate more excitation over the whole stimulus presentation. It may also occur simply as the result of the inherent noise in the system, which may accumulate excitation in one channel so that it remains dominant even when it is not being actively stimulated. Therefore, in some instances, an intermediate filter will contain the information necessary for the auditory system to determine what percept is heard, in others the percept heard is dependent upon channel-switching between the two channels. Three examples are offered here to illustrate how this mechanism operates.

In the first example, the frequency of tone A (fA = 1000 Hz) is close to the frequency of tone B (fB = 1060 Hz), with a tone-repetition time of 50 msec. Figure 4 shows the output of the excitation paths of the three channels. After 10 sec, Channel 2, the channel with a centre frequency midway between the stimulus frequencies, is consistently the channel with the highest excitation level. This arises because Channel 2 is strongly excited by both tones. It has a CF of 1030 Hz and an ERB of 136 Hz. Both stimulating tones are close to the CF of this channel and receive little attenuation by its bandpass filter. As a consequence, Channel 2 is the most excited for most of the stimulus presentation. It therefore dominates the other two channels, which are attenuated.

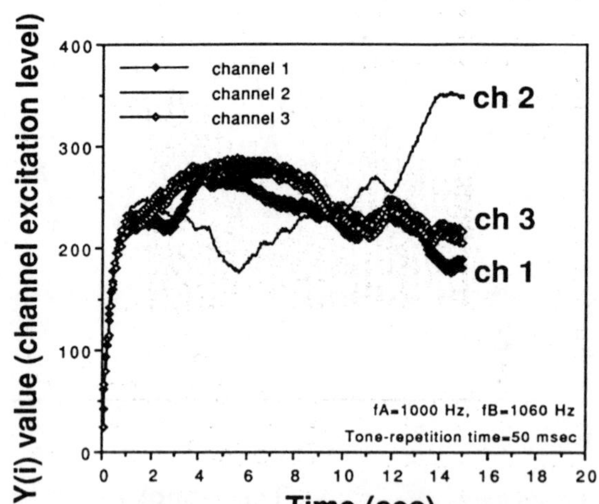

FIG. 4. Excitation levels of all three channels when fA = 1000 Hz, fB = 1060 Hz, and tone-repetition time = 50 msec. The model parameters were $M = 0.004$, $Z_{crit} = 5.0$, and $\gamma = 300$ msec.

This middle channel responds equally strongly to both tones A and B. As a consequence, the output level of tone A will equal the level of tone B in the system output. The amplitude ratio (Z) will equal approximately one, and the model output will contain alternating frequencies at equal amplitudes. In other words, the tone sequence is "perceived" as temporally coherent, and the percept would be a single sound image changing in frequency. The random-bias function makes the initial percept uncertain, but eventually Channel 2 comes to dominate the picture because of the greater overall stimulation of that channel.

In the second example (Figure 5), fA (1000 Hz) is substantially less than fB (1240 Hz), with a long tone-repetition time (250 msec). Because the tone duration is only 40 msec, there is a silence of 210 msec between one tone and the next. This silent period allows the signal strength in each channel to decline by a large amount—due to the "leaky integrator", which has a time constant (γ) of 300 msec. This decline in excitation level between tone presentation produces the overlapping excitation levels found in Figure 5.

On this occasion, Channel 2 receives relatively little excitation, because the two frequencies are distant from the CF of Channel 2, which is approximately 1114 Hz. The strongest channel, therefore, alternates between Channel 1 (when tone A is playing) and Channel 3 (when tone B is active). This means that when each tone is playing, it is being relayed faithfully through its own channel without attenuation. Here the system output would be tempor-

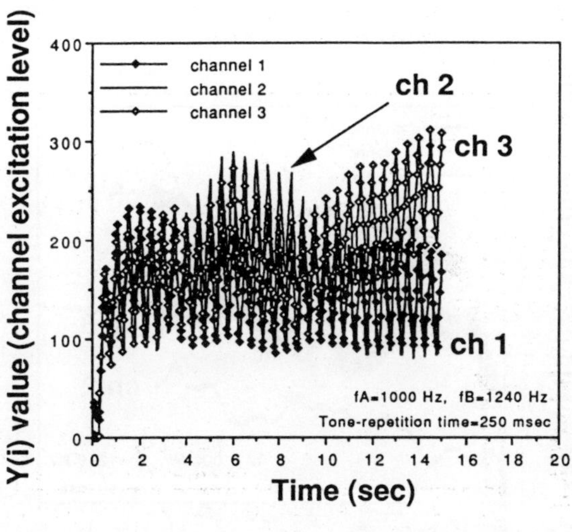

FIG. 5. The excitation levels of all three channels when fA = 1000 Hz, fB = 1240 Hz, and tone-repetition time = 250 msec. The model parameters were $M = 0.004$, $Z_{crit} = 5.0$, and $\gamma = 300$ msec. The trace for Channel 2 is buried in those of Channels 1 and 3 due to their similar excitation levels.

ally coherent and very similar to Example 1, despite the fact that the signal is coming via a different route. This effect is found in the first 10 sec of the model output shown in Figure 5.

However, the random bias applied to the channel excitation levels can destabilize this effect, sometimes causing only one channel to predominate for a sustained period. When this is the case, then the system output would be dominated by the output of only onc of the channels. If it were Channel 1 or 3, this would result in a marked level difference between frequencies A and B at the model output. This creates the percept of streaming as only one frequency predominates in the output.

In Figure 5 the channel excitation values are roughly the same for the first 10 sec of the sequence, that is, the sequence is temporally coherent because the system switches back and forth between the two dominant channels. However, after 10 sec Channel 3 predominates, and streaming occurs because the system output is dominated by the output of Channel 3. When this happens, tone A is attenuated relative to tone B, and Z_{crit} is exceeded, giving rise to the percept of figure (tone B) and ground (tone A).

In the third example (Figure 6), *f*A (1000 Hz) is again substantially less than *f*B (1240 Hz), but the stimulus has a shorter tone-repetition time, with a 50-msec interval between tone onsets. Note that this makes the rise- and decay-cycles shorter and the vertical excursions of the excitation level function much less than in Example 2. After a few seconds, Channel 1 becomes dominant, and streaming will occur with tone A as foreground and

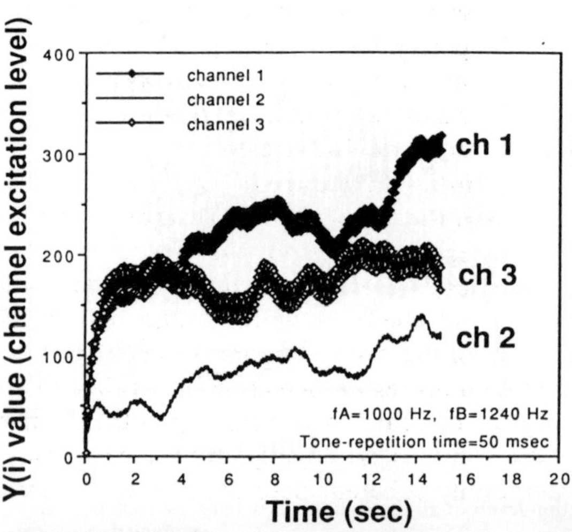

FIG. 6. The excitation levels of all three channels when *f*A = 1000 Hz, *f*B = 1240 Hz, and tone-repetition time = 50 msec. The model parameters were $M = 0.004$, $Z_{crit} = 5.0$, and $\gamma = 300$ msec.

tone B as background. Because the excitation of a given channel does not vary much within a single stimulus cycle, the differences between the channels are accentuated in this condition. In this example, streaming occurs after only 4 sec and continues for the rest of the stimulus.

From these examples we can see that temporal coherence occurs either when the middle channel is predominant (fA is approximately equal to fB) or when the dominant channel alternates between fA and fB (this is facilitated when the tone-repetition time is longer). When channel alternation takes place, the vertical excursions of the excitation levels overlap so that one channel peaks first—that is, dominates the output—followed by the other channel (as in Figure 3). This effect is found in the first 10 sec of Example 2 (Figure 5) and the first 4 sec of Example 3 (Figure 6). Streaming occurs when the middle channel cannot be used (fA is not equal to fB) and when rapid switching between Channel 1 (fA) and Channel 3 (fB) does not take place—that is, the vertical excursions of the excitation levels do not overlap.

EXPERIMENT

Van Noorden (1975) has described the existence of two perceptual boundaries that are dependent on frequency separation and tone-repetition time. He presented subjects with a sequence of two alternating 40-msec tones and plotted streaming vs. temporal coherence responses as a function of the frequency difference between the tones and the tone-repetition time (Figure 7; after McAdams & Bregman, 1979). Above his "temporal coherence boundary" it is impossible to integrate the two tones comprising the sequence into a single perceptual stream. The listener typically hears two separate pulsing tones, one clearly louder than the other. The choice of which one is louder seems to be a matter of chance. Below his "fission boundary" it is impossible to hear more than one stream.

If one tone is held constant in frequency (fA, base tone) whereas the other (fB) varies in frequency, the fission boundary above and below fA is fairly constant across tone-repetition period and approximately equal to one semitone. This corresponds to half an equivalent rectangular bandwidth (ERB) and suggests that the bandwidth of the basilar membrane filter influences the location of the fission boundary. The region between the two boundaries is an ambiguous region perceptually, as either a segregated or an integrated percept may be heard, depending upon the attentional set of the observer. While the stimulus is playing, the listener typically hears both streaming and temporally coherent percepts in a slow, apparently random alternation.

Van Noorden's (1975) results imply that if fA were kept constant, we would expect a low probability of coherence whenever fB is above the

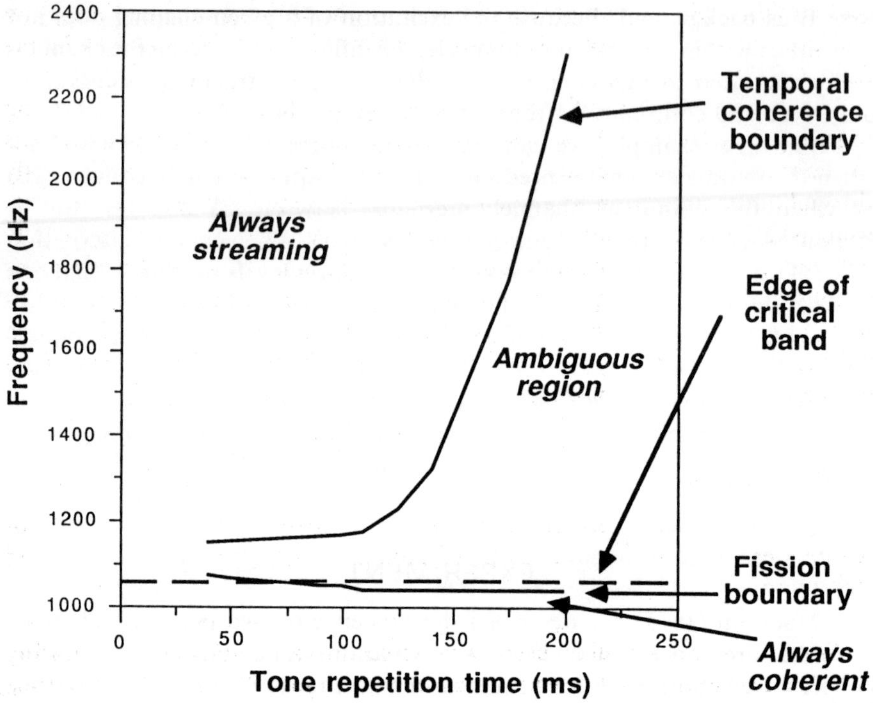

FIG. 7. The temporal coherence boundary (upper curve) and the fission boundary (lower curve) for two alternating pure tones of 40-msec duration played in an A B A B sequence redrawn from McAdams and Bregman (1979). Three perceptual regions are present. The percept of the listener is determined by the frequency separation between the two tones and the tone-repetition time (see text).

temporal coherence boundary and a high probability of coherence whenever *f*B is below the fission boundary. Intermediate probability values would result if *f*B were in the ambiguous region.

An experiment was devised in order to see whether the model simulated the effects of the temporal coherence and fission boundaries as described by Van Noorden (1975) and to provide data in a form readily comparable to the output of the computer model. Unfortunately, his procedure used a frequency-separation adjustment method to find the frequency difference needed for a specific tone-repetition time, which gave a reliable, continuous streaming percept. We found that this methodology was not suitable for constructing an adequate simulation using the computer model. We therefore made observations using listeners involving a number of combinations of frequency differences (*f*B − *f*A) and tone-repetition times in an attempt to establish the probability of temporal coherence as a function of these variables. This approach had the advantage that the results were in a form that could readily be compared with the output of the computer simulation and used to verify the probability-of-coherence implications of Van Noorden's (1975) results.

In the experiment itself subjects were required to listen to an alternating tone sequence (A B A B) for 15 sec and asked to follow the changing percepts of temporal coherence and streaming as they changed spontaneously throughout the duration of the sequence. At the end of the sequence subjects were asked to press a button indicating whether the percept was temporally coherent (a tone changing in frequency) or streaming (two unrelated streams of pulses) just as the sequence ended. The procedure used in the experiment was suggested by the results of Anstis and Saida (1985, Figure 2), which indicated that the percept of streaming builds up over time but has stabilized by the time 15 sec has passed.

Method

Subjects. There were six subjects aged betweeen 26 and 45, four of whom were already familiar with the concepts of temporal coherence and streaming.

Stimuli. The stimulus used was 15 sec of a continuously repeating A B A B sequence of 40-msec pure tones (see Figure 8). Each 40-msec tone had a 5-msec rise and fall time—implemented using raised cosine ramps—in order to prevent onset and offset clicks. The pitch of *f*A was kept constant at 1000 Hz, and that of *f*B was varied between stimuli. The subjects were presented with tone sequences where the frequency difference values were 60, 120, 180, 240, 300, 360, and 420 Hz, and the tone-repetition time values (i.e.

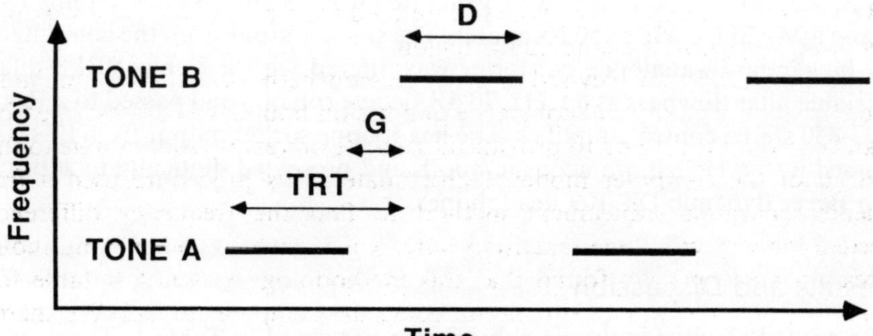

FIG. 8. A sequence of four tones that illustrates the basic stimulus pattern used in the experiment. D is the duration of each tone, G is the duration of the gap between successive tones, and TRT is the tone-repetition time.

time between the onset of successive tones) were 50, 90, 130, 170, 210, and 250 msec. Each combination of frequency difference and tone-repetition time was presented to the subjects once in each experimental block. All stimuli were presented diotically at 35 dB above each listener's absolute threshold for the base tone (*f*A).

Procedure. The subjects were seated in a sound-attenuating booth and listened to as many practice example sequences (drawn at random from the above pools) as were necessary to make them familiar with the percepts of temporal coherence and streaming, and also to notice the way that these percepts alternated with time over the course of the sequence. When they were satisfied with and understood the examples, they were then asked to listen to the various tone sequences and follow the changing percepts over time whilst trying to preserve a sense of temporal coherence in the tone sequence. They were told that at the end of the sequence they should press a button indicating whether the *last* percept they heard was temporal coherence or streaming. There was a silent gap of 3 sec between the end of one sequence and the beginning of the next. Subjects were prompted to make their decision and warned of the next trial by a computer terminal present in the booth. It is important to note that each subject was asked to respond in terms of the period *immediately prior* to signal cessation, and this point was stressed to the subjects.

Design. All six subjects completed 5 blocks, each of which contained all 42 frequency-difference and tone-repetition time combinations presented in random order. The total number of coherence responses for each combination was then converted to a percentage. Each percentage is, therefore, based on 30 observations.

Apparatus. The stimuli were generated using a 40,000-Hz sampling rate using a MASSCOMP 5450 computer. The signal output from the computer's 12-bit digital-to-analogue converter was filtered with a Kemo VBF8 dual-variable filter (lowpass at 5 KHz, 90 dB/octave roll off) and passed to a Rotel RC-850 stereo control amplifier. The headphone socket output from this was passed into a Hedemora acoustic booth and presented diotically to subjects via Beyer dynamic DT 109 headphones.

Results and Discussion

The pooled results for the six subjects are presented in Table 1. The results show broadly the expected trend that, at the end of a 15-sec stimulus, there is a decreasing probability of temporal coherence as the frequency difference between the two tones is increased. In addition to this, the probability of

TABLE 1
The Percentage of Coherent Responses out of 30 Trials as a Function of Tone Repetition Time[a] and Frequency Difference[b]

Frequency Difference		*Tone Repetition Time*					
fA (Hz)	*fB (Hz)*	*50 msec*	*90 msec*	*130 msec*	*170 msec*	*210 msec*	*250 msec*
1000	1060	83	87	97	97	93	90
1000	1120	77	80	83	90	100	97
1000	1180	53	60	67	53	80	90
1000	1240	50	27	57	57	57	83
1000	1300	30	30	30	47	63	80
1000	1360	30	20	27	40	47	60
1000	1420	23	20	43	37	53	83

[a] In msec.
[b] In Hz.

coherence rises with long tone-repetition times. These two findings confirm the probability-of-coherence implications of Van Noorden's (1975) results, which were obtained by using a variable frequency adjustment technique with two subjects.

One implication that emerges from our results is that the percepts of streaming and temporal coherence are essentially probabilistic in nature—that is, if the probability of coherence is below a certain critical value, then the percept is classified as a streaming percept. Similarly, if the probability of coherence is above a certain critical value, then the percept is classified as being temporally coherent. The ambiguous region would then result from having probability of coherence values that lay between these two critical values. This would imply that the temporal coherence and fission boundaries define regions of extreme probability values, which serve to "force" the subjective percept of the listener towards either temporal coherence or streaming.

Model Evaluation

First Evaluation

We now use these empirical results for the purpose of testing the model. The same stimuli as used in the experiment described above were presented to the model. Because the model, like human listeners, generates a probabilistic output, 500 trials for each of the 42 frequency-difference/repetition-time combinations were carried out. The "streaming or coherent" decision was based on the last second of the model output, imitating the task given to the subjects. On each trial the model was required to decide whether the sequence was streaming or temporally coherent as described above.

The range value for the random bias module (M) was 0.004, the critical ratio value (Z_{crit}) was 1.22, and the time constant of the leaky integrator (γ) was 200 msec. The model results were compared directly with those of the subjects by plotting the percentage of coherent responses against fB for each tone-repetition time value used (Figure 9).

As can be seen, the model-subject responses in each tone-repetition time graph are similar to each other, with the exception of the 250-msec function. Despite this anomaly, however, the general trends are similar. As the frequency difference increases, the probability of coherence becomes less. However, the slope of this trend becomes shallower at longer tone-repetition intervals.

Second Evaluation

Anstis and Saida (1985) systematically studied the probability of coherence as a function of the total length of the stimulus. They showed that all stimuli begin by sounding coherent. Later in the sequence, however, the perception is more likely to have a streaming quality. The probability of coherence declines apparently as a function of total duration. Their methodology was already suitable for computer simulation. Accordingly, we collected no data from listeners but simply recorded the response of the model to the stimuli used in their experiment.

The stimuli replicated were A B A B sequences 30 sec long, which consisted of two tones (fA = 800 and fB = 1200 Hz) with tone-repetition times of either 62.5 or 125 msec. The duration of each tone was equal to the tone-repetition time. Each sequence was played 250 times. During the presentation of the stimulus, decisions by the model in favour of temporal coherence were totalled for each second along the length of the sequence and expressed as a percentage. The results were then plotted and matched with those of Anstis and Saida (1985). The three parameters of the model (M, Z_{crit}, and γ) were unchanged from the previous evaluation.

A comparison of the model output and the results of Anstis and Saida (1985) is shown in Figure 10. The model is clearly successful in replicating the build-up of streaming over time found by Anstis and Saida (1985).

GENERAL DISCUSSION

The model behaves in a manner that suggests that it may contain the seeds of an explanation of our own experimental results—and hence those of Van Noorden (1975)—and also those of Anstis and Saida (1985), because both studies were successfully replicated by the model using only one particular set

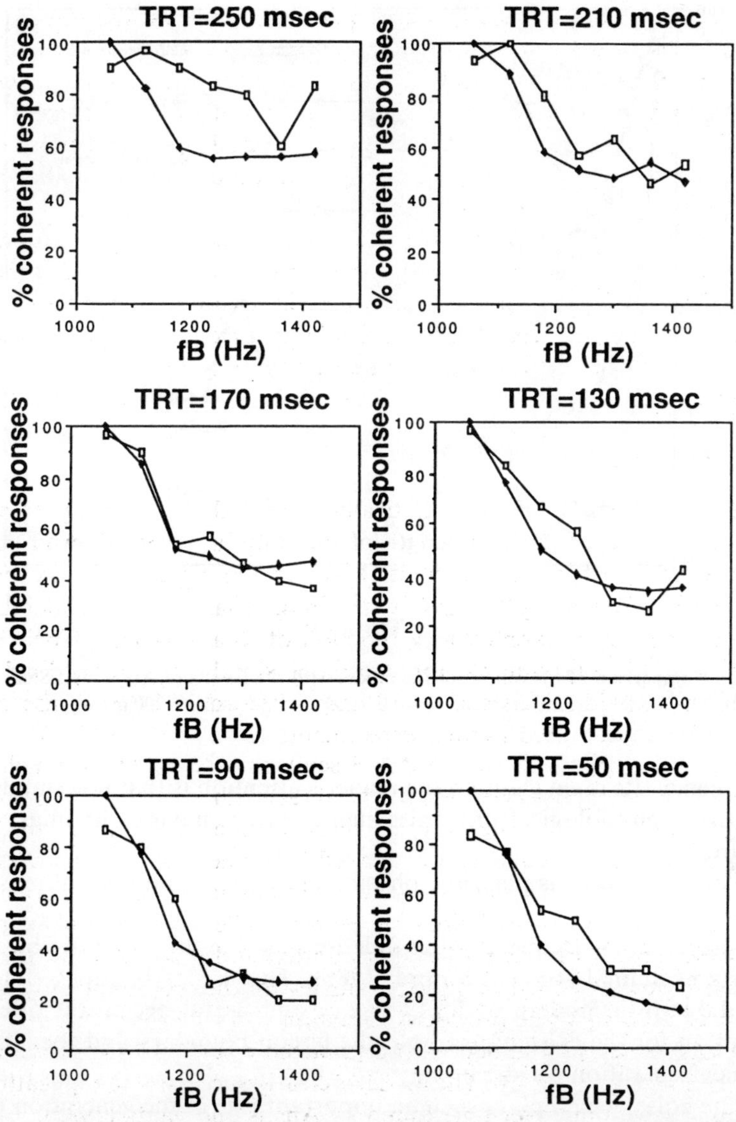

FIG. 9. Comparisons of model and subject results for each tone-repetition time value used (diamonds = model responses, squares = subject responses). The model parameters were $M = 0.004$, $Z_{crit} = 1.22$, and $\gamma = 200$ msec.

of parameters. This would indicate that for these particular stimuli the model is imitating the responses of human listeners fairly accurately.

To the best of our knowledge, this is a novel approach to the problem of accounting for perceptual coherence among successive pure tones of chang-

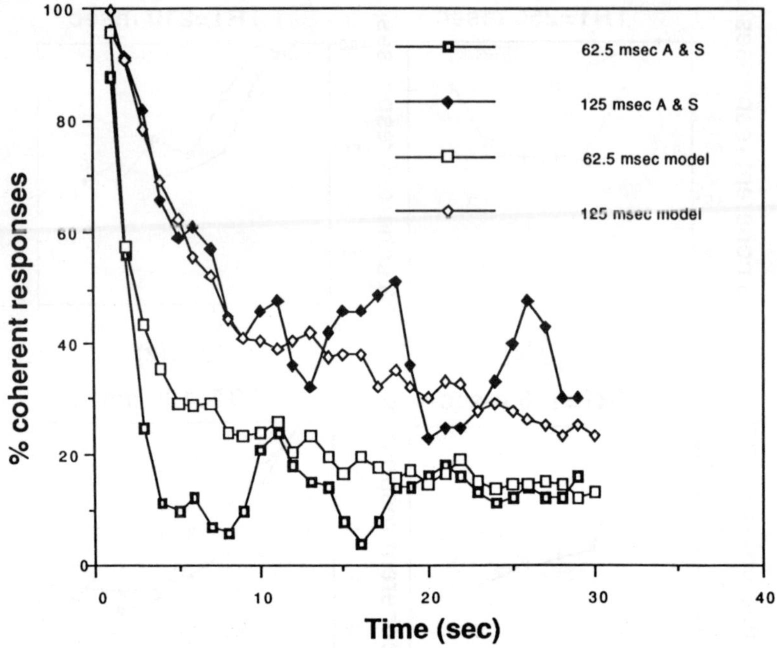

FIG. 10. Comparison of the output of the model with the results of Anstis and Saida (1985, Figure 2). The model parameters were $M = 0.004$, $Z_{crit} = 1.22$, and $\gamma = 200$ msec.

ing frequency. Its main claim to the reader's attention is that it is simple and works using physiological principles suggested by previous findings in the literature.

The current model is plausible physiologically for a number of reasons:

1. The bandpass frequency filter functions used in the model are based on human and animal studies (Moore, 1986). The use of bandpass filters is unavoidable in a modern auditory theory and useful because it offers an explanation for the existence of both the fission boundary and the effect of frequency separation on streaming.
2. The noise, which plays such an important role in the generation of the streaming effects, is a prominent feature of auditory nerve activity. Fibres in the auditory nerve operate in a stochastic manner where the probability of firing is determined by the signal level. As the signal level increases, the variance associated with this probability will also increase.
3. The ventral cochlear nucleus has chopper units whose rate of firing reflects stimulus amplitude, which are tonotopically arranged and could be used for channel-selection purposes (Oertel et al., 1988). Our excitation-level path is intended to reflect this function.

4. The use of a temporal integration principle, suggested by the study of Anstis and Saida (1985), has been demonstrated in the ventral cochlear nucleus (Oertel et al., 1988). Stellate cells appear to be particularly well suited, both anatomically and physiologically to this function.

5. The cochlear nucleus has lateral inhibitory networks in both ventral and dorsal sections, suggesting competition between channels (Oertel et al., 1988). This model explores the possibility that mutual inhibition of channels may be a critical component in the physiological basis of selective attention.

Bregman and Campbell (1971) define a stream as "a sequence of auditory events whose elements are related perceptually to one another, the stream being segregated perceptually from other co-occurring auditory events". Similarly, Bregman and Pinker (1978) define a stream as a psychological organization whose function is to represent mentally the acoustic activity of a single source over time. These are high-level theoretical constructs. However, we would argue that streaming could equally be understood in terms of physiological factors as utilized in the model. Our model suggests that auditory events are temporally coherent whenever the system output transmits both tones with equal amplitude. This occurs whenever an intermediate filter has more excitation than the others. It also happens whenever the choice of the strongest channel oscillates between channels with CFs at the frequencies of the two tones. In both cases, the signal strength ratio (Z) of the two tones is approximately equal to 1.0 or is less than the critical ratio (Z_{crit}) when temporal coherence occurs.

Our model has the considerable virtue of simplicity. By using only the intrinsic randomness of the activity of the auditory nerve and a leaky integrator, we have managed to replicate not only the experimental findings of Anstis and Saida (1985) but have also been able to reproduce our own experimental results, which in turn replicate Van Noorden's results. These replications justify the potential value of a low-level analysis, such as ours, for explaining high-level psychological phenomena.

It is appropriate, then, to use the principles by which the model works to address the findings of other studies that have investigated more complex auditory phenomena. In the following examples we assume that a multi-channel version of the model is in operation rather than the abbreviated three-channel model demonstrated above.

Dannenbring and Bregman (1976b) presented subjects with 20-sec sequences composed of alternating pure tones and bursts of band-passed noise (Figure 11) and found that the sequence exhibited marked streaming—that is, there seemed to be no relationship between the pure tones and the noise bursts and subjects could attend to only one type of stimulus at a time. When this type of stimulus is presented to subjects, we would expect streaming to occur due to the action of the leaky integrator. When the pure tone is initially

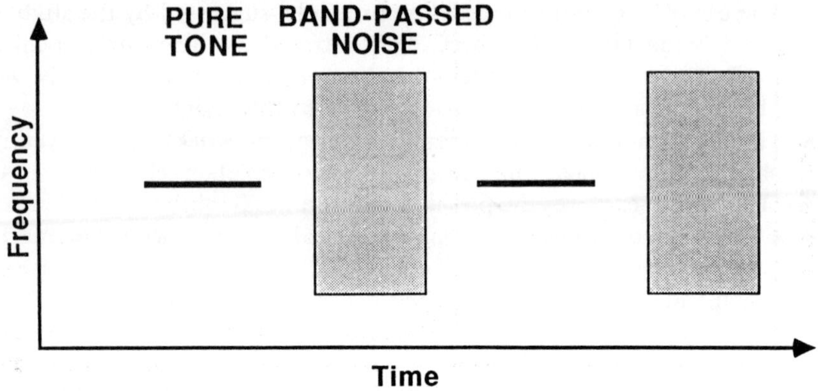

FIG. 11. The stimulus configuration used in the study of Dannenbring and Bregman (1976b).

sounded, an excitation peak is created in the channel with a corresponding CF. When this tone is followed by a noise burst, the stimulus energy of the noise "tops up" the excitation level in this channel, maintaining the excitation peak initially created by the pure tone. This causes this channel to have the highest excitation level, as there is no silent period long enough to allow excitation levels to decay significantly because another pure tone almost immediately follows the noise burst. However, the excitation levels in the other channels stimulated by the noise burst *will* decay during the time the next pure tone is on as they are not directly stimulated. The resulting excitation-level imbalance between the pure tone channel and the other channels will increase the value of Z above the critical streaming value, resulting in the formation of a stream centred on the CF of the pure tone. This characteristic behaviour of the model can also give us an insight into the possible mechanism behind the Gestalt perceptual principle of "proximity".

Ciocca and Bregman (1987) presented subjects with stimuli composed of an initial sinusoidal tone glide and a steady-state tone (A or B), which were separated by a noise burst (Figure 12). Their results indicated that frequency proximity dominated over trajectory alignment in determining the perceived continuity between the glide and the tone—that is, in Figure 12 tone B will give the best integration with the glide. This, according to our model, will be due to the residual excitation left in the system at the last frequency channel stimulated prior to the noise burst. Although the noise burst adds excitation to all frequency regions, this excitation is uniform in nature, and the last channel stimulated prior to the noise burst (i.e. the channel with a CF corresponding to tone B) will still have a higher excitation level than the other channels due to the "topping-up" principle and hence become the dominant channel. This will lead to the system being primed for a recurrence of a tone corresponding to the CF of the dominant channel (or one of a

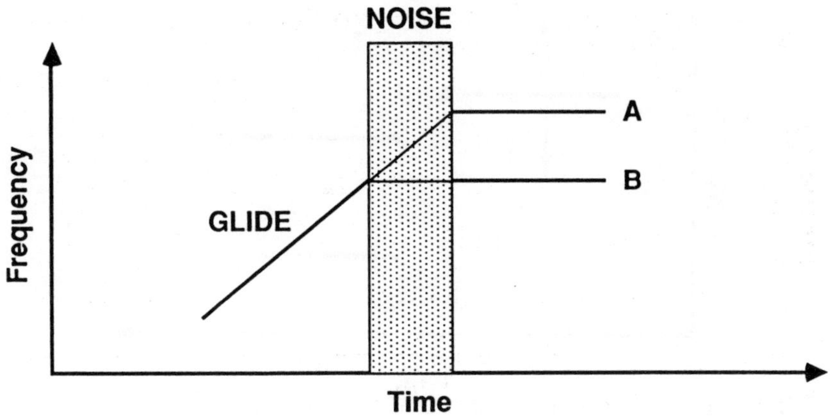

FIG. 12. The stimulus configuration used in the study of Ciocca and Bregman (1987).

similar frequency). Hence, the best continuity between stimuli will occur when the next stimulus starts at a frequency at or near the CF of this dominant channel as the excitation pattern will then be unbroken, resulting in an integrated, unified percept. This explanation accords well with the findings of Ciocca and Bregman (1987).

The phenomenon of an unbroken excitation pattern is also found in another study by Bregman and Dannenbring (1973). They found that joining the component tones of a repeating A B A B tone sequence with frequency glides increased the integration of the sequence, causing temporal coherence. In our model a glide will cause a sweep of excitation going from the channel corresponding to tone A to the channel corresponding to tone B and back again. The model takes the channel with the highest excitation level as the dominant channel. In this experimental situation, dominance would follow the sweep from tone A to tone B and back again, making the sequence temporally coherent. This is because the excitation integration in the A and B channels and all channels between will not get high enough for any one channel to dominate for a long period because the applied channel excitation is transient in nature. As no particular channel dominates the overall output, the value of Z will be close to one, and the sequence will therefore be judged as temporally coherent.

We do not wish to exaggerate the power of the model presented here. So far we can only claim to have made a start in our efforts to complement and perhaps explain the formation of auditory Gestalt perceptual phenomena by attempting to find a physiological origin for psychological phenomena. Only a limited range of data has been considered in this paper as the model has been deliberately simplified to form a secure basis for further investigations and extensions (such as a hair-cell model and a cross-channel grouping

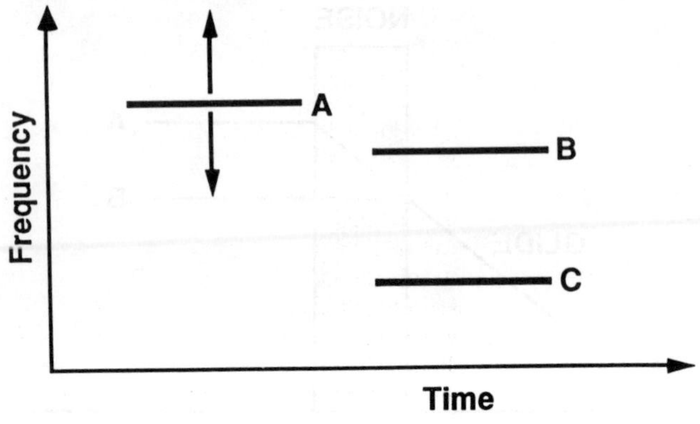

FIG. 13. The stimulus configuration used in the study of Bregman and Pinker (1978).

mechanism). The addition of a cross-channel grouping mechanism will allow the model to process more complex perceptual effects. For example, Bregman and Pinker (1978) presented subjects with a tone dyad (BC) that was alternated repeatedly with a captor tone (A), which was near to one of the tones (B) in frequency (Figure 13). Their results indicated that the perceived richness of the BC dyad was reduced due to the captor tone stripping tone B out of the dyad, causing the formation of an AB stream, and that this effect was related to the frequency proximity of the A and B tones. From the results of this study we can see that there is an interaction between a stream-formation mechanism and a cross-channel grouping mechanism that works on the basis of common onsets and offsets. Hence, any computer model that seeks to reproduce this effect and others of a similar nature (e.g. Bregman & Tougas, 1989) must include both mechanisms. The current version of the model described in this paper lacks a cross-channel grouping mechanism, although parallel studies are addressing this issue (Meddis & Hewitt, submitted). Even without this addition, it is possible that the principles upon which the existing model is based can successfully be extended to explain more complex auditory phenomena.

REFERENCES

Anstis, S. & Saida, S. (1985). Adaptation to auditory streaming of frequency-modulated tones. *Journal of Experimental Psychology: Human Perception and Performance*, *11* (3), 257–271.

Bregman, A.S. (1978). Auditory streaming is cumulative. *Journal of Experimental Psychology: Human Perception and Performance*, *4* (3), 380–387.

Bregman, A.S. (1984). Auditory scene analysis. In *Proceedings of the Seventh International Conference on Pattern Recognition.* Silver Spring, MD: IEEE Computer Society Press.

Bregman, A.S. (1990). *Auditory scene analysis.* Cambridge, MA: MIT Press.

Bregman, A.S. & Campbell, J. (1971). Primary auditory stream segregation and perception of order in rapid sequences of tones. *Journal of Experimental Psychology*, *89*, 244–249.

Bregman, A.S. & Dannenbring, G.L. (1973). The effect of continuity on auditory stream segregation. *Perception and Psychophysics*, *13*, 308–312.

Bregman, A.S. & Pinker, S. (1978). Auditory streaming and the building of timbre. *Canadian Journal of Psychology*, *32*, 19–31.

Bregman, A.S. & Tougas, Y. (1989). Propagation of constraints in auditory organisation. *Perception and Psychophysics*, *46*, 395–396.

Ciocca, V. & Bregman, A.S. (1987). Perceived continuity of gliding and steady-state tones through interrupting noise. *Perception and Psychophysics*, *42*, 476–484.

Dannenbring, G.L. & Bregman, A.S. (1976a). Effect of silence between tones on auditory stream segregation. *Journal of the Acoustical Society of America*, *59*, 987–989.

Dannenbring, G.L. & Bregman, A.S. (1976b). Stream segregation and the illusion of overlap. *Journal of Experimental Psychology: Human Perception and Performance*, *2*, 544–555.

Frisina, R.D., Smith, R.L., & Chamberlain, S.C. (1985). Differential encoding of rapid changes in sound amplitude by second-order auditory neurons. *Experimental Brain Research*, *60*, 417–422.

Glasberg, B.R. & Moore, B.C.J. (1990). Derivation of auditory filter shapes from notched-noise data. *Hearing Research*, *47*, 103–138.

McAdams, S. & Bregman, A.S. (1979). Hearing musical streams. *Computer Music Journal*, *3*, 26–43, 60.

Meddis, R. & Hewitt, M.J. (submitted). Modelling the identification of concurrent vowels with different fundamental frequencies. *Journal of the Acoustical Society of America*.

Moore, B.C.J. (1986). Parallels between frequency selectivity measured psychophysically and in cochlear mechanics. *Scandinavian Audiological Supplement*, *25*, 139–152.

Oertel, D., Wu, S.H., & Hirsch, J.A. (1988). Electrical characteristics of cells and neuronal circuitry in the cochlear nuclei studied with intracellular recording from brain slices. In G.M. Edelman, W.E. Gall, & W.M. Cowan (Eds.), *Auditory function*. New York: John Wiley.

Patterson, R.D. & Moore, B.C.J. (1986). Auditory filters and excitation patterns as representations of frequency resolution. In B.C.J. Moore (Ed.), *Frequency selectivity in hearing*. London: Academic Press.

Rose, J.E., Hind, J.E., Anderson, D.J., & Brugge, J.F. (1971). Some effects of stimulus intensity on response of auditory nerve fibres in the squirrel monkey. *Journal of Neurophysiology*, *34*, 685–699.

Van Noorden, L.P.A.S. (1975). *Temporal coherence in the perception of tone sequences*. Unpublished doctoral dissertation, Institute for Perception Research, Eindhoven, The Netherlands.

Williams, S.M. (1989). *A prototype tool for computational modelling of auditory grouping effects*. Department of Computer Science Research Report, University of Sheffield.

Revised manuscript received 3 December 1990

THE QUARTERLY JOURNAL OF EXPERIMENTAL PSYCHOLOGY, 1991, *43A* (3) 543–564

Frequency Selectivity for Hearing-impaired and Broadband-noise-masked Normal Listeners

Judy R. Dubno and Amy B. Schaefer
UCLA School of Medicine, Los Angeles, CA, U.S.A.

When evaluating frequency selectivity, it is difficult to determine if the deviation from normal performance observed for hearing-impaired listeners reflects abnormal cochlear function or normal, level-dependent changes in frequency selectivity. This experiment was designed to investigate the dependence of frequency-selectivity measures on threshold and signal level. Auditory-filter characteristics, critical ratios, forward-masked psychophysical tuning curves, and narrowband-noise masking patterns were obtained from normal-hearing listeners in quiet and in the presence of broadband noise at five levels. These findings were then compared to previously obtained frequency-selectivity measurements for subjects with mild-to-moderate sensorineural hearing loss whose absolute thresholds are comparable to the normal-hearing listeners' masked thresholds. The results suggest that frequency selectivity deteriorates as threshold increases for all subjects. However, the poor frequency selectivity exhibited by hearing-impaired listeners may not be explained entirely by the effects of threshold and signal level. Nevertheless, because frequency selectivity is poorer in the normal auditory system at higher stimulus levels, the deviation from normal performance observed for hearing-impaired listeners may not be as large as previously suggested.

Fundamental to the study of sensorineural hearing impairment and its consequences is a clear understanding of the capabilities of the hearing-impaired listener relative to those of the normal listener. Toward this goal, frequency selectivity by individuals with normal and impaired auditory

---

Requests for reprints should be sent to Judy R. Dubno, UCLA School of Medicine, Division of Head and Neck Surgery, Los Angeles, CA, U.S.A. 90024–1794.

This work was supported by grants from the National Institute on Deafness and Other Communication Disorders (National Institutes of Health), the Hope for Hearing Foundation, and the Victor Goodhill Ear Center. The authors would like to acknowledge the invaluable suggestions and comments offered by Donald D. Dirks, Brian C.J. Moore, and Quentin Summerfield.

systems has been measured in many experiments. Frequency selectivity refers to the ability of the auditory system to separate the various frequency components of complex sounds, and has been estimated by measuring the change in the threshold of audibility of a sound that results from the presence of another sound. Results of psychophysical studies suggest that (1) frequency selectivity of normal-hearing listeners decreases as signal level increases (e.g. Zwicker & Schorn, 1978), and (2) frequency selectivity of listeners with sensorineural hearing loss is poorer than that of normal subjects (Wightman, McGee, & Kramer, 1977; Florentine, Buus, Scharf, & Zwicker, 1980; Ritsma, Wit, & van der Lans, 1980). However, because hearing-impaired subjects' auditory thresholds are elevated, frequency selectivity of hearing-impaired subjects is sometimes measured at higher signal or masker levels relative to normal-hearing subjects. Consequently, if frequency selectivity is poorer in the normal auditory system at higher stimulus levels, the deviation from normal performance observed for hearing-impaired listeners may not be as large as previously suggested.

There is considerable evidence that measurements of frequency selectivity for hearing-impaired individuals are not independent of signal or masker levels, or the listener's auditory threshold. In a detailed review, Humes (1982) compares frequency selectivity for normal-hearing and hearing-impaired listeners obtained from several experiments and finds that hearing-impaired listeners' poorer selectivity occurs when signal or masker sound-pressure levels are significantly higher for hearing-impaired than for normal-hearing subjects. Humes concludes that the deterioration in frequency selectivity observed for hearing-impaired listeners may be a representation of the capabilities of the normal auditory system when measured at high signal levels, rather than the consequence of cochlear pathology. Auditory-filter characteristics estimated from masked thresholds obtained in notched noise have been shown to be dependent on the magnitude of hearing loss (Glasberg & Moore, 1986). More recent results from a large group of hearing-impaired listeners also demonstrate that estimates of auditory-filter characteristics vary with absolute threshold (Dubno & Dirks, 1989). Thus, in previous psychophysical studies, differences in signal and/or masker levels and auditory thresholds among listeners have made it difficult to determine the effect of cochlear pathology on frequency selectivity.

In the present experiment to differentiate the effects of threshold elevation and signal levels on estimates of frequency selectivity, performance of normal-hearing subjects has been evaluated under conditions in which their thresholds have been elevated by the addition of broadband noise. The rationale for such an experimental design is that performance of normal-hearing and hearing-impaired listeners may be compared at equal signal and masker sound-pressure and sensation levels. Broadband noise also simulates the reduced dynamic range and more closely approximates the loudness-growth function of listeners with sensorineural hearing loss. A weakness of the design is the high level of activity in the auditory system produced by the noise to elevate thresholds is not equivalent to a reduction in gain in the auditory system. Nevertheless, the primary differences between the two groups of listeners are the presence of cochlear pathology for the hearing-impaired subjects and the presence of background noise for the masked normal-hearing subjects.

In an early study of the effects of noise on frequency selectivity, Green, Shelton, Picardi and Hafter (1981) demonstrate that shapes of psychophysical tuning curves (PTCs) obtained in noise do not change as a function of probe level, as do those obtained in quiet. Results of other studies (e.g. Pick, 1980; Nelson & Freyman, 1984) suggest that frequency selectivity is level dependent. Furthermore, studies of frequency selectivity (Humes, Espinoza-Varas, & Watson, 1988; Jesteadt, Stelmachowicz, & Callaghan, 1987; Nelson, 1988) and temporal resolution (Florentine & Buus, 1984; Florentine, Fastl, & Buus, 1988) do not consistently demonstrate equivalent performance for masked normal-hearing and hearing-impaired listeners. A model has been proposed recently in a retrospective analysis by Humes et al. (1988) to account for differences in frequency selectivity and temporal resolution observed among normal-hearing and hearing-impaired listeners. In this study, sensorineural hearing loss is modeled as threshold elevation due to an internal noise and is simulated by assuming that thresholds of *hypothetical* noise-masked normal-hearing listeners are equal to actual thresholds of hearing-impaired subjects. Using this model, frequency selectivity for hearing-impaired listeners is accurately predicted for measurement paradigms using fixed masker levels. However, frequency selectivity for hearing-impaired subjects measured using fixed, low-sensation level signals (e.g. PTCs) is not accurately predicted by the model, nor are results of several temporal-resolution paradigms. Thus, the influence of threshold and signal-level differences on frequency selectivity and the magnitude of the difference in frequency selectivity between normal-hearing and hearing-impaired listeners have not been clearly defined.

In an effort to provide more accurate estimates of frequency selectivity for hearing-impaired listeners, the dependence of frequency-selectivity measures on threshold and signal level is investigated in the current experiment using normal-hearing listeners whose thresholds were elevated by masking with broadband noise. Auditory-filter characteristics, PTCs, and narrowband-noise masking patterns are obtained from normal-hearing listeners whose thresholds are elevated by the addition of broadband noise. Measurements of frequency selectivity previously obtained from 24 hearing-impaired listeners (Dubno & Dirks, 1989) are then compared to results for the masked normal-hearing listeners. Residual differences in frequency selectivity that may be observed between masked normal-hearing listeners and individuals with sensorineural hearing loss are independent of threshold elevation or signal-level differences and, therefore, may provide more accurate estimates of the influence of cochlear pathology on frequency selectivity.

Method

Observers. Nineteen young (18–31 years of age) normal-hearing listeners participated in this study. Each subject passed a hearing screening at 15 dB HL (ANSI, 1969) at octave frequencies from 250 to 8000 Hz; normal tympanometric measures were observed in all cases. Subjects were randomly assigned to one of three groups corresponding to the three experimental tasks. Testing consisted of measurements of thresholds and one of three frequency-selectivity tasks (auditory-filter characteristics estimated using a symmetric notched-noise masker, forward-masked PTCs, or narrowband-noise masking patterns) in quiet and in the presence of a broadband noise at five overall sound-pressure levels. Testing was completed in four or five 2-hr sessions. The subjects did not have experience with psychophysical procedures, and were paid for their participation. Details regarding the frequency-selectivity measurements for 24 hearing-impaired subjects may be found in Dubno & Dirks (1989).

Apparatus and Stimuli. Signals were digitally generated pure tones ranging in frequency from 250 to 5000 Hz. One of these signals (1200 Hz) was used as the probe signal in the auditory-filter and PTC measurements. Eleven pure-tone signals (630, 800, 1000, 1200, 1250, 1400, 1600, 2000, 2500, 3150, and 4000 Hz) were used in the measurement of narrow-band-noise masking patterns. Pure-tone signals were 350 msec in duration, with rise and fall times of 25 msec. The probe signal for the PTC measurements was 20 msec in duration, with rise and fall times of 5 msec. Signal amplitude was controlled by a programmable attenuator (Matrix Systems Model 6153/1956). The signal was then added to the appropriate masker, mixed with broadband noise, and delivered to a TDH-49P earphone mounted in a supra-aural cushion. The amplitude of the signal for PTC measurements was fixed at 10 dB above the subject's absolute threshold for the 20-msec, 1200-Hz signal (for measurements in quiet) or 10 dB above their broadband threshold[1] (for measurements in noise).

The masker was (1) a 350-msec broadband noise with a variable-width spectral notch surrounding the pure-tone signal, for the auditory-filter measurements, (2) 200-msec pure tones for the forward-masked PTCs, or (3)

[1] The term "broadband threshold" refers to thresholds measured in the continuous broadband noise used to elevate normal-hearing listeners' thresholds. The term "masked threshold" refers to thresholds measured in the notched-noise or narrowband-noise maskers.

a 350-msec narrowband noise for the masking patterns. For the auditory-filter measurements, there were nine spectral-notch widths, as specified by the deviation from the probe frequency divided by the probe frequency, ranging from 0 to 0.4. For the forward-masked PTC measurements, ten maskers were used (600, 800, 1000, 1050, 1100, 1150, 1200, 1250, 1300, and 1400 Hz); masker-probe separation was 2 msec. For the masking patterns, the narrow-band-noise masker had a bandwidth of 200 Hz, and was centred at 1200 Hz. In addition to these maskers, a continuous broadband noise was present under some conditions. Broadband noise was produced by a Grason-Stadler Model 901B Noise Generator, attenuated (Hewlett-Packard Model 350D), mixed with the signal and masker and delivered to the earphone. Spectrum levels were 40 dB/Hz for the notched-noise and narrowband-noise maskers. Overall sound-pressure levels of the broadband noise were 30, 40, 50, 60, and 70 dB SPL. The maximum masker level for the PTC measurements was set to 100 dB SPL.

Procedure. For all tasks, thresholds (or masker levels for the PTCs) were obtained using a two-interval forced-choice adaptive psychophysical procedure with feedback, converging on 71% correct performance (Levitt, 1971). First, thresholds for 10 pure-tone signals, spaced at one-third octave centre frequencies from 250 to 5000 Hz, were measured in quiet. Second, thresholds were measured for these signals in five levels of broadband noise. Third, auditory-filter, PTC, or masking-pattern measurements were obtained without broadband noise. Fourth, these same measurements were made in four or five levels of broadband noise.

For auditory-filter measurements, thresholds for the 1200-Hz signal were measured in notched-noise maskers as a function of notch width. For forward-masked PTCs, the level of the pure-tone masker necessary to just mask the low-level 1200-Hz probe was determined. An additional set of PTCs was obtained without the broadband noise and with the probe sound-pressure levels set equal to the levels used for the broadband-noise conditions (i.e. 10 dB above the broadband threshold for the 20-msec, 1200-Hz probe). For masking-pattern measurements, thresholds for eleven pure-tone signals were measured in the presence of a narrowband-noise masker. The 30-dB SPL broadband-noise condition was omitted for the masking-pattern measurements because essentially no additional masking occurred with broadband noise at this level.

Results and Discussion

Thresholds. Figure 1 shows mean thresholds for 10 pure-tone signals ranging in frequency from 250 to 5000 Hz for the 19 normal-hearing listeners in quiet and in five levels of broadband noise. As expected, the broadband

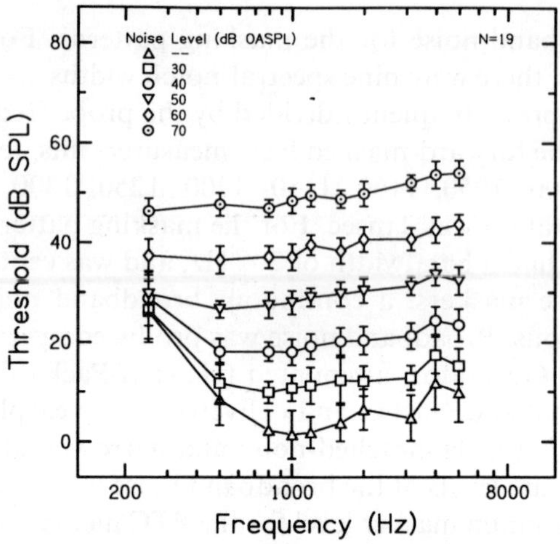

FIG. 1. Mean thresholds (in dB SPL) for 10 pure-tone signals ranging in frequency from 250 to 5000 Hz for 19 normal-hearing subjects in quiet (triangles) and in five levels of broadband noise (other symbols). Error bars encompass ± 1 *SD* from the mean.

noise yields thresholds that are relatively uniform across frequency, and equivalent to a mild-to-moderate magnitude of hearing loss. At 1200 Hz, the frequency of the probe signal used in the frequency-selectivity measurements, mean thresholds ranged from 1.4 dB SPL (in quiet) to 49.5 dB SPL (in 70-dB SPL broadband noise).

Auditory-Filter Characteristics. Figure 2 contains results for the frequency-selectivity measurement from which parameters describing auditory-filter characteristics are derived. Data in the upper left panel are mean masked thresholds for a 1200-Hz signal in notched noise as a function of notch width for six normal-hearing listeners. Each of the remaining panels includes results obtained in notched noise and broadband noise. The broken, horizontal line in each panel is plotted at the mean absolute (or broadband) threshold at the signal frequency for each condition. In each panel, as notch width increases, masked threshold decreases and approaches the broadband threshold for the widest notches. Masked thresholds in the zero-notch condition remain constant as broadband-noise level increases. However, in the wider-notch conditions, masked thresholds increase as the broadband-noise level increases and are limited by the broadband threshold. Therefore, the slope of the curve relating threshold to notch width appears to be dependent on the threshold at the signal frequency.

Auditory-filter characteristics were derived from the masked thresholds by assuming the rounded exponential (or roex) model (Patterson, Nimmo-Smith, Weber, & Milroy, 1982), using the two-parameter (*p,r*) model in

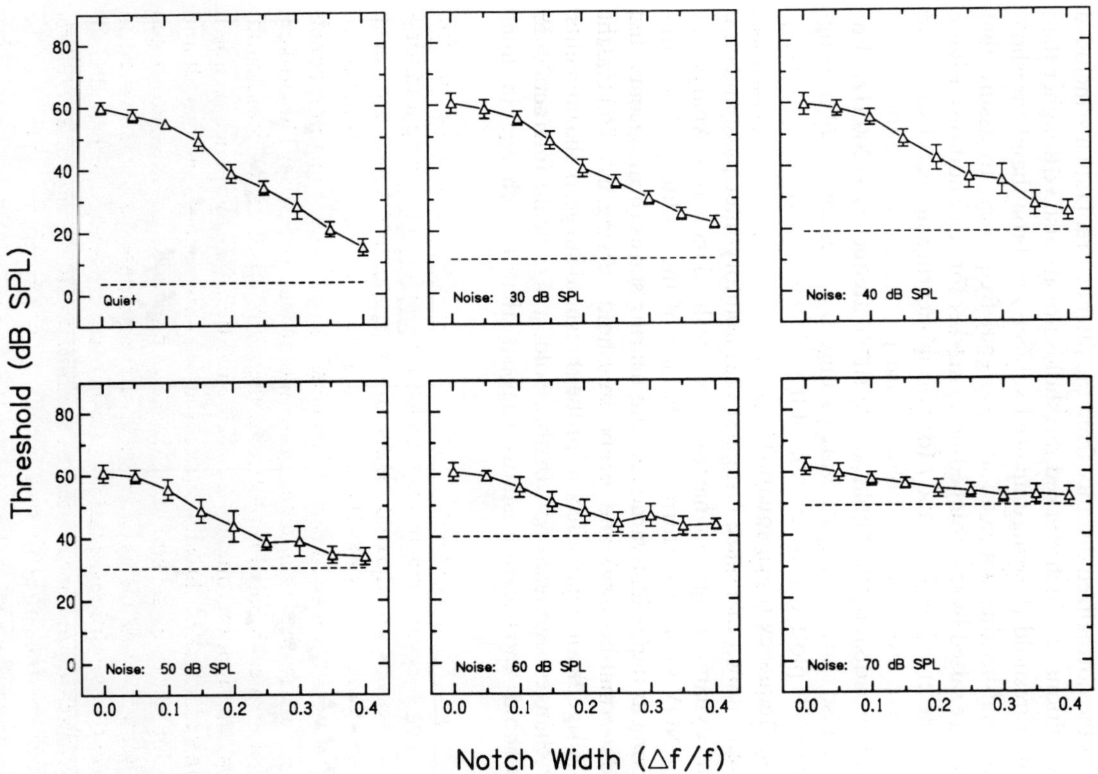

FIG. 2. Mean masked thresholds (in dB SPL) for a 1200–Hz signal in notched noise as a function of the width of the notch for six normal-hearing subjects. Masked thresholds in the upper left panel were obtained with the notched-noise masker only. Each of the remaining panels includes results obtained in notched noise and broadband noise. Overall broadband noise level is identified in the lower left-hand corner of each panel. Error bars encompass ± 1 *SD* from the mean. The broken, horizontal line in each panel is plotted at the mean absolute (or broadband) threshold at the probe frequency for each condition.

which p determines the degree of selectivity of the filter and r is the filter's dynamic range. The two-parameter roex model has the form

$$W(g) = (1 - r)\,(1 + pg)\,e^{-pg} + r$$

in which g is the normalized distance from the filter centre. Data are included only for conditions in which masked thresholds are at least 3 dB higher than the absolute threshold (hearing-impaired subjects) or broadband threshold (masked normal-hearing subjects) at the signal frequency, to assure that thresholds were raised by the notched-noise masker for all conditions. Figure 3 shows parameter values for p and r for normal-hearing subjects listening in quiet and in five levels of broadband noise plotted as a function of the absolute (or broadband) threshold at the signal frequency (1200 Hz). For comparison, also shown in Figure 3 are parameter values for the 24 hearing-impaired subjects plotted as a function of these listeners' absolute thresholds at the signal frequency (open squares).

The results shown in Figure 3 suggest that auditory-filter passbands are broader and dynamic ranges are narrower as threshold increases. Analyses of variance (ANOVA) were performed with each of the auditory-filter parameters serving as dependent variables, and hearing status (hearing-impaired or masked normal-hearing) and probe threshold serving as independent variables. A significant main effect of probe threshold suggests that the filter parameter changes significantly with threshold; a significant interaction of probe threshold and hearing status suggests that the change in filter

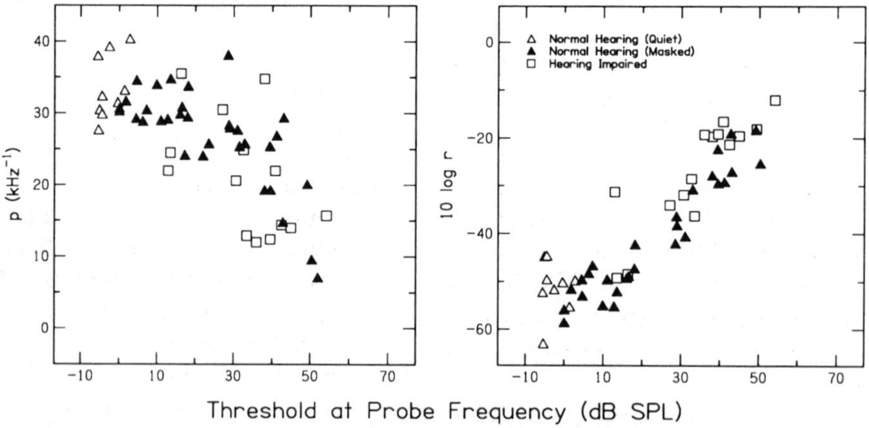

FIG. 3. Auditory-filter passband (left panel) and dynamic range (right panel) as a function of the threshold for the 20-msec, 1200-Hz probe. Data are included for normal-hearing (open triangles) and hearing-impaired (open squares) subjects listening in quiet, and for normal-hearing subjects listening in five levels of broadband noise (filled triangles).

parameter as a function of hearing loss for hearing-impaired listeners is significantly different than the change in filter parameter as a function of broadband threshold for masked normal-hearing listeners. For these data, whereas p and r vary significantly with probe threshold ($p < 0.01$), the interactions between each filter parameter and hearing status are not significant ($p > 0.05$).

Two factors should be noted regarding these results. First, because the spectral notch is positioned symmetrically around the signal, differences in the asymmetry of the auditory-filter shape among subjects will not be observed. Glasberg & Moore (1986) found that the lower-frequency branch of the auditory filter is shallower than normal for hearing-impaired listeners, and that the slopes of the branches vary systematically with threshold. It is not known whether differences in the asymmetry of the auditory-filter shape, and differences in the more steeply-sloping, high-frequency branch of the filter, will remain when comparisons are made between hearing-impaired and masked normal-hearing listeners. Second, the reduction in auditory-filter dynamic range with increased threshold is expected with the roex model. The representation of the "tails" of the auditory filter, determined in the model by masked thresholds at wide notch widths, has been shown previously to be limited by the absolute threshold (Glasberg, Moore, Patterson, & Nimmo-Smith, 1984).

In spite of these weaknesses, the results of the current experiment suggest that comparisons of hearing-impaired and *masked* normal-hearing listeners may more closely reflect changes in frequency selectivity associated with cochlear pathology, rather than comparisons with normal subjects' performance in quiet. Auditory-filter characteristics are associated with threshold and stimulus levels. However, when masked normal-hearing and hearing-impaired subjects' thresholds are equivalent, residual differences observed in their auditory-filter parameters will be independent of the effects of threshold elevation or signal level.

Critical Ratios. Critical ratios for normal-hearing subjects were computed from masked thresholds at 1200 Hz obtained in five levels of broadband noise. Critical ratios for hearing-impaired subjects were computed from masked thresholds at 1200 Hz obtained in the zero-notch condition of auditory-filter measurements (Dubno & Dirks, 1989). As shown in Figure 4, critical ratios remain relatively constant as threshold increases for both masked normal-hearing listeners and hearing-impaired listeners. The results of ANOVAs, conducted as described for the auditory-filter parameters, reveal that critical ratios do not change significantly with probe threshold ($p > 0.05$), and the interaction of probe threshold and hearing status (hearing-impaired or masked normal-hearing) is not significant ($p > 0.05$). That is, critical ratios do not change significantly with absolute threshold for hearing-

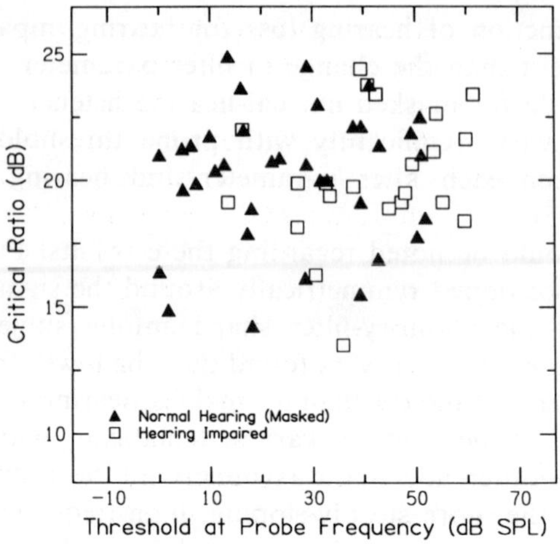

FIG. 4. Critical ratios (masked threshold minus noise spectrum level, in dB) as a function of the absolute (or broadband) threshold at 1200 Hz. Critical ratios for normal-hearing subjects (filled triangles) were computed from thresholds at 1200 Hz obtained in five levels of broadband noise. Critical ratios for hearing-impaired subjects (open squares) were computed from the masked thresholds obtained in the zero-notch condition of auditory-filter measurements (Dubno & Dirks, 1989).

impaired listeners or with broadband threshold for masked normal-hearing listeners. For masked normal-hearing listeners, this result is consistent with the masked thresholds obtained in the zero-notch condition of the auditory-filter measurements in various levels of broadband noise. These masked thresholds remain constant as broadband-noise level increases (see Figure 2).

The results for both groups are similar to those reported for hearing-impaired subjects by Tyler, Fernandes, & Wood (1982) and are also consistent with the predictions of the Humes et al. (1988) model based on masked normal-hearing listeners' thresholds and absolute thresholds of hearing-impaired listeners. It has been suggested that the critical ratio may increase slightly with threshold in some subjects (Tyler et al., 1982). However, the thresholds at which the critical ratio tends to increase are somewhat higher than those obtained in the current experiment (>60 dB SPL). Results from the current experiment suggest that critical ratios for hearing-impaired listeners are equivalent to normal-hearing listeners when measured using comparable signal levels.

Forward-masked Psychophysical Tuning Curves. Figure 5 presents mean PTCs for seven normal-hearing subjects. The triangles are mean masker levels for each masker frequency required to mask the 1200-Hz signal in quiet and in five levels of broadband noise. The filled circles are the listeners' mean

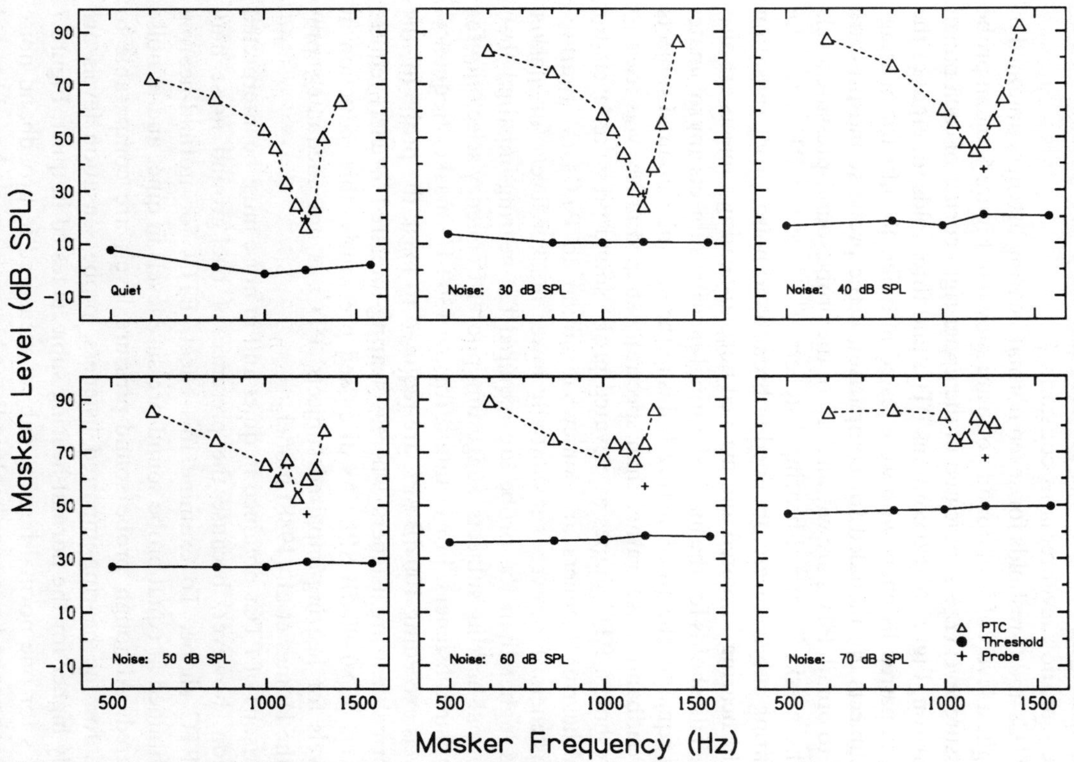

FIG. 5. Mean forward-masked psychophysical tuning curves (open triangles) and thresholds (filled circles) for seven normal-hearing subjects measured in quiet (upper left-hand panel) and in five levels of broadband noise (remaining panels). Overall broadband noise level is identified in the lower left-hand corner of each panel. In each panel, the plus symbol (+) indicates the frequency (1200 Hz) and mean sound-pressure level of the probe. Missing symbols indicate that masker levels are required that exceed the limits set for this experiment.

absolute (or broadband) thresholds at each masker frequency. The plus symbol (+) indicates the frequency and level of the probe, which was set 10 dB above the absolute (or broadband) threshold for the 20-msec probe in each condition. Substantial changes are observed in some aspects of the shape of the PTCs as broadband-noise level increases. These changes could result from increasing probe sound-pressure level or probe threshold; however, probe sensation level remains constant.

Mean PTCs and thresholds for seven normal-hearing listeners obtained in the four highest levels of broadband noise are shown in Figure 6; mean probe sound-pressure level (L_p) is indicated in the upper right corner of each panel. For comparison, Figure 6 also contains PTCs and thresholds for eight of the 24 hearing-impaired listeners who were tested in quiet. Results for hearing-impaired subjects are included for comparison if the probe sound-pressure levels used to obtain PTCs are within 2 dB of the probe sound-pressure levels used for the masked normal-hearing listeners. Because the PTCs for the normal-hearing subjects were obtained in broadband noise, probe sensation levels for the hearing-impaired and masked normal-hearing subjects are also equivalent. Thresholds for the masked normal-hearing subjects approximate, but are not equal to, the absolute thresholds of the hearing-impaired subjects because broadband noise, rather than spectrally shaped noise, was used to elevate thresholds. PTC shapes at elevated probe sound-pressure levels for the normal-hearing listeners are somewhat similar to PTCs for hearing-impaired listeners. However, substantially lower masker levels for masker frequencies higher than the probe are required for hearing-impaired than masked normal-hearing subjects, suggesting poorer frequency selectivity for hearing-impaired listeners. For example, for the 1300-Hz masker frequency, masker levels exceeding 100 dB SPL are required to mask the probe for the masked normal-hearing listeners, whereas hearing-impaired listeners require masker levels of 80–90 dB SPL. As discussed previously, this reduction in masker levels for hearing-impaired subjects' PTCs is not adequately predicted by the Humes et al. (1988) model.

Comparisons of PTCs obtained in quiet and in noise must be interpreted with caution, however, because the presence of background noise may influence PTC shape. To examine this effect, PTCs for normal-hearing listeners obtained at equal probe sound-pressure levels in quiet and in noise are compared. Although probe sound-pressure levels are comparable to levels used for the hearing-impaired listeners, probe sensation levels are significantly higher for the normal-hearing subjects tested in quiet. Figure 7 shows PTCs for one normal-hearing subject measured in broadband noise using the probe sound-pressure levels indicated in each panel. An additional set of PTCs was obtained using these probe levels but without broadband noise. Filled symbols display the absolute (or broadband) thresholds at each masker frequency. As probe sound-pressure and sensation levels increase,

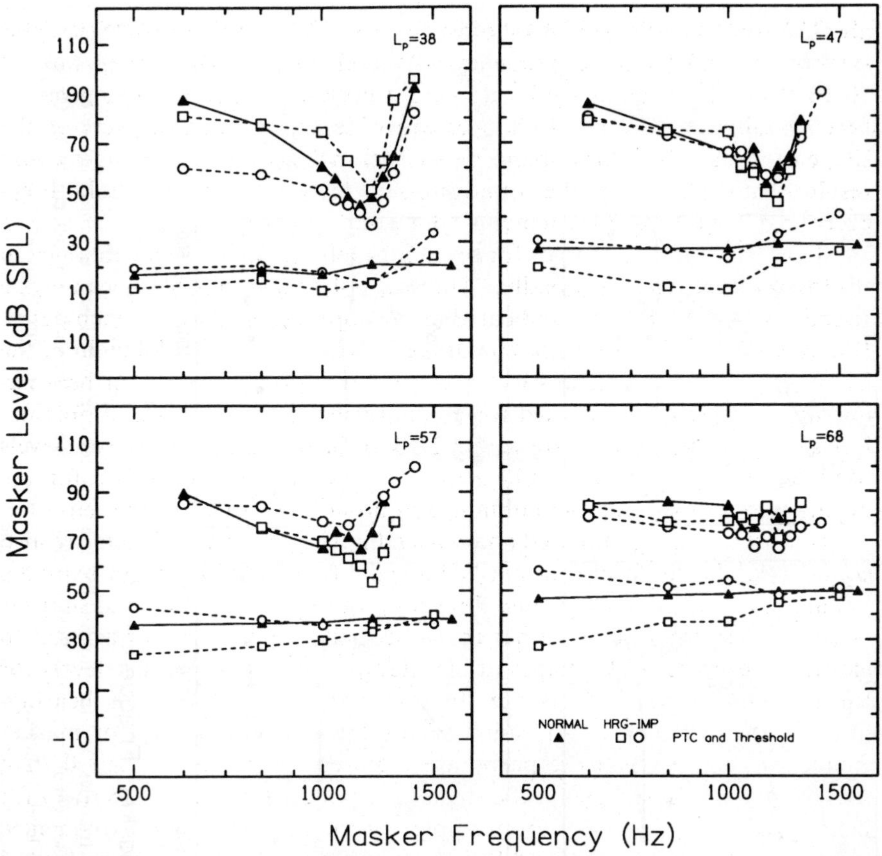

FIG. 6. Forward-masked psychophysical tuning curves and thresholds for seven normal-hearing listeners obtained in the four highest levels of broadband noise (filled symbols). Open symbols are psychophysical tuning curves and thresholds obtained in quiet for eight hearing-impaired listeners (two subjects in each panel). Mean probe levels (L_p, in dB SPL) for the normal-hearing listeners are shown for each noise condition; probe levels for the hearing-impaired subjects are within 2 dB of these levels. Missing symbols indicate that masker levels are required that exceed the limits set for this experiment.

significantly higher masker levels are required to mask the probe in quiet, and somewhat narrower PTCs are obtained relative to those obtained in noise. As is the case for comparisons of masked normal-hearing and hearing-impaired subjects in Figure 6, differences in masker levels are largest for masker frequencies higher than the probe frequency. It is likely that the apparent difference in tuning observed between the quiet and noise conditions is due to the availability of off-frequency cues in quiet as the probe level increases (Green et al., 1981).

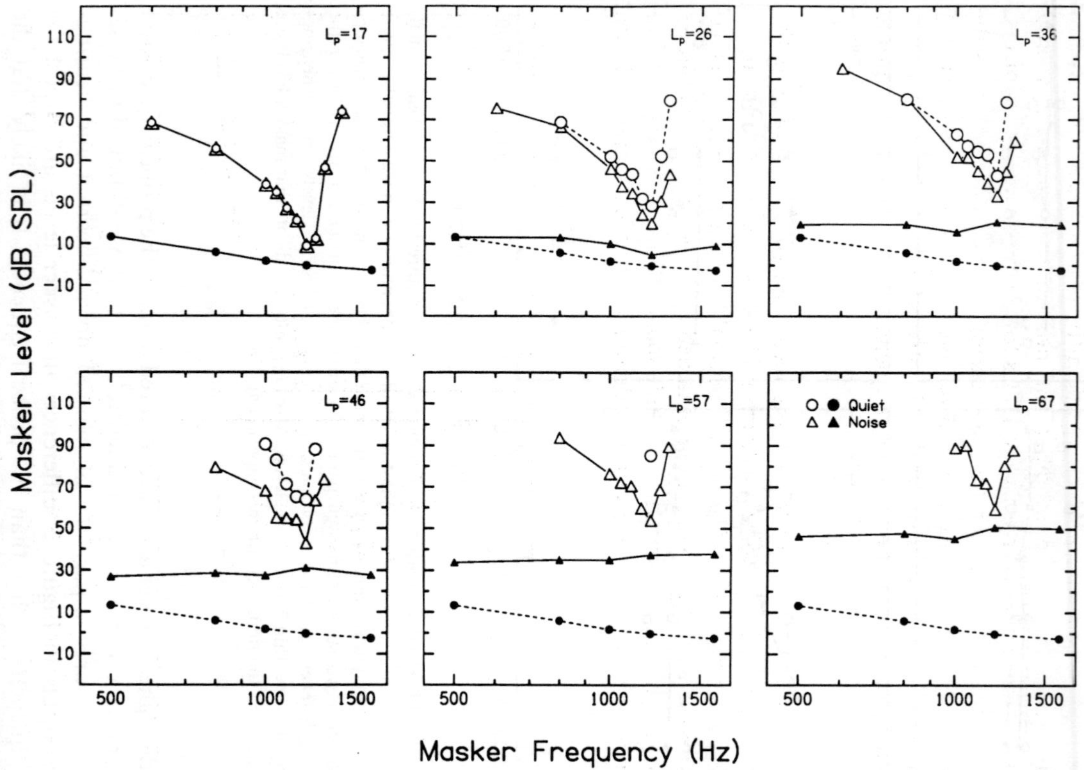

FIG. 7. Forward-masked psychophysical tuning curves (open triangles) and thresholds (filled triangles) for one normal-hearing subject measured in quiet (upper left-hand panel) and in five levels of broadband noise (remaining panels). Probe levels (L_p, in dB SPL) are shown for each condition. Open circles are psychophysical tuning curves obtained at the probe levels indicated but without broadband noise. Filled circles are absolute thresholds. Missing symbols indicate that masker levels are required that exceed the limits set for this experiment.

A final comparison of PTCs was made between normal-hearing and hearing-impaired subjects tested in quiet. In Figure 8, PTCs for one normal-hearing subject tested at two probe sound-pressure levels are compared to PTCs for four of the 24 hearing-impaired listeners. Absolute thresholds are also shown for each subject. Within each panel, probe sound-pressure levels are equal for all subjects, but probe sensation levels are higher for normal-hearing listeners. As noted above, significantly higher masker levels are required to mask the probe in quiet for normal-hearing listeners, and narrower PTCs are obtained relative to PTCs for hearing-impaired subjects. Masker-level differences between normal-hearing and hearing-impaired subjects increase substantially as probe level increases; for normal-hearing subjects, masker levels exceeding 100 dB SPL are required to mask high-level probe signals, even when the masker frequency is adjacent to the probe frequency.

Masking Patterns. Figure 9 contains mean masked thresholds in the presence of a narrowband-noise masker for 11 pure-tone signals ranging in frequency from 630 to 4000 Hz for six normal-hearing subjects. Masked thresholds in the upper left panel were obtained with the narrowband-noise masker alone. The remaining panels include masked thresholds obtained in narrowband noise and four levels of broadband noise. Mean thresholds are

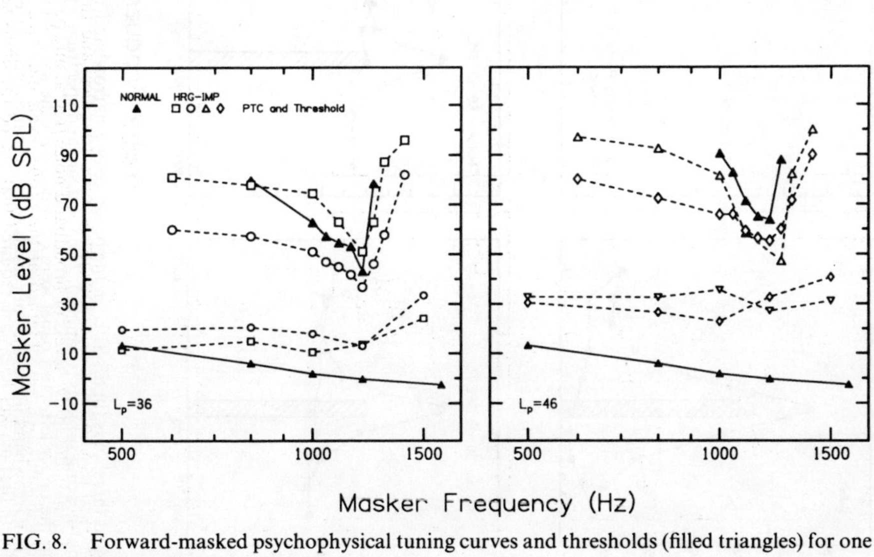

FIG. 8. Forward-masked psychophysical tuning curves and thresholds (filled triangles) for one normal-hearing subject measured in quiet at two probe levels (L_p, in dB SPL). Open symbols are psychophysical tuning curves and thresholds obtained in quiet for four hearing-impaired listeners (two subjects in each panel); probe levels for the hearing-impaired subjects are within 2 dB of probe levels indicated. Missing symbols indicate that masker levels are required that exceed the limits set for this experiment.

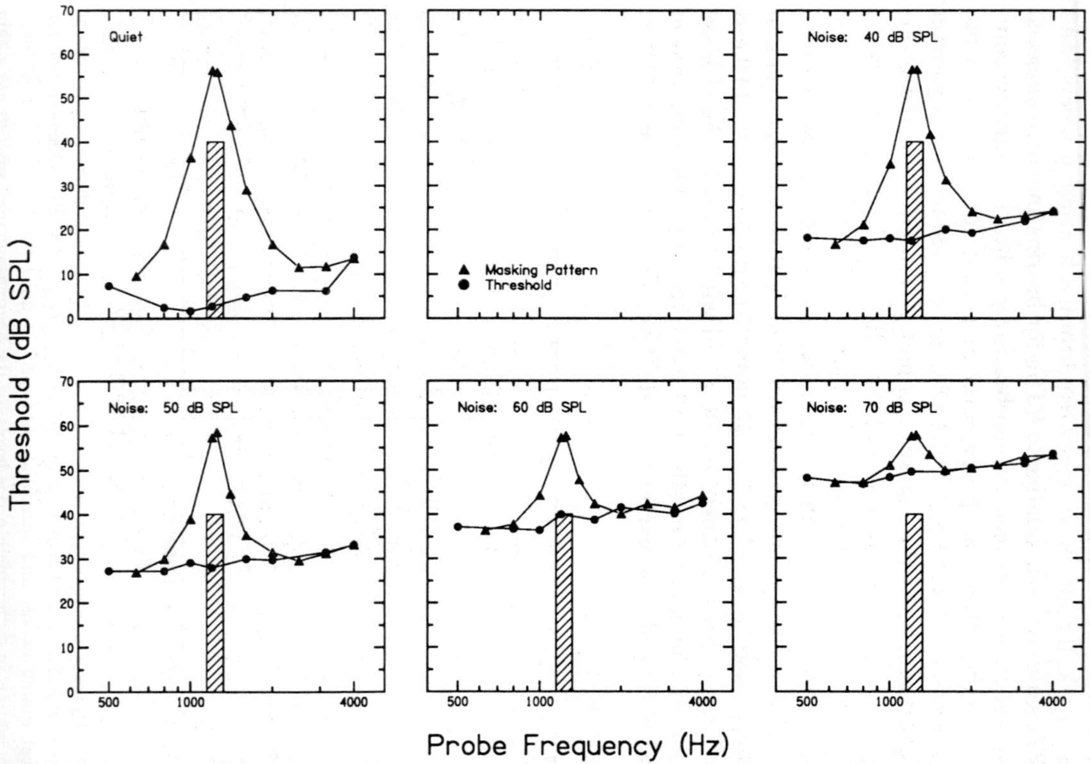

FIG. 9. Mean masked thresholds (in dB SPL) in the presence of a narrowband-noise masker for 11 pure-tone signals ranging in frequency from 630 to 4000 Hz for six normal-hearing subjects (triangles). The spectrum and spectrum level of the narrowband-noise masker are illustrated by the hatched bars. Masked thresholds in the upper left-hand panel were obtained with the narrowband-noise masker only. Each of the remaining panels includes masked thresholds obtained in narrowband noise and four levels of broadband noise. Overall broadband-noise level is identified in the upper left-hand corner of each panel. Thresholds (circles, in dB SPL) for pure-tone signals ranging in frequency from 500 to 4000 Hz were obtained in quiet and in four levels of broadband noise.

also shown for pure-tone signals ranging in frequency from 500 to 4000 Hz in quiet and in broadband noise. In each panel, masked thresholds for signal frequencies within the narrowband-noise passband remain constant as broadband-noise level increases. These results supply further evidence that critical ratios do not change significantly with broadband threshold. For signal frequencies just outside the passband, masked threshold increases slightly with broadband threshold, whereas thresholds at frequencies remote from the masker are equal to the broadband thresholds.

Analogous to the comparisons made for auditory-filter characteristics and PTCs, masking patterns for masked normal-hearing listeners may be compared to those obtained from hearing-impaired listeners. However, this comparison is limited by two factors: (1) The magnitude of hearing loss for frequencies within the masker passband cannot exceed the masker level. (2) To make appropriate comparisons with broadband-noise masked normal-hearing listeners, hearing-impaired listeners' audiometric configuration should be relatively uniform. Furthermore, because masked thresholds were measured across a wide frequency range (630 to 4000 Hz), it is important that the absolute thresholds for the hearing-impaired listeners not exceed the normal-hearing listeners' broadband thresholds in this range. With these restrictions, masking patterns obtained for noise-masked normal listeners in three levels of broadband noise (50, 60, and 70 dB SPL) can be appropriately compared to results for 3 of the 24 hearing-impaired listeners. These 3 subjects have moderate hearing loss and uniform audiometric configurations. A typical masking pattern for a hearing-impaired subject is shown in Figure 10, together with the masking pattern obtained for the masked normal-hearing listeners in the presence of the 60-dB SPL broadband noise. This masking pattern was selected for comparison to the hearing-impaired subject's results because broadband thresholds obtained in this broadband-noise level closely approximate the hearing-impaired listener's absolute thresholds. Masked thresholds within the narrowband-noise passband for the hearing-impaired subject are equal to the masked normal-hearing listeners' thresholds, resulting in equal critical ratios. However, despite the similarity between the absolute and broadband thresholds, the narrowband noise yields higher masked thresholds at frequencies above and (in one instance) below the masker passband for the hearing-impaired listener relative to the masked normal-hearing listeners.

These findings suggest that the narrowband-noise masker produces more upward and downward spread of masking for hearing-impaired listeners than would be predicted from their absolute thresholds. However, these preliminary results are limited to a few individuals with similar uniform audiometric configurations. In comparing masking patterns for normal-hearing and hearing-impaired subjects, listeners with more steeply sloping audiometric configurations, who may be more vulnerable to spread-of-

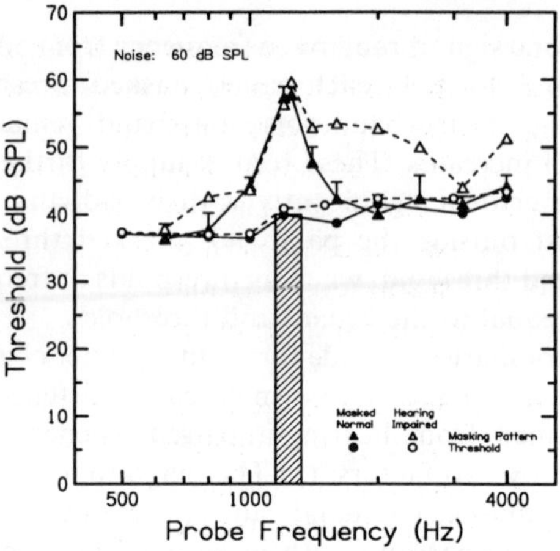

FIG. 10. Mean masked thresholds and +1 *SD* (in dB SPL) obtained in the presence of a narrowband-noise masker and a 60-dB SPL broadband noise for six normal-hearing subjects (filled triangles). Masked thresholds obtained with the narrowband-noise masker for one hearing-impaired subject are shown by the open triangles. Filled circles are the mean thresholds for the normal-hearing subjects obtained with the 60-dB SPL broadband noise only. Open circles are absolute thresholds for the hearing-impaired subject.

masking effects, should be examined. Increased upward spread of masking has been demonstrated in mildly-impaired listeners with sloping configurations (Smits & Duifhuis, 1982; Humes, 1982; Trees & Turner, 1986; Gagne, 1988).

In addition, threshold differences between the hearing-impaired and masked normal-hearing listeners may have influenced the masking-pattern results. Ideally, thresholds for noise-masked normal-hearing listeners and hearing-impaired listeners should be matched exactly. Based on these preliminary results, an experiment (Dubno & Schaefer, 1990) has been conducted comparing masking patterns for hearing-impaired listeners and masked normal-hearing listeners whose thresholds have been precisely matched using spectrally shaped broadband noise. In that experiment, masked thresholds at frequencies above (and in some cases below) the narrowband-noise masker passband are consistently higher for six hearing-impaired subjects than for their masked normal-hearing counterparts.

GENERAL DISCUSSION

The results of this experiment suggest that measurements of frequency selectivity are strongly influenced by signal level and the listener's thresholds. For each of the measurement paradigms used in this experiment, frequency selectivity appears poorer as threshold increases in the presence of either cochlear pathology (hearing-impaired listeners) or broadband noise (normal-hearing listeners). Critical ratios, however, do not change significantly as a function of threshold for either group of listeners. Therefore, with the exception of critical ratios, if frequency selectivity for normal-hearing and hearing-impaired subjects is compared without controlling for the confounding effects of threshold and signal level, the magnitude of the difference in frequency selectivity between normal-hearing and hearing-impaired subjects may be exaggerated.

Frequency selectivity, as determined by masked thresholds measured in broadband noise (i.e. critical ratios), is equivalent for hearing-impaired and masked normal-hearing listeners at moderate signal levels. However, for PTC and masking pattern measurements, frequency selectivity is poorer for hearing-impaired listeners than for masked normal-hearing listeners, even when thresholds and signal levels are equated. Thus, the poor frequency selectively exhibited by hearing-impaired listeners (as observed previously by Florentine et al., 1980, and others) may not be explained entirely by the effects of threshold and signal level. Nevertheless, residual differences in frequency selectivity observed between individuals with sensorineural hearing loss and *masked* normal-hearing listeners may be more directly related to the effects of cochlear pathology.

It has been suggested that residual differences in frequency selectivity may be related to reductions in speech-recognition ability observed in some hearing-impaired subjects that are unaccounted for by elevated thresholds (e.g., Dubno, Dirks, & Schaefer, 1989; Pavlovic, Studebaker, & Sherbecoe, 1986). A reduction in frequency selectivity at higher signal levels may have a differential effect on speech recognition for normal and hearing-impaired listeners. For example, under most listening conditions, spread of masking observed for normal-hearing listeners does not adversely affect speech recognition. However, at normal conversational-speech levels, sensation levels within important spectral regions of the speech signal are reduced for many hearing-impaired individuals. Normal or increased spread of masking at higher signal levels could reduce these sensation levels even further, effectively negating the benefit of increased speech-presentation level. Furthermore, if the speech signal is amplified to assure maximal audibility, speech recognition may not improve as expected if the auditory system does not function optimally at the signal levels provided by the amplification system.

Finally, an additional factor to be considered in comparing performance of hearing-impaired and masked normal-hearing subjects is the effect of the broadband noise used to elevate the thresholds of the normal-hearing listeners. Whereas a single masker is used to obtain the hearing-impaired listeners' masked thresholds, the normal listeners' results are obtained with a combination of two maskers (e.g. a narrowband-noise masker combined with broadband noise). There is considerable disagreement concerning the amount of masking that should result from pairs of temporally and spectrally overlapping maskers, and the role of intermasker suppression (Lutfi, 1983; Humes & Jesteadt, 1989). Additivity-of-masking models will be used to determine whether the effectiveness of the broadband noise is reduced by the more intense second masker, resulting in apparently lower masked thresholds for the masked normal-hearing listeners relative to the hearing-impaired subjects. Finally, for the narrowband-noise masking patterns, the detection of intermodulation distortion products may have also differentially affected masked thresholds for hearing-impaired and masked normal-hearing listeners (Smoorenburg, 1972; Gagne, 1988).

In conclusion, appropriate comparisons of frequency selectivity among normal-hearing and hearing-impaired individuals have been limited as a result of differences in thresholds and stimulus levels among these listeners. Experimental designs that control the confounding effects of threshold and signal level are essential for interpreting differences in frequency selectivity among normal-hearing and hearing-impaired listeners. The current findings suggest that frequency selectivity deteriorates at higher stimulus levels for all subjects. However, in some conditions, frequency selectivity is poorer than normal for hearing-impaired subjects, even when thresholds and signal levels are equated.

REFERENCES

ANSI (1969). *Specifications for audiometers* (ANSI S3.6–1969). New York: American National Standards Institute.

Dubno, J.R. & Dirks, D.D. (1989). Auditory filter characteristics and consonant recognition for hearing-impaired listeners. *Journal of the Acoustical Society of America*, *85*, 1666–1675.

Dubno, J.R. & Schaefer, A.B. (1990). Frequency resolution and consonant recognition for hearing-impaired and masked normal-hearing listeners. *Abstracts of the Thirteenth Midwinter Meeting, Association for Research in Otolaryngology*, *13*, 113.

Dubno, J.R., Dirks, D.D., & Schaefer, A.B. (1989). Stop-consonant recognition for normal-hearing and hearing-impaired listeners with high-frequency sensorineural hearing loss. II. Articulation index predictions. *Journal of the Acoustical Society of America*, *85*, 355–364.

Florentine, M., Buus, S., Scharf, B., & Zwicker, E. (1980). Frequency selectivity in normally-hearing and hearing-impaired observers. *Journal of Speech and Hearing Research*, *23*, 646–669.

Florentine, M. & Buus, S. (1984). Temporal gap detection in sensorineural and simulated hearing impairments. *Journal of Speech and Hearing Research*, *27*, 449–455.

Florentine, M., Fastl, H., & Buus, S. (1988). Temporal integration in normal hearing, cochlear impairment, and impairment simulated by masking. *Journal of the Acoustical Society of America*, *84*, 195–203.

Gagne, J-P. (1988). Excess masking among listeners with a sensorineural hearing loss. *Journal of the Acoustical Society of America, 83*, 2311–2321.

Glasberg, B.R. & Moore, B.C.J. (1986). Auditory filter shapes with unilateral and bilateral cochlear impairments. *Journal of the Acoustical Society of America, 79*, 1020–1033.

Glasberg, B.R., Moore, B.C.J., Patterson, R.D., & Nimmo-Smith, I. (1984). Dynamic range and asymmetry of the auditory filter. *Journal of the Acoustical Society of America, 76*, 419–427.

Green, D.M., Shelton, B.R., Picardi, M.C., & Hafter, E.R. (1981). Psychophysical tuning curves independent of signal level. *Journal of the Acoustical Society of America, 69*, 1758–1762.

Humes, L.E. (1982). Spectral and temporal resolution by the hearing impaired. In G.A. Studebaker & F.H. Bess (Eds.), *The Vanderbilt hearing aid report: State of the art—Research needs* (pp. 16–31). Upper Darby, PA: Monographs in Contemporary Audiology.

Humes, L.E., Espinoza-Varas, B., & Watson, C.S. (1988). Modeling sensorineural hearing loss. I. Model and retrospective evaluation. *Journal of the Acoustical Society of America, 83*, 188–202.

Humes, L.E. & Jesteadt, W. (1989). Models of the additivity of masking. *Journal of the Acoustical Society of America, 85*, 1285–1294.

Jesteadt, W., Stelmachowicz, P.G., & Callaghan, B.P. (1987). Predicting masked thresholds in impaired listeners from combinations of normal masked thresholds and hearing loss. *Journal of the Acoustical Society of America, 81* (Supplement 1), S77.

Levitt, H. (1971). Transformed up-down methods in psychoacoustics. *Journal of the Acoustical Society of America, 49*, 467–477.

Lutfi, R. (1983). Additivity of simultaneous masking. *Journal of the Acoustical Society of America, 73*, 262–267.

Nelson, D.A. (1988). Frequency selectivity at equivalent sound-pressure levels in normal-hearing and hearing-impaired listeners. *Journal of the Acoustical Society of America, 83* (Supplement 1), S75.

Nelson, D.A. & Freyman, R.R. (1984). Broadened forward-masked tuning curves from intense masking tones: Delay-time and probe-level manipulations. *Journal of the Acoustical Society of America, 75*, 1570–1577.

Patterson, R.D., Nimmo-Smith, I., Weber, D.L., & Milroy, R. (1982). The deterioration of hearing with age: Frequency selectivity, the critical ratio, the audiogram, and speech threshold. *Journal of the Acoustical Society of America, 72*, 1788–1803.

Pavlovic, C.V., Studebaker, G.A., & Sherbecoe, R.L. (1986). An articulation index based procedure for predicting the speech recognition performance of hearing-impaired individuals. *Journal of the Acoustical Society of America, 80*, 50–57.

Pick, G.P. (1980). Level dependence of psychophysical frequency resolution and auditory filter shape. *Journal of the Acoustical Society of America, 68*, 1085–1095.

Ritsma, R.J., Wit, H.P., & van der Lans, W.P. (1980). Relations between hearing loss, maximal word discrimination score and width of psychophysical tuning curves. In G. van den Brink & F.A. Bilsen (Eds.), *Psychophysical, physiological and behavioural studies in hearing* (pp. 175–182). Delft, Holland: Delft University Press.

Smits, J.T.S. & Duifhuis, H. (1982). Masking and partial masking in listeners with a high-frequency hearing loss. *Audiology, 21*, 310–324.

Smoorenburg, G.F. (1972). Audibility region of combination tones. *Journal of the Acoustical Society of America, 52*, 603–614.

Trees, D.E. & Turner, C.W. (1986). Spread of masking in normal subjects and in subjects with high-frequency hearing loss. *Audiology, 25*, 70–83.

Tyler, R.S., Fernandes, M., & Wood, E.J. (1982). Masking of pure tones by broad-band noise in cochlear pathology. *Journal of Speech and Hearing Research, 25*, 117–124.

Wightman, F.L., McGee, T., & Kramer, M.C. (1977). Factors influencing frequency selectivity in normal and hearing-impaired listeners. In E.F. Evans & J.P. Wilson (Eds.), *Psychophysics and physiology of hearing* (pp. 295–306). London: Academic Press.

Zwicker, E. & Schorn, K. (1978). Psychoacoustical tuning curves in audiology. *Audiology*, *17*, 120–140.

Revised manuscript received 30 October 1990

THE QUARTERLY JOURNAL OF EXPERIMENTAL PSYCHOLOGY, 1991, *43A* (3) 565–583

Binaural Loudness Matches in Unilaterally Impaired Listeners

Fan-Gang Zeng and Christopher W. Turner

Syracuse University, Syracuse, N.Y., U.S.A.

Binaural loudness matching data using a 2IFC adaptive procedure were obtained in high-frequency, unilateral cochlear-impaired listeners. The matches were obtained at frequencies where both ears had similarly normal thresholds, and also at other frequencies where the impaired ear had various degrees of hearing loss. In these listeners, one presumed difference between the ears is the limited or altered spread of excitation in the impaired ear. In agreement with previous studies using other approaches (Hellman, 1974, 1978; Hellman & Meiselman, 1986; Moore, Glasberg, Hess & Birchall, 1985; Schneider & Parker, 1987), the results of the present study suggest that both the range and the slope of loudness growth function are not dependent on the spread of excitation, but instead are related primarily to the degree of threshold elevation at the test frequency. Following this suggestion, a spread-of-excitation-independent model, based upon a group of neurons with the same characteristic frequency (CF) but different thresholds, is proposed to account for loudness growth in both normal and recruitment cases. In particular, it is shown quantitatively that a compressed distribution of thresholds due to threshold elevation may be responsible for loudness recruitment in sensorineural hearing loss.

Loudness is formally defined as "that attribute of auditory sensation in terms of which sounds may be ordered on a scale extending from soft to loud" (ANSI, 1973). In a normal-hearing listener, loudness sensation for a pure tone can extend across an enormous dynamic range of energy—sometimes exceeding 10^{12}, or 120 dB (Stevens, 1970). How the auditory system encodes such a wide operating range while individual peripheral neurons have a relatively limited operating range (about 30–50 dB in most cases, Evans,

---

Requests for reprints should be sent to Fan-Gang Zeng, House Ear Institute, 2100 West Third Street, Los Angeles, CA 90057, U.S.A.

This research was supported in part by Grants DC00377 and DC00380 from National Institute on Deafness and other Communication Disorders. The authors are grateful to J. J. Zwislocki for a critical reading of an earlier version of this manuscript. The authors would also like to acknowledge the helpful comments from two anonymous reviewers on additional physiological and psychophysical aspects of intensity coding.

1981; Kiang, Watanabe, Thomas, & Clark, 1965) has long been a focus of many psychophysical and physiological studies. Attempts to resolve this dynamic range mismatch have focused primarily on two types of peripheral neural coding schemes that might serve to encode intensity: spread of excitation along the frequency continuum and a distribution of thresholds along the intensity continuum.[1] Following this line of inquiry, the goal of the present study is to investigate the relative importance of these two population responses for the coding of the large range of loudness.

Let us begin by defining the two types of neural population responses considered here and how they are capable of encoding the large range of loudness. Suppose a pure tone stimulus with a level barely above threshold is presented to the auditory system; it would only excite a small group of auditory neurons whose characteristic frequency is similar to the stimulus frequency. As the stimulus level increases, other neurons whose CF is remote from the stimulus frequency will respond (Kim, Chang & Sirianni, 1990, Figures 3 and 4). This type of "spread of excitation" along the basilar membrane (or frequency continuum) has long been viewed as the important coding scheme for loudness. The hypothesis that the loudness of a pure tone is proportional to the summation of its excitation along the frequency continuum forms the basis for Zwicker's loudness coding model (Zwicker, 1975). Recently, this coding scheme has been challenged by the psychophysical finding that the magnitude of loudness for a pure tone is not decreased in cases for which contribution from the tone's spread of excitation is eliminated by using a high-pass and/or low-pass noise as a masker (Hellman, 1974, 1978; Moore, Glasberg, Hess, & Birchall, 1985; Schneider & Parker, 1987). However, the physiological validity of using a masking noise to eliminate the spread of excitation is questionable; recent neurophysiological evidence shows that such a noise does not produce a distinct high- or low-pass edge in the normalized-rate profiles of auditory neurons, especially at high masking levels (Hellstrom, 1989). Avoiding the use of masking noise to restrict the spread of excitation, Hellman and Meiselman (1986) conducted a study in which loudness functions at low frequencies were obtained in sloping high-frequency, bilateral cochlear-impaired subjects using the methods of absolute magnitude estimation and production. The obtained loudness functions for these subjects were similar to those of normal-hearing subjects in terms of the dynamic range and the steepness of loudness growth. This result is incompatible with the idea that loudness is related to the spread of excitation.

---

[1] Other single units properties such as phase locking to the stimulus frequency and the onset response have been shown to play a minor role in accounting for the large psychophysical dynamic range (Viemeister, 1983; Carlyon & Moore, 1984).

An alternative explanation may be found in another type of population coding scheme that is independent of the spread of excitation: CF-neurons with a distribution of thresholds along the intensity continuum. Many physiological studies (Liberman, 1978, Figure 3; Sachs & Abbas, 1974, Figure 3) have shown that there exist a group of neurons originating from a narrow region on the basilar membrane (i.e. similar CF) but with thresholds distributed across approximately a 60-dB range. Such a distribution of thresholds can extend the physiological dynamic range of the auditory system beyond the range offered by a single neuron and potentially yield a range comparable to that of loudness sensation. Such a CF-neuron population coding scheme has been proposed to encode the large range of loudness (Moore et al., 1985) and also applied to models addressing the dynamic range of intensity discrimination as well (e.g. Delgutte, 1987; Viemeister, 1988; Winslow & Sachs, 1988).

A related issue is the phenomenon of loudness recruitment observed in cochlear-impaired ears. Loudness recruitment is an abnormality of intensity coding whereby the growth of loudness of a sound with increases in intensity is steeper than that measured in normal ears. Although loudness recruitment was first described more than 70 years ago by Fowler (1928), its physiological mechanism still remains controversial. By one popular model, loudness recruitment is viewed as a by-product of deteriorated frequency selectivity in cochlear-impaired listeners, which in turn results in an abnormal or more rapid spread of excitation with intensity among auditory neurons of different characteristic frequencies (Evans, 1975; Kiang, Moxon, & Levine, 1970). There is evidence, both psychophysically (Pick, Evans, & Wilson, 1977; Florentine, Buss, Scharf, & Zwicker, 1980) and physiologically (Evans, 1975; Leonard & Khanna, 1984), that frequency selectivity is reduced in hearing impairment of cochlear origin. Nevertheless, this mechanism for loudness recruitment has been challenged by the previously mentioned studies of Hellman (1974, 1978) and Moore et al. (1985), which suggest that loudness recruitment may be due to a physiological abnormality that exists within a narrow range on the basilar membrane.

In the present study, we use listeners with high-frequency hearing loss to investigate the underlying neural mechanisms for loudness coding. This approach is justified because Liberman and Dodds (1984b, Figure 14) showed that the tuning curves of the eighth nerve fibres originating from an impaired region of a cochlea will have elevated sensitivities in the sensitive tip regions. In the specific case of outer-hair-cell loss, the tails of the tuning curves are often hypersensitive, but this hypersensitivity does not exceed 10–20 dB and is limited to frequencies at least 1–2 octaves below the CF of the neuron. Thus, a localized hearing loss would most probably result in an abnormal excitation pattern for stimuli at frequencies just below or above those at which a listener has a sensitivity loss. Thus, the sensation of loudness in these listeners for tones adjacent to the hearing loss might be expected to be abnormal at low and medium stimulus levels, if loudness depends upon the spread of excitation. Therefore, measurement of loudness at these frequencies may shed light on the question: is loudness dependent or independent of the spread of excitation along the basilar membrane? (1) Binaural loudness matches were obtained as a function of intensity at frequencies of hearing loss to verify that loudness recruitment exists. (2) Loudness matches were obtained at other frequencies, where both ears have similar (normal) thresholds, so that one presumed difference between the two ears is the limited or altered spread of excitation in the impaired ear. We also described a modified 2IFC adaptive procedure for obtaining loudness matches, and the results of a validation experiment for this 2IFC procedure (monaural loudness matching). In the discussion, a physiological model based upon a group of CF-neurons with different thresholds is proposed to account the loudness growth functions in both normal and impaired ears.

Methods

Procedure. Many procedures have been used to obtain loudness balances over the years, among which are magnitude balance and cross-modality techniques (Stevens, 1958; Hellman & Zwislocki, 1961; Hellman, 1974, 1978; Hellman & Meiselman, 1986), method of adjustment (Fletcher & Munson, 1933; Ross, 1967), and method of constant stimuli (Robinson & Dadson, 1956). Recently, adaptive procedures have been incorporated into loudness judgements (Jesteadt, 1980; Lim, Rabinowitz, Braida, & Durlach, 1977; Schlauch & Wier, 1987). An adaptive procedure is one in which the stimulus on each trial is a function of the preceding stimuli and responses. This type of procedure has been shown to have many advantages, particularly in terms of speed and efficiency, over the above-mentioned traditional techniques (Zwislocki, Maire, Feldman, & Rubin, 1958; Levitt, 1971; Robinson & Watson, 1972).

We modified Jesteadt's adaptive procedure in order to yield greater efficiency in our loudness-matching experiment. Briefly, Jesteadt procedure is actually a 1IFC procedure and requires the subject on each trial to listen to two consecutively presented tones, a reference tone followed by a comparison tone, and then to judge whether the comparison tone is louder or softer than the reference. The key modification made in the current 2IFC procedure is the realization of the interchangeable concept between the two equivalent statements that *a 250-Hz tone sounds softer than a 1000-Hz tone* and *a 1000-Hz tone sounds louder than a 250-Hz tone*. Put in another way, in contrast to Jesteadt's procedure, we do not need to identify a reference stimulus for the subject at the start of the experiment and ask him/her to judge whether the matching tone is louder or softer than the reference. Rather, the subject is asked to identify the interval that contains the stimulus sounding louder—the 250-Hz tone interval or the 1000-Hz tone interval. If the 250-Hz tone is judged the louder of the pair, then the procedure rule can decrease its intensity. Otherwise, if the 1000-Hz tone sounds louder, then the procedure can increase the 250-Hz tone's intensity. In this case, the 1000-Hz tone serves as a "hidden reference", which doesn't change its intensity during the experiment. One advantage associated with this modification is that a simple instruction to the subject is possible, as well as an easier task or response from the subject—"which one is louder." This task, in which the two intervals for listening also correspond to the two possible responses, is similar to a typical 2IFC procedure to which subjects may be accustomed. Another modification made in this 2IFC procedure is the decision rule. We used a majority decision rule, or the best of three trials, to estimate the point of subjective equality (PSE) directly. The majority rule is defined in such a way that, if a subject gives the "louder" response to the 250-Hz tone in any two consecutive or two out of three trials, then the intensity of the 250-Hz tone is decreased, whereas if the subject gives the "louder" response to the 1000-Hz tone in the same pattern, then the intensity of the 250-Hz tone is increased. The probability of a 250-Hz tone sounding louder than a 1000-Hz tone at a fixed intensity level will converge to 50% when the level of the 250-Hz tone is adjusted by this majority decision rule (see Levitt, 1971, p. 471, entry 8). By so doing, each run will give two estimates of PSE (we are using two interleaving sequences).

A single trial consisted of a pair of successively presented tones, the reference and the comparison. The order of the reference and comparison was randomized across trials. Each of the two intervals in a single trial was 204 msec in duration. The listening intervals were indicated by lights located on the subject's response box. The inter-stimulus interval was 400 msec. No trial-by-trial feedback or any other kind of feedback regarding the matched loudness was given to the subject. Because it was desirable that the judgement for the subject should be very easy for the first several trials, the procedure always started by presenting the comparison tone to the subject at a much higher estimated loudness level than the reference tone in one sequence and much lower in the other sequence. The decrement or increment step for the comparison tone's intensity was 6 dB until the fourth reversal; after that it was changed to a 2-dB step. The procedure automatically terminated following the 14th reversal for each sequence. The intensity value for matched loudness in each run was estimated from the mean of the last 10 reversals. In the binaural matching procedure we always obtained the binaural loudness matching functions with two stimulus paradigms. In one paradigm, the intensity level of a tone to the left ear was fixed and that to the right ear changed according to the subject's response. In the other paradigm, the fixed and variable ears were interchanged. In general, the estimates from both sequences were consistent, without any tendency for one to be greater or smaller than the other. The testing time for a single run (yielding two PSE estimates) usually took 5–6 min.

Subjects. One normal-hearing female, RB, 26 years of age, served as the subject in a methodological validation experiment, in which the 2IFC adaptive procedure was used to obtain equal loudness contours.

Three unilateral cochlear-impaired listeners, ER, MG, and RP, who have moderate to severe high-frequency loss were also employed as subjects. They were 19, 45, and 54 years of age, respectively. Standard audiometric evaluations, including bone-conduction thresholds, tympanometry, acoustic reflex tests, and tone decay measures, indicated that the hearing losses were of cochlear origin. Air-conduction thresholds for 204-msec pure tones were determined using an adaptive threshold-tracking procedure that tracked the 71% level of correct responses. Appropriate masking noise was presented to the normal ear when testing the thresholds in the impaired ears. The thresholds of the normal ears in all three subjects were better than 20 dB (ANSI, 1969) at the test frequencies from 125 Hz to 8000 Hz.

Stimuli. All the test tones were stored on a LSI-11/23 computer's hard disk in digitized form and were output by a digital-to-analog converter (Data Translation 3366) at a sampling rate of 20 kHz. All tones were 204 msec in duration, including a linear 25-msec rise and fall time. The synthesized tones were smoothed by a 10-kHz low-pass filter and presented to the subject via a TDH-49 headphone mounted in an MX-41/AR cushion. The TDH-49 headphone had a relatively flat frequency response up to 5–6 kHz, above which the headphone response decreased. Attenuation was achieved by a Charybdis Model D unit under control of the laboratory computer. Sound levels were expressed as the values measured with the headphone in an NBS-9A coupler.

Results

Validation of the 2IFC Adaptive Procedure. Equal loudness contours from the normal-hearing subject, RB, measured by the 2IFC adaptive procedure, are shown in Figure 1, in which each solid line represents equal loudness levels at the different testing frequencies. The 1000-Hz tone served as the reference tone. The standard deviation for most measurements was about 2–3 dB, with a range of 1.33 dB to 4.74 dB. The slopes derived from the linear regression of the loudness growth functions for all the comparison frequencies are displayed on the table to the right of Figure 1. It can be noted that the slopes for those tones with higher thresholds, especially low frequencies, are 15–22% steeper than 1. The finding that the steep loudness

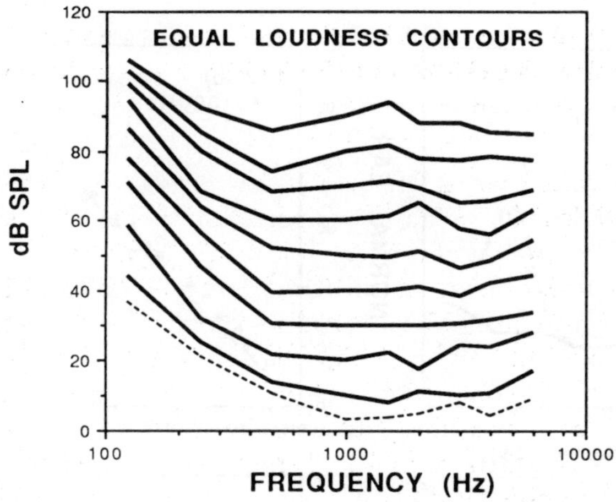

F (Hz)	SLOPE
125	1.22
250	1.20
500	1.15
1000	1.00
1500	0.98
2000	1.03
3000	1.10
4000	1.10
6000	1.17

FIG. 1. Equal loudness contours measured by a 2IFC adaptive procedure in a normal-hearing subject. The thick solid lines represent equal loudness levels at different frequencies. The thin dashed line shows the quiet thresholds of the subject. The table at the right shows the derived slopes (in dB/dB) of loudness matching functions as compared to the 1000-Hz tone.

functions are associated with the elevated low-frequency thresholds has been consistently observed in previous studies using other procedures (Fletcher & Munson, 1933; Ross, 1967; Robinson & Dadson, 1956). The comparable results between the current modified 2IFC adaptive procedure and other previous procedures indicated that the current procedure can be used reliably in our loudness-matching experiment.

Loudness Matching in Unilaterally Impaired listeners. Results from three unilateral cochlear-impaired subjects are presented in Figures 2, 3, and 4, respectively. Each figure displays the results from one subject and has a panel (a) showing that subject's thresholds of audibility in dB HL in both ears (the solid line represents thresholds in the normal ear, and the dashed line represents the impaired ear). The remainder of the panels in each individual figure shows the binaural loudness matching data between ears at frequency regions of normal or elevated thresholds. For reference, the dashed diagonal lines on each loudness-matching function represent a perfect match in intensity between ears.

Binaural loudness matching data at five frequencies, which were obtained in subject MG, are shown in Figure 2. Figure 2 (a) plots the thresholds of audibility in dB HL of both ears. Because the intensity needed for the impaired ear to match the loudness is the same as in the normal ear at high levels—see the matching points lying on the diagonal in Figure 2 (d) and 2 (e)—"complete" loudness recruitment is indicated at the frequencies of

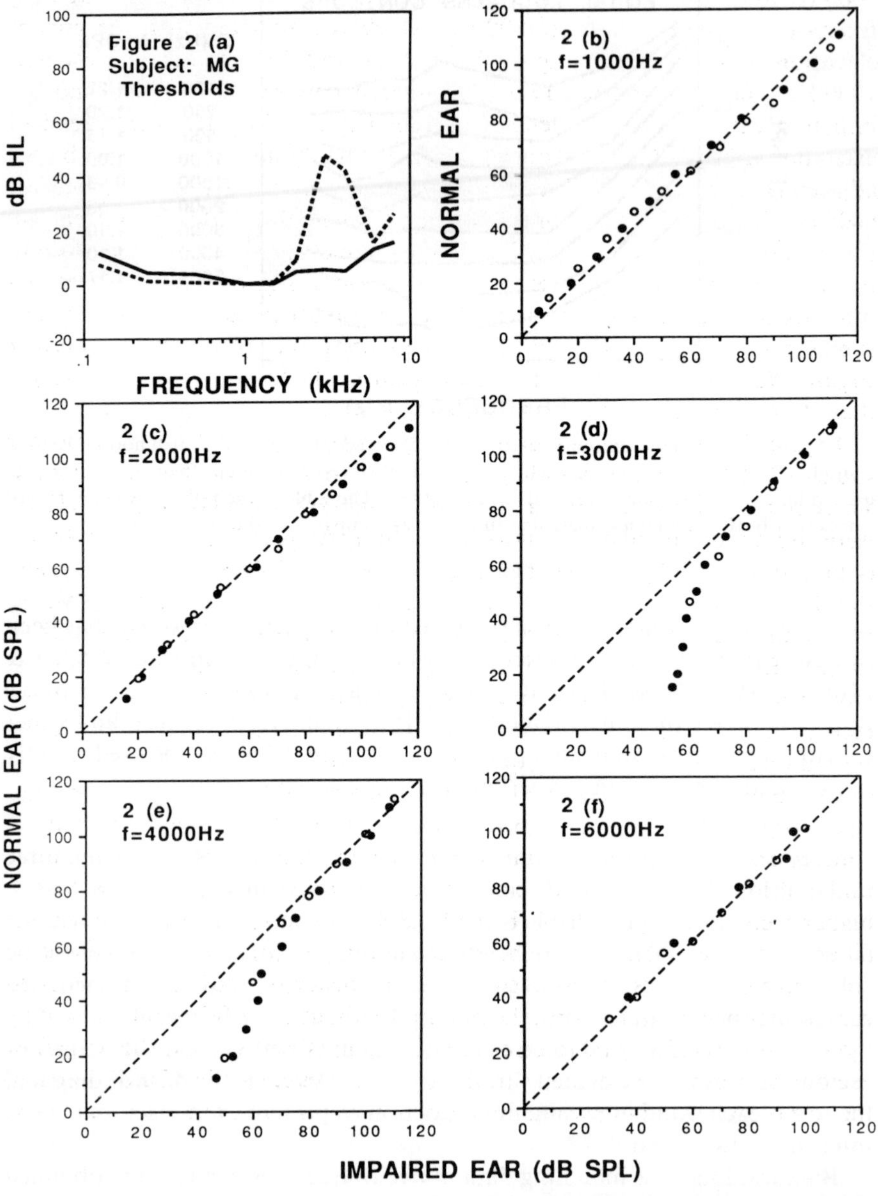

FIG. 2. Binaural loudness matching data set from subject MG. Panel (a) shows the thresholds in dB HL of the normal ear (solid line) and the impaired ear (dashed line). Panels (b)–(f) display the intensities in dB SPL required for both ears to have a matched loudness at five different frequencies. For reference, the dashed diagonal lines represent a perfect loudness match in intensity between the ears. Solid circles are data from conditions under which the reference tone in the normal ear had a fixed intensity during the matching experiment, whereas open circles are the reverse conditions.

3000 Hz and 4000 Hz. Also noted is a steeper slope of loudness—matching function at 3000 Hz than at 4000 Hz, which is associated with the greater elevation of threshold. In Figure 2 (b), 2 (c), and 2 (f), loudness growth at 1000 Hz, 2000 Hz, and 6000 Hz is compared between the normal and the impaired ears. At the frequencies of 1000 Hz and 2000 Hz, the spread of excitation towards higher frequencies is presumably limited or altered by the adjacent hearing loss, whereas that towards lower frequencies is limited for 6000 Hz. However, at these three frequencies, where thresholds are normal, yet the spread of excitation is limited, both the loudness growth range and slope in the impaired ear are very close to normal. Loudness growth functions at two other frequencies, 250 Hz and 1500 Hz, were also obtained and shown to have similar results. A secondary effect on the loudness function may be noticed in Figure 2 (c): the loudness in the impaired ear at 2000 Hz increases less steeply than it does in the normal ear at highest intensities.

Figure 3 shows the binaural loudness-matching results from another subject, ER, who has an audiogram similar to the previous subject, MG. Three points on subject ER's audiogram—1000 Hz, 1500 Hz, and 2000 Hz—were chosen as the binaural loudness-matching frequencies, because 1000 Hz is at the lower edge of the hearing loss region, 1500 Hz is at the rising shoulder of the hearing loss contour, and 2000 Hz is at the point where maximum hearing loss occurs. Basically, it can be seen that the results of subject ER replicate the findings that have been described in Figure 2. However, an additional point in Figure 3 (c) demonstrates complete loudness recruitment at 1500 Hz (where some hearing loss existed), although the spread of excitation at this frequency is limited.

Compared with subjects MG and ER, subject RP has a more severe high-frequency hearing loss, as shown in Figure 4 (a). Again, the same general conclusions are reached from this subject's data. In other words, the dynamic range of loudness appears to be relatively unaffected by the hearing loss at higher frequencies—Figure 4 (b) and (c). Let us also consider some subtle differences in this subject. It can be noticed in Figure 4 (c) and (d) that there is an "incomplete" loudness recruitment at the frequency of 1000 Hz (the impaired ear can not catch up the normal ear, lagging about 7–8 dB behind). This may indicate that loudness recruitment may depend slightly upon the spread of excitation. However, compared to the significant effect of threshold elevation, the role of the spread of excitation in loudness recruitment would be secondary.

DISCUSSION

Empirical Issues

The current results from the binaural loudness matching in unilateral cochlear-impaired listeners suggest that both the range and the steepness of loudness growth may not be dependent on the spread of excitation, but

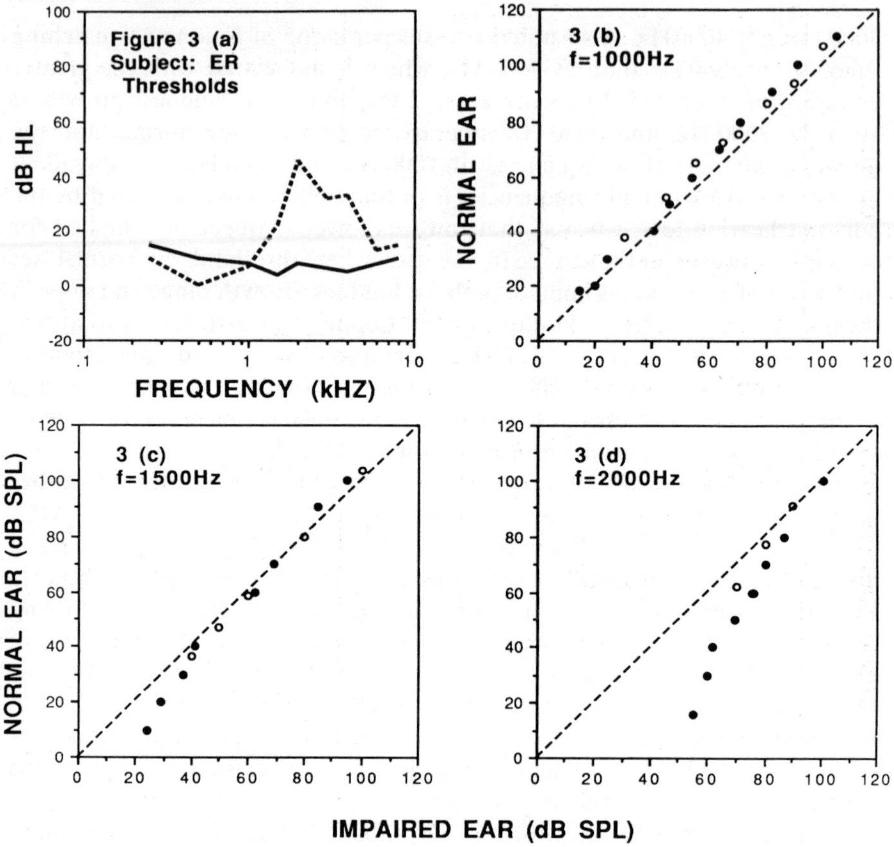

FIG. 3. Binaural loudness matching data set from subject ER. Symbols are the same as those in Figure 2.

instead be related primarily to the degree of threshold elevation. Our finding in terms of the role of the spread of excitation in loudness coding supports previous studies using high- and/or low-pass noise masking (Hellman, 1974, 1978; Moore et al., 1985; Schneider & Parker, 1987) and that using absolute magnitude estimation/production technique in bilateral cochlear-impaired listeners (Hellman & Meiselman, 1986). The present results suggest that alterations in the pattern of spread of excitation, as caused by cochlear hearing loss, have little if any effect upon the sensation of loudness. This result holds true for cases in which spread is limited in either the upward (basal) or downward (apical) direction. Therefore, it appears reasonable to accept the conclusion put forth by other investigators that loudness of a pure tone can be encoded within a narrow range along the basilar membrane. Similar conclusions for the mechanisms of intensity discrimination have also been postulated (Moore & Raab, 1974; Viemeister, 1974, 1983).

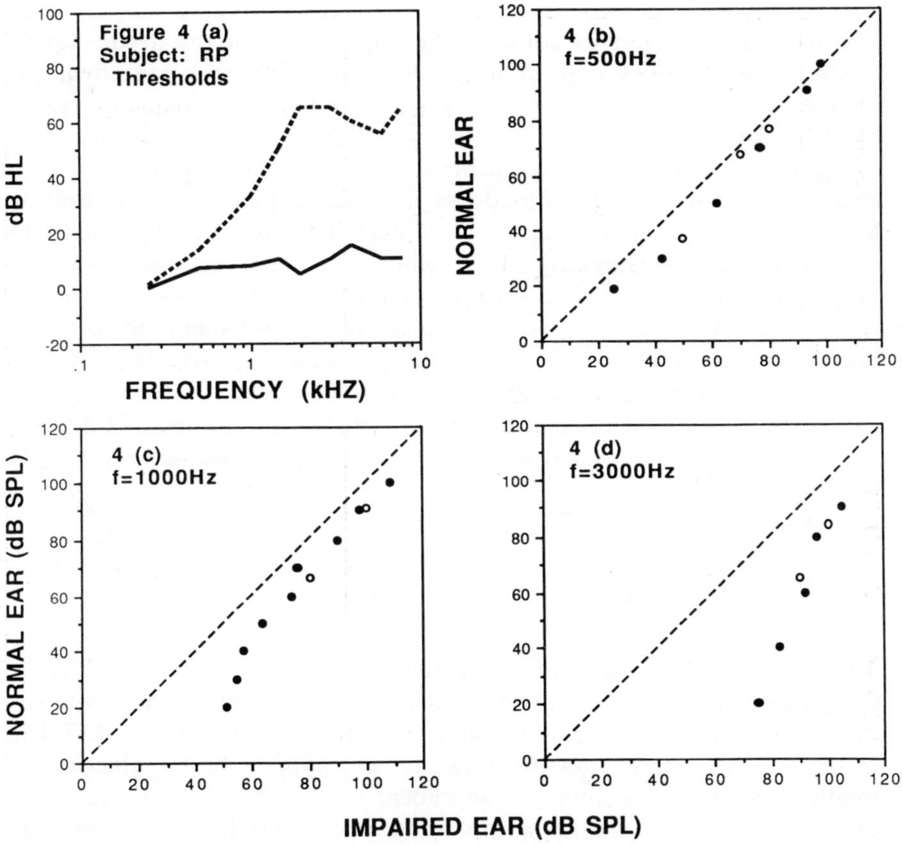

FIG. 4. Binaural loudness matching data set from subject RP. Symbols are the same as those in Figure 2.

Clinical Implications. Loudness recruitment and associated phenomena, such as intensity discrimination, have been used widely as a clinical diagnostic tool to distinguish between the hearing loss of cochlear origin and retrocochlear origin (for a summary, see Hallpike, 1976). One of the most valuable tests for loudness recruitment is the ABLB (Alternate Binaural Loudness Balance: Fowler, 1937). The test requires a unilaterally hearing-impaired listener to match the loudness of two tones that have the same frequency and are presented alternately to the two ears. Thus, the test is limited to listeners with unilateral hearing loss. Reger and Kos (1952), among others, have suggested the use of a monaural loudness balance technique when the patient has a bilateral symmetrical hearing loss. This technique has been applied to the hearing loss population when there is a substantial difference in the thresholds at neighbouring frequencies, such as in presbycusic hearing-loss cases. Let us consider the implications of this technique. If loudness coding does depend upon the spread of excitation, then the loudness growth for the tone in the normal-threshold, low-frequency region of a high-frequency hearing loss listener would be reduced. One consequence of a shallower growth at low frequencies is that the intensity level required to produce the same amount of loudness at higher frequencies, where hearing loss is present, would be reduced accordingly. This would lead to the result that loudness as measured by a monaural balance technique seems to grow more steeply at the high frequencies, namely the phenomenon of loudness recruitment. However, this may not actually be the case, due to the fact that loudness at high frequencies would not really grow more steeply itself, but, rather, the loudness of the low-frequency reference tone, to which the high-frequency is balanced grows less steeply. On the other hand, the present study has demonstrated that loudness at the lower frequencies, where the sensitivity is normal, grows in a normal fashion. Thus the present results provide additional validation for the use of a monaural balance technique to test for recruitment.

Theoretical Models

To our knowledge, most theoretical loudness models incorporating physiological data have used the spread of excitation to account for the power law of loudness functions (e.g. Goldstein, 1974; Howes, 1974; Lachs & Teich, 1981). As the current and previous studies support the hypothesis that loudness coding is essentially independent of the spread of excitation, a quantitative model, based upon a distribution of neural thresholds, similar to those used by Delgutte (1987), Viemeister (1988), and Winslow and Sachs (1988) in predicting intensity discrimination data, seems more reasonable.

Degree of Spread of Excitation and Loudness. Neither the present study nor the previous ones can quantitatively define the width of the region on the basilar membrane needed to encode the sensation of loudness. Information available from using hearing-impaired subjects is limited by the fact that one hearing-impaired subject only provides one type of alteration in the spread of excitation—usually high-frequency hearing loss. Using high- and low-pass noise masking may be questionable due to both the lack of supporting physiological evidence and the undefined non-linear interactions between the masker and tone, especially when the bandwidth of the noise notch is narrow. To answer this question requires further study, in which the degree of the spread of excitation can be precisely controlled without the above-mentioned limitations. For the present, we make the simplifying assumption that loudness can be encoded from the neural outputs originating from a single hair cell. The model that is described in the following section can be easily modified to assume a larger distance along the basilar membrane simply by including a multiplicative constant.

Single Hair-Cell Loudness Coding Model. We consider only a single hair cell case in the current model. Liberman (1978) suggested that each inner hair cell, which receives an average of 26 neurons, has about 16 high-, 6 medium-, and 4 low-SR neurons. The maximum rate change (the difference between saturation and spontaneous rate), taken from Winslow and Sachs (1988), is in the order of 100, 180, and 130 spike per sec for high-, medium-, and low-SR neurons, respectively. For the sake of visual convenience, two simplifying assumptions concerning these physiological data were made without changing the model in principle: (1) As the medium- and low-SR neurons share many properties in terms of rate-intensity functions, we have combined them as one group of neurons. (2) We have normalized the maximum rate change to 100 spike per sec for all neurons and assumed that the number of the combined medium- and low-SR neurons increases to 16 accordingly. This is because the overall maximum rate change for the new group of neurons (medium/low-SR) is $6*180+4*130 \sim 1600$ spikes per sec. The rate-intensity functions for these neurons follow the descriptive equations of Sachs and Abbas (1974), and Winslow and Sachs (1988, pp. 172, 175, and 187). Figure 5 (a) displays 6 such rate-intensity functions[2] for each group of neurons, with high-SR neurons having solid lines, and medium/low-SR neurons having dashed lines. Three obvious differences between these two groups of neurons can immediately be observed in Figure 5 (a). (1) Threshold differences: high-SR neurons have low thresholds, whereas medium/low have high thresholds; (2) dynamic range differences: high-SR neurons have a relatively limited dynamic range of about 35 dB, whereas medium/low may have up to 100 dB of dynamic range because of the sloping saturation characteristic; (3) threshold distribution differences: high-SR neurons have a narrow threshold distribution (about 10 dB), whereas medium/low have a distribution of about 40 dB. These differences are in general consistent with the physiological data of Liberman (1978) and Winslow and Sachs (1988), though some secondary differences such as an overlapping of the threshold distribution between two groups of SR neurons is not included in the present model.

Supposing that loudness is directly proportional to the overall driven rate of this group of auditory neurons, the linear summation of the driven rate from each neuron as a function of intensity is plotted as the filled squares in

[2] In addition to the spontaneous and maximum rate, three more parameters were needed to specify the rate-intensity functions in the present model: Saturating function constant $N = 1.77$; compression threshold $\theta_I = 100$ dB SPL; and the range of excitatory threshold θ_E for high-SR neurons was from 30 to 40 dB SPL, while that for medium/low-SR neurons was from 60 to 100 dB SPL.

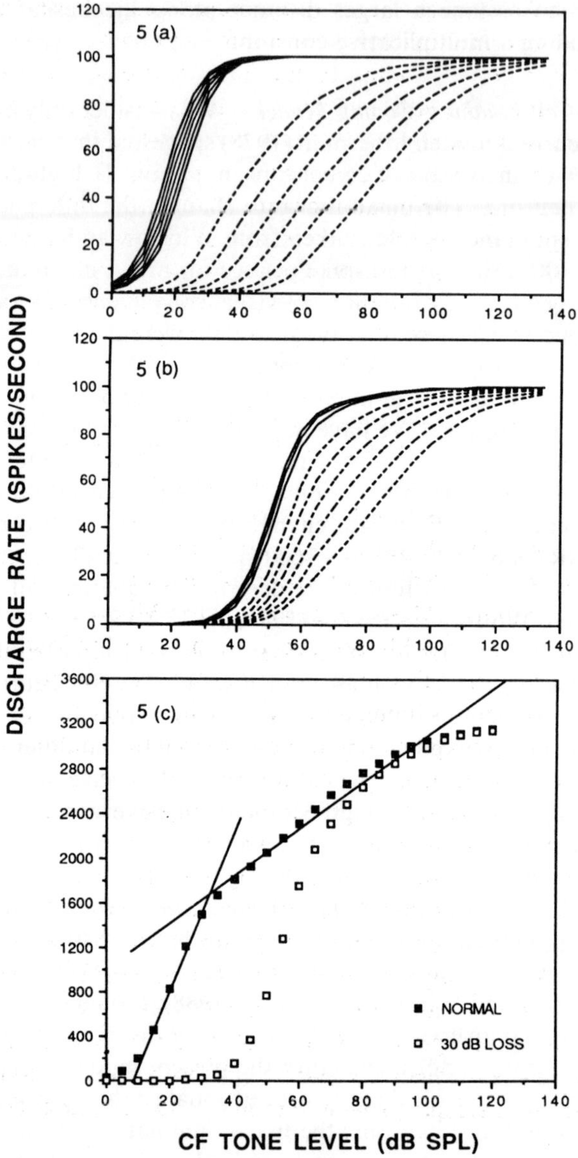

FIG. 5. One hair-cell loudness coding model. Panel (a) shows the simplified normal rate–intensity functions from two groups of auditory neurons with same CF but different thresholds. The low-threshold neurons, associated with high-SR, are plotted as the solid lines, whereas the high-threshold neurons with medium/low-SR are plotted as the dashed lines; Panel (b) shows same functions for those neurons as in Panel (a) in a case of 30-dB hearing loss; Panel (c) shows the overall driven rate from the two groups of neurons as a function of intensity, with the solid squares representing the normal case and the open squares representing the 30-dB loss case. Two solid straight lines are plotted as a typical loudness growth function, with the steeper line having a slope of 1 and the shallower line having 0.5.

Figure 5 (c). The two straight lines across those filled squares represent the two segments on a typical loudness function for a pure tone. The steeper line has a slope of one corresponding to the well-described phenomenon that loudness grows linearly with intensity at low levels (Zwislocki, 1965); whereas the shallower line represents the power function of loudness growth for mid- to high-intensities.[3] The close correspondence between the predicted overall driven rate change from all the neurons innervating one hair cell and the psychophysical data regarding the shape of loudness function suggests that, at least in theory, it is physiologically feasible to encode the enormous dynamic range of loudness within a very narrow CF range on the basilar membrane.

Mechanisms of Recruitment and Other Implications. Liberman and his colleagues have reported a series of studies regarding the effects of chronic cochlear pathology (either noise- or drug-induced) on auditory neurons' response properties such as threshold, spontaneous rate, and rate-intensity functions (Liberman, 1984; Liberman and Dodds, 1984a; Liberman and Kiang, 1984). One of the effects of cochlear hearing loss is a compressed distribution of thresholds. Moore et al. (1985) and Moore (1989, p. 78) have discussed this effect as possibly serving a mechanism for loudness recruitment in cochlear-impaired listeners. We quantitatively implement this effect in the current model by assuming an upward shift of all neurons' thresholds by an amount linearly proportional to their original thresholds: the lower the original threshold of a neuron, the greater the shift applied to that neuron. Figure 5 (b) demonstrates such an effect of a compressed threshold distribution among these neurons in the case of a 30-dB hearing loss. Compared with Figure 5 (a), the highest-threshold neuron (rightmost dashed line) shows little change, whereas the low-threshold neurons are shifted towards higher thresholds. The compression effect on these low-threshold, high-SR neurons is so strong that we can only visibly plot 3 of them in this figure, as compared to 6 in the normal case—panel (a). The corresponding "loudness", expressed as the summed neural outputs, in the case of the 30 dB hearing loss is shown in Figure 5 (c) as open squares. Figure 5 (c) shows that "loudness" in the hearing loss ear has a steeper growth than in the normal ear at first and then

---

[3] The slope of the shallower line is 0.5, when referenced to the steeper line representing a linear growth of loudness as a function of intensity at low levels. Such a two-stage function shape was also observed in the basilar membrane input–output curves (Sellick, Patuzzi, & Johnstone, 1982; Robles, Ruggero, & Rich, 1986), which were in turn suggested to determine the rate-intensity functions of different SR neurons (Yates, Winter, & Robertson, 1990). In other words, loudness sensation, related to the firing rate of different SR neurons, may already have been determined at the level of basilar membrane.

catches up; in other words, loudness recruitment is simulated in our single-hair-cell model.

Two physiological features are considered as most likely to account for the success of predicting loudness function in the current model: a distribution of different thresholds among all neurons, and the sloping saturation characteristic for medium/low-SR neurons. It is interesting to note that both high-SR neurons and medium/low-SR neurons are able to provide an equal overall rate of approximately 1600 spikes per sec, respectively. As the high-SR neurons cover a narrow dynamic range about 30–40 dB, whereas the medium/low neurons cover the remainder of the loudness growth range (about 80 dB), this leads to the steeper growth of loudness at low levels and shallower growth as level increases. This is an interesting prediction, because it is the collective behaviour of this group of neurons (due to the distribution of thresholds and sloping saturation) that gives rise to this characteristic of loudness function, which is also present in the basilar membrane input–output curves (Sellick, et al., 1982; Robles, et al., 1986). In contrast to Phillips' (1987) suggestion, the current model indicates that the steepened rate-intensity function is not critical in accounting for the loudness recruitment, especially for those high-SR neurons. As one can see in Figure 5 (b), the rate-intensity functions' slopes of the high-SR neurons have changed little as compared with normal case—Figure 5 (a). While the rate-intensity functions for the medium/low-SR neurons are steepened, it is the compressed distribution of thresholds that has the greatest effect on the slope of the loudness growth function. This argument may provide a consistent explanation for the loudness recruitment in both cases of cochlear-impairment and noise-masking, as Costalupes, Young, and Gibson (1984) showed that simultaneous noise masking produces a similar horizontal shift towards higher levels on the rate-intensity functions. In summary, the loudness function predicted by the current model is consistent with the present and previous experimental results and their conclusions: that is, loudness function may be primarily dependent on the threshold elevation (or hearing loss) within a narrow region on basilar membrane, whereas the effect of the spread of excitation may be secondary.

REFERENCES

ANSI (1969). *American National Standard Specifications for Audiometers.* [ANSI S3.6–1969 (R1973)]. New York: American National Standard Institute.

ANSI (1973). *Psychoacoustical terminology.* New York: American National Standard Institute.

Carlyon, R.P. & Moore, B.C.J. (1984). Intensity discrimination: A severe departure from Weber's law. *The Journal of the Acoustical Society of America*, *76*, 1369–1376.

Costalupes, J. A., Young, E.D., & Gibson, D.J. (1984). Effects of continuous noise backgrounds on rate response of auditory nerve fibers in cat. *Journal of Neurophysiology*, *51*, 1326–1344.

Delgutte, B. (1987). Peripheral auditory processing of speech information: Implications from a physiological study of intensity discrimination. In M.E.H. Schouten (Ed.), *The psychophysics of speech perception* (pp. 333–353). Utrecht, Netherlands: Martinus Nijhoff.

Evans, E.F. (1975). The sharpening of cochlear frequency selectivity in the normal and abnormal cochlea. *Audiology, 14*, 419–442.

Evans, E.F. (1981). The dynamic range problem: place and time coding at the level of cochlear nerve and nucleus. In J. Syka & L. Aitkin (Eds.), *Neural mechanisms of hearing* (pp. 69–85). New York/London: Plenum Press.

Fletcher, H.F. & Munson, W.A. (1933). Loudness, its definition, measurement and calculation. *Journal of the Acoustical Society of America, 5*, 82–108.

Florentine, M., Buss, S., Scharf, B., & Zwicker, E. (1980). Frequency selectivity in normal-hearing and hearing-impaired observers. *Journal of Speech and Hearing Research, 23*, 646–669.

Fowler, E.P. (1928). Marked deafened areas in normal ears. *Archives of Otolaryngology, 8*, 151–155.

Fowler, E.P. (1937). The diagnosis of diseases of the neural mechanism of hearing by the aid of sounds well above threshold. *Laryngoscope (St. Louis), 47*, 289–300.

Goldstein, J.L. (1974). Is the power law simply related to the driven spike response rate from the whole auditory nerve? In H.R. Moskowitz (Ed.), *Sensation and measurement* (pp. 223–229). Dordrecht: Reidel.

Hallpike, C.S. (1976). Sensorineural deafness and derangements of the loudness function: their nature and clinical investigation. In W.D. Keidel & W.D. Neff (Eds.), *Auditory system: Clinical and special topics* (pp. 1–35). Berlin: Springer-Verlag.

Hellman, R.P. (1974). Effect of spread of excitation on the loudness function at 250 Hz. In H.R. Moskowitz (Ed.), *Sensation and measurement* (pp. 241–249). Dordrecht: Reidel.

Hellman, R.P. (1978). Dependence of loudness growth on skirts of excitation patterns. *The Journal of the Acoustical Society of America, 63*, 1114–1119.

Hellman, R.P. & Meiselman, C.H. (1986). Is high-frequency hearing necessary for normal loudness growth at low frequencies? *Proceedings of the Twelfth International Congress on Acoustics*, (Vol. 1, pp. B11–15), Toronto: Beauregard Press.

Hellman, R.P. & Zwislocki, J.J. (1961). Some factors affecting the estimation of loudness. *The Journal of Acoustical Society of America, 33*, 687–694.

Hellstrom, L.I. (1989). Physiological responses to the pulsation threshold paradigm. I: Pulsation threshold patterns do not reproduce physiological rate profiles of high-pass and low-pass noise maskers. *The Journal of the Acoustical Society of America, 85*, 230–242.

Howes, W.L. (1974). Loudness function derived from data on electrical discharge rates in auditory nerve fibers. *Acoustica, 30*, 247–259.

Jesteadt, W. (1980). An adaptive procedure for subjective judgments. *Perception and Psychophysics, 28*, 85–88.

Kiang, N.Y.-S., Moxon, E.C., & Levine, R.A. (1970). Auditory-nerve activity in cats with normal and abnormal cochleae. In G.E.W. Wolstenholme, J. Knight, & A. Churchill (Eds.), *Sensorineural hearing loss, Ciba Symposium* (pp. 241–273). London: Churchill.

Kiang, N.Y.-S., Watanabe, T., Thomas, E.C., & Clark, L.F. (1965). *Discharge patterns of single fibers in the cat's auditory nerve*. Cambridge, MA: M.I.T. Press.

Kim, D.O., Chang, J.G., & Sirianni, J.G. (1990). A population study of auditory-nerve fibers in unanesthetized decerebrate cats: Response to pure tones. *The Journal of the Acoustical Society of America, 87*, 1648–1655.

Lachs, G. & Teich, M.C. (1981). A neural-counting model incorporating refractoriness and spread of excitation. II. Application to loudness estimation. *The Journal of the Acoustical Society of America, 69*, 774–782.

Leonard, D.G.B. & Khanna, S.M. (1984). Histological evaluation of damage in cat cochlea used for measurement of basilar membrane mechanics. *The Journal of the Acoustical Society of America, 75*, 515–527.

Levitt, H. (1971). Transformed up-down methods in psychoacoustics. *The Journal of the Acoustical Society of America, 49*, 467–477.

Liberman, M.C. (1978). Auditory-nerve response from cats raised in a low-noise chamber. *The Journal of the Acoustical Society of America, 63*, 442–455.

Liberman, M.C. (1984). Single-neuron labeling and chronic cochlear pathology. I. Threshold shift and characteristic-frequency shift. *Hearing Research, 16*, 33–41.

Liberman, M.C. & Dodds, L.W. (1984a). Single-neuron labeling and chronic cochlear pathology. II. Stereocilia damage and alterations of spontaneous discharge rates. *Hearing Research, 16*, 43–53.

Liberman, M.C. & Dodds, L.W. (1984b). Single-neuron labeling and chronic cochlear pathology. III. Stereocilia damage and alterations of thresholds tuning curves. *Hearing Research, 16*, 55–74.

Liberman, M.C. & Kiang, N.Y.-S. (1984). Single-neuron labeling and chronic cochlear pathology. IV. Stereocilia damage and alterations in rate- and phase-level functions. *Hearing Research, 16*, 75–90.

Lim, J.S., Rabinowitz, W.M., Braida, L.D., & Durlach, N.I. (1977). Intensity perception VIII. Loudness comparisons between different types of stimuli. *The Journal of the Acoustical Society of America, 62*, 1256–1267.

Moore, B.C.J. (1989). *An introduction to the psychology of hearing* (3rd ed.). London: Academic Press.

Moore, B.C.J., Glasberg, B.R., Hess, R.F., & Birchall, J.P. (1985). Effects of flanking noise bands on the rate of growth of loudness of tones in normal and recruiting ears. *The Journal of the Acoustical Society of America, 77*, 1505–1513.

Moore, B.C.J. & Raab, D.H. (1974). Pure-tone intensity discrimination: Some experiments relating to the "near-miss" to the Weber's law. *The Journal of the Acoustical Society of America, 55*, 1049–1054.

Phillips, D.P. (1987). Stimulus intensity and loudness recruitment: Neural correlates. *The Journal of the Acoustical Society of America, 82*, 1–12.

Pick, G.F., Evans, E.F., & Wilson, J.P. (1977). Frequency resolution in patients with hearing loss of cochlear origin. In E.F. Evans & J.P. Wilson (Eds.), *Psychophysics and physiology of hearing*. London: Academic Press.

Reger, S.N. & Kos, C.M. (1952). Clinical measurements and implications of recruitment. *Annals of Otolaryngology, 61*, 810.

Robinson, D.E. & Watson, C.S. (1972). Psychophysical methods in modern psychoacoustics. In J.V. Tobias (Ed.), *Foundations of modern auditory theory* (Vol. 2, pp. 99–131). New York: Academic Press.

Robinson, D.W. & Dadson, R.S. (1956). A re-determination of the equal-loudness relations for pure tones. *British Journal of Applied Physics, 7*, 166–181.

Robles, L., Ruggero, M.A., & Rich, N.C. (1986). Basilar membrane mechanics at the base of the chinchilla cochlea. I. Input-output functions, tuning curves, and response phases. *The Journal of the Acoustical Society of America, 80*, 1364–1374.

Ross, S. (1967). Matching functions and equal-sensation contours for loudness. *The Journal of the Acoustical Society of America, 42*, 778–793.

Sachs, M.B. & Abbas, P.J. (1974). Rate versus level functions for auditory-nerve fibers in cats: tone bursts stimuli. *The Journal of the Acoustical Society of America, 60*, 1157–1163.

Schlauch, R.S. & Wier, C.C. (1987). A method for relating loudness-matching and intensity-discrimination data. *Journal of Speech and Hearing Research*, *30*, 13–20.

Schneider, B.A. & Parker, S. (1987). Intensity discrimination and loudness for tones in notched noise. *Perception and Psychophysics*, *41*, 253–261.

Sellick, P.M., Patuzzi, R., & Johnstone, B.M. (1982). Measurement of basilar membrane motion in the guinea pig using the Mossbauer technique. *The Journal of the Acoustical Society of America*, *72*, 131–141.

Stevens, S.S. (1958). Problems and methods of psychophysics. *Psychological Bulletin*, *54*, 177–196.

Stevens, S.S. (1970). Neural events and the psychophysical law. *Science*, *170*, 1043–1050.

Viemeister, N.F. (1974). Intensity discrimination of noise in the presence of band-reject noise. *The Journal of the Acoustical Society of America*, *56*, 1594–1600.

Viemeister, N.F. (1983). Auditory intensity discrimination at high frequencies in the presence of noise. *Science*, *221*, 1206–1208.

Viemeister, N.F. (1988). Psychophysical aspects of auditory intensity coding. In G.M. Edelman, W.E. Gall & W.M. Cowan (Eds.), *Auditory functions: Neurobiological bases of hearing* (pp. 213–241), New York: John Wiley.

Winslow, R.L. & Sachs, M.B. (1988). Single-tone intensity discrimination based on auditory-nerve rate responses in backgrounds of quiet, noise, and with stimulation of the crossed olivocochlear bundle. *Hearing Research*, *35*, 165–190.

Yates, G.K., Winter, I.M., & Robertson, D. (1990). Basilar membrane nonlinearity determines auditory nerve rate-intensity functions and cochlear dynamic range. *Hearing Research*, *45*, 203–220.

Zwicker, E. (1975). Scaling. In W.D. Keidel & W.D. Neff (Eds.), *Handbook of sensory physiology. Auditory system* (Vol. V/2, pp. 401–448). Berlin/New York: Springer-Verlag.

Zwislocki, J.J. (1965). Analysis of some auditory characteristics. In R.D. Luce, R.R. Bush, & E. Galanter (Eds.), *Handbook of mathematical psychology* (pp. 80–96). New York: John Wiley.

Zwislocki, J.J., Maire, F., Feldman, A.S., & Rubin, H. (1958). On the effect of practice and motivation on the threshold of audibility. *The Journal of the Acoustical Society of America*, *30*, 254–262.

Revised manuscript received 31 December 1990

THE QUARTERLY JOURNAL OF EXPERIMENTAL PSYCHOLOGY, 1991, *43A* (3) 585–601

Vowel and Consonant Recognition with the Aid of a Multichannel Cochlear Implant

Michael F. Dorman
Arizona State University, Tempe, Arizona, U.S.A.

Korine Dankowski
Richards Medical, Memphis, Tennessee, U.S.A.

Geary McCandless, James L. Parkin
University of Utah School of Medicine, Salt Lake City, Utah, U.S.A.

Luther Smith
Sinai Samaritan Medical Center Milwaukee, Wisconsin, U.S.A.

In this report we review the vowel and consonant recognition ability of patients who use a multichannel cochlear implant and who achieve relatively good word identification scores. The results suggest that vowel recognition is accomplished by good resolution of the frequency of the first formant (F1) combined with poor resolution of the frequency of the second formant (F2). The results also suggest that consonant recognition is accomplished (1) by using information from the amplitude envelope, including periodicity/aperiodicity, as cues to manner and voicing, (2) by using F1 as an aid to the identification of manner and voicing, and (3) by using information from cochlear place of stimulation to provide a very crude indication of the shape of the frequency spectrum above 1 kHz.

In this report we describe the word, consonant, and vowel recognition ability of patients who use the Ineraid multichannel cochlear implant. The patients were individuals who had lost all functional hearing bilaterally following insult to the peripheral auditory system. The implant was designed to stimulate electrically elements of the auditory nerve and, in so doing, to

Requests for reprints should be sent to: Prof. M.F. Dorman, Department of Speech and Hearing Science, Arizona State University, Tempe, Arizona 85287–0102 U.S.A.

Support for this research was provided by the National Institute for Deafness (RO1–00654).

restore to the patients a measure of auditory sensitivity and some degree of speech and non-speech recognition. Our aim in this report is to infer from the results of several experiments the information in the speech signal that is used by these patients to identify the elementary units of speech, that is, the consonants and vowels. In the first part, we review previous research. In the second, we present the results of two new experiments.

Implant Design

The Ineraid prosthesis consists of (1) 6 monopolar electrodes implanted in the scala tympani with remote reference; (2) a percutaneous pedestal to which the electrode wires are attached, and (3) a portable speech processing and electrode stimulation system (Eddington, 1980). The most apical electrode is located about 22 mm from the round window. The electrodes are spaced at 4 mm intervals. The four most apical electrodes are activated in most patients.

Each electrode is driven by an analogue signal derived from the input signal after the operation of an automatic gain control (AGC) circuit and bandpass filtering. The AGC circuit has a very rapid attack time and a relatively slow release time. The centre frequencies of the filters for channels 1–4 (most-apical to most-basal electrodes) are 0.5 1, 2, and 3.4 kHz. The filters roll off at 6 dB/octave.

Given the depth of insertion of the electrodes and their spacing, the bandpassed input to each electrode may be a half octave or more lower in frequency than the corresponding place of cochlear stimulation (see Greenwood, 1990, for a discussion of cochlear frequency position functions).

Coding of Information

Information about consonant and vowel identity is present in the time, amplitude, and frequency domains of an acoustic signal. Shannon (1986) demonstrated in a variety of tasks that temporal resolution can be similar for implant patients and for normal hearing listeners when signals are presented at similar loudness levels. However, Hochmair-Desoyer, Hochmair, and Stiglbrunner (1985) and Tyler, Moore and Kuk (1989a) have found large individual differences among implant patients when temporal resolution is assessed by gap detection.

All implant patients evidence a very reduced dynamic range for signal amplitude (dynamic range is the difference in signal levels sufficient to elicit a response at threshold and to elicit a response of uncomfortable loudness). Hochmair-Desoyer et al. (1985) report dynamic ranges as small as 3 dB and only as large as 25 dB. Dankowski and McCandless (1990) report dynamic ranges between 6 and 17 dB for patients who use the Ineraid.

Implant patients extract only a limited amount of information about stimulus frequency from the acoustic signal. For implant patients, frequency is specified by "rate" and/or "place" codes.

Rate coding is accomplished by auditory fibers discharging in synchrony, or phase locking, to the period of an electrically delivered stimulus. Significant phase locking has been reported for frequencies greater than 1 kHz (Dynes, 1989; Hartmann & Klinke, 1990). However, psychophysical studies with implant patients who use a single electrode prosthesis indicate that pitch increases with pulse rate to only approximately 1000 pulses per sec (pps). For some patients, the perception of pitch may asymptote at a rate as low as 175 pps (Hochmair-Desoyer, Hochmair, Burian, & Stiglbrunner, 1983; Townshend, Cotter, Van Campernolle, & White, 1987). Difference limens for pitch can be very small (10%) for pulse rates up to 300 pps but are much larger (15–40%) for pulse rates near 1000 pps.

The spectral properties of a signal can also be encoded along a scale of relative frequency by information about the *place* of cochlear stimulation. Eddington (1980) assessed the relative pitch of signals presented to a series of monopolar electrodes arrayed from basal to apical locations in the scala tympani. For a given repetition rate, relative pitch increased in a non-linear fashion as more basal electrodes were stimulated. Thus, if signals are bandpass filtered, as in the Ineraid prosthesis, and the energy in the bands is directed to an array of intracochlear electrodes, the rank ordering of the frequency bands can be preserved.

For many Ineraid patients, the number of pitch percepts at frequencies greater than 1 kHz is not limited to the number of channels in the prosthesis or electrodes in the cochlea. For example, when signals are presented in 300-Hz increments between 1 and 2 kHz, patients report hearing changes in pitch. We may account for this in the following way: Recall that signals are delivered to the electrodes after bandpass filtering at 6 dB/octave. The shallow skirts of the filters ensure that a given signal will present energy to more than one electrode. Thus, as signals are varied between 1 kHz and 2 kHz, the distribution of current at electrodes 1–4 will vary. The changes in the distribution of current along the cochlea may be the mechanism that underlies the changes in pitch (see Townshend et al., 1987).

Patients who use the Ineraid prosthesis appear to use a combination of rate and place coding for frequency analysis. Smith (1988) reported that when pure tone signals were directed to a single electrode, pitch estimates reached asymptote at stimulation rates between 400 Hz and 1 kHz. When pure tones were directed through the signal processing system of the Ineraid to all four electrodes, pitch estimates increased with stimulation rate up to 2–3 kHz. Presumably, the increase in range of pitch estimates resulted from place coding of frequencies higher than 1 kHz.

Word Recognition

Patients who use the Ineraid prosthesis have been tested with a variety of word lists. Dorman, Dankowski, Smith, and McCandless (1989b) reported scores ranging from 0 to 100% correct for 50 patients tested with two-syllable (or spondee) words. The median score was 44% correct. Dorman et al. also reported scores ranging from 0 to 60% correct for a more difficult single-syllable word test (the NU-6 word list). The median score on this test was 14% correct. The relatively high scores posted by the best patients suggests that a significant amount of information about consonant and vowel identity can be extracted from the auditory representation of the speech signal (see also Gantz et al., 1988, and Tyler et al., 1989a, for discussions of word recognition by implant patients).

Recognition of Vowels

For normal hearing listeners, the principal cues to vowel identity are the frequencies of the first, second, and third formants of the speech signal. These formant frequencies cover a range of approximately 3.0 kHz. For the "front" vowels in English, the vowels in "beet", "bit", "bait", "bet", "bat", good resolution of low-frequency information (under 600 Hz) combined with poor resolution of higher-frequency information is sufficient for recognition (Dubno & Dorman, 1987). In the extreme condition of having *only* F1 present in the signal, some vowels can still be identified with accuracy greater than chance by some listeners. Dorman and Dubno reported that two of ten normal hearing patients scored greater than 90% correct for a set of five front vowels created with only F1.

The data reviewed above suggest that vowel identification scores for multichannel implant patients would be better than chance if F1 frequency were well resolved and some information about F2 frequency were available.

We have conducted several experiments to assess the ability of implantees to recognize vowels. Our first experiment was conducted with a single subject who had achieved high scores on tests of word recognition (Dorman et al., 1988). The stimuli were 12 computer-synthesized words that shared a common initial and final consonant (/b/ and /t/, respectively), and which differed in the medial vowel (e.g. "beet", "bit", "bet"). Three sets of the 12 stimuli were created. For one, all five formants were synthesized. For a second, only the first formant was synthesized. For a third, only F2–F5 were synthesized. Vowel duration was constant for all sets. The patient was 79% correct for the signals with five formants, 33% correct for the signals synthesized with only F1, and 41% correct for the signals synthesized with only F2–F5. These results indicate that information about both the first and higher formants can be available for use by patients in the task of vowel identification (see also Tyler, Tye-Murray, & Otto, 1989b, for an elegant demonstration of the use of the first and second formants in vowel identification).

In a second experiment, eight patients who had achieved scores of greater than 70% correct on a test of word recognition were presented the 12 synthesized words for identification (Dorman, Dankowski, Smith, & McCandless, 1989a). The combined confusion matrix for the patients is shown in Figure 1. The range of scores was 49 to 79% correct. The mean score was 60% correct. The vowels in "beet", "bit", "bait", "bite", "bet", "bat", "Bert", "boot" were relatively well identified (mean score = 70% correct). The vowels in "but", "bought", "boat" were not well identified (mean score = 29% correct). These vowels were characterized by relatively low-frequency F2s (858–1200 Hz) and relatively high-frequency F1s (greater than 625 Hz starting frequency). Overall, error responses for a given vowel

RESPONSE

STIMULUS	beet	bit	bait	bet	Bert	bat	but	bought	bout	boat	bite	boot
beet	95											5
bit	11	64	4	4	11	1	2					3
bait	11	9	49	3	12	1	1			3	1	9
bet		8		76		8	6				2	
Bert		4	4	3	82	4			1		1	1
bat				4		67	16	2	9	2		
but	1	3		16	5	28	29	17			1	
bought				7		12	22	35	6		13	
bout		1	1			3	2		23	66	4	
boat		1	1	3	4		9	7	6	54	6	7
bite			5	6	1	1		3	4	11	69	
boot		3		7			3	2	3	1		80

FIG. 1. Percent response to synthetic "bVt" stimuli by implant patients.

were vowels with similar F1 and F2. In most instances, the error responses were not widely distributed but, rather, were the one or two vowels with the most similar formant pattern. Errors in which vowels with high F2s were heard as vowels with low F2s, for example "boot" for "beet", were relatively uncommon.

The small number of cases in which a vowel with a high F2 was confused with a vowel with a low F2 suggests that information about extreme values of F2 was available for use in identification. This information is probably specified by a place code. Electrode 2 would be maximally activated by low F2s (near 1 kHz) and Electrode 3 would be maximally activated by high F2s (near 2 kHz).

The relatively good identification of front vowels suggested that F1 was well resolved. This follows from the view that the principal cue to vowel "height" is F1. To assess this directly, four patients were tested in a same–different task to determine the difference limen for an isolated F1. The "standard" F1 was at 400 Hz, and the "comparison" F1s ranged from 400 to 500 Hz. A mean level of 75% correct was achieved with a difference of 60 Hz (Dorman et al., 1989a). This degree of resolution is sufficient for the differentiation of most F1s in English and is most probably the result of rate coding (although it is not possible from the present data to rule out an account based on the relative distribution of current along the cochlea).

Recognition of Consonants

Information about consonant identity exists in the time, amplitude, and frequency domains of the acoustic signal. If implant patients extract time-intensity (envelope) information from the signal with fidelity, then certain manner distinctions among consonants should be well marked (Summerfield, 1985). In a vowel–consonant–vowel (vCv) environment, stop consonants are marked by a period of relative silence and so should not be confused with semivowels, nasals, or fricatives, which lack the distinctive silent interval. By similar logic, the stop-initiated fricative in "chin" should not be confused with the fricatives in "sin" or "fin".

Envelope information could also contribute to the distinction between voiced and voiceless stop consonants (see, for example, Van Tassel, Soli, Kirby & Widin, 1987). In a vCv environment, voiced stops are characterized by the presence of a low-amplitude voicing signal during the period of stop closure. Voiceless stops are characterized by a period of silence during closure. However, the voiced–voiceless distinction is also marked by a number of other cues. Rosen (1989) suggests that the voiced–voiceless distinction may be signalled, most generally, by the presence of periodicity or aperiodicity, which in the Ineraid occurs most commonly in low and high channels, respectively, of the implant.

Finally, envelope cues can aid in the identification of the fricatives in "fin" and "thin" on the one hand, and in "sin" and "shin" on the other. The two pairs of voiceless fricatives are normally marked by large differences in the amplitudes of the fricative noises—the fricatives in "fin" and "thin" can be 15 dB less intense than the fricatives in "sin" and "thin", which in turn may be 5–10 dB less intense than an accompanying vowel.

As we noted above, resolution of cues in the frequency domain is constrained by the upper limit of rate coding and by limited information about place of cochlear stimulation. Most generally, these constraints will limit the resolution of cues to *place* of articulation. As a consequence, we should expect that information about place will be transmitted with less fidelity than information about manner or voicing.

The results of a consonant identification task for 10 implantees who had relatively good word identification scores are shown in Figures 2 and 3

STIMULUS \ RESPONSE	b	d	g	p	t	k	s	sh	th	ch	z	m	n	w	l	y
b	100															
d	7	60	33													
g		20	80													
p				60	33	7										
t				7	80	7	7									
k					20	80										
s							100									
sh							7	93								
th	20	13					40		20		7					
ch										100						
z	7	7				7			13		47	7				13
m									7			53	27	7		7
n												20	60		7	13
w												20	13	47	13	7
l												7		27	60	7
y											13					87

FIG. 2. Percent response to "vCv" stimuli by "better" patients.

RESPONSE

STIMULUS	b	d	g	p	t	k	s	sh	th	ch	z	m	n	w	l	y
b	51	20	6	11	3								3	3	3	
d	14	48	28			6							3			
g	3	31	48	6	3	9										
p				46	43	6		3		3						
t				23	28	46					3					
k	3			11	26	57	3									
s	9	6	3	17	6		26		14		6	6			9	
sh								97		3						
th	20	3	3	9			17		37			3	3	3	3	
ch					6		11			83						
z	6						3		3		11			60	14	3
m	6	3							3		3	60		6	20	
n												14	57	14		14
w									3					74	17	6
l									6			3		60	23	9
y																100

FIG. 3. Percent response to "vCv" stimuli by "poorer" patients.

(Dorman et al., 1990). The stimuli were naturally produced consonants in "vCv" format.

The mean score, averaged over all subjects, was 58% correct. Three subjects achieved scores better than 60% correct. The confusion matrix for these "better" subjects is shown in Figure 2. Seven subjects achieved scores less than 60% correct. The confusion matrix for these "poorer" subjects is shown in Figure 3.

The results were analysed in term of conditional information transmitted (Soli, 1990) for envelope features of the signals and for the more traditional features of place, manner, and voicing. The envelope features were those defined by Van Tassel et al. (1987). Voicing envelope cues distinguish voiced from voiceless consonants and were described earlier in this section. Amplitude envelope cues distinguish voiced consonants with a high amplitude, /mnwrly/, from all other consonants. Burst amplitude cues distinguish voiceless stops from other consonants on the basis of the high intensity, burst/affrication segment at signal onset.

The analyses indicate that the better patients received 75% or more of the information about the features of burst envelope, amplitude envelope, voicing envelope, and frication. In contrast, the poorer subjects received only 47 to 62% of the available information about those features. Thus, the better subjects received about 30% more information than the poorer subjects for the burst envelope, amplitude envelope, and frication features. Much smaller differences (10 to 17%) were seen for the features voicing envelope, place, and nasality (see Tye-Murray & Tyler, 1989, for another feature analysis of consonant identification by Ineraid patients).

EXPERIMENT 1
Cues to Stop Consonant Place of Articulation

In the study described above, stop consonant place of articulation was recognized at an above-chance level of performance. Three cues influence the identification of place: The onset frequency and direction of the second and third formant transitions (Liberman, Delattre, Cooper, & Gerstman, 1954), the "tilt" of the spectrum at signal onset [high frequency emphasis for /d/, "peaked", middle frequency emphasis for /g/ and low frequency emphasis for /b/ (Blumstein, Issacs, & Mertus, 1982)], and the abruptness of spectral change following onset (abrupt for /b/ and /d/, non-abrupt for /g/) (Kewley-Port, 1983; Lindholm, Dorman, Taylor, & Hannley, 1988).

Our aim in Experiment 1 was to assess the contribution of these cues to the identification of stop consonants by our patients and by a group of normal-hearing listeners. To accomplish this, we created a set of stimuli in which the three stimulus factors were crossed (3 types of formant transition × three types of spectral tilt; and 3 types of formant transition × two levels of abruptness).

Method

Subjects. The subjects were 18 normal-hearing adults and three implantees. The normal-hearing listeners ranged in age from 22 to 56 years. The implantees ranged in age from 31 to 53 years. The implantees were chosen for participation in the experiment on the basis of consonant recognition scores greater than 50% correct (on the 16-item test described in the previous experiment) and on availability for testing. Patient 1 lost his hearing following a skull fracture and had been deaf for 1 year before implantation. Patient 2 lost her hearing following a progressive hearing loss of unknown origin. She had been deaf for 28 years before implantation. Patient 3 lost his hearing following Meniere's Disease. He had been deaf for 5 years before implantation.

Stimuli. The prototype stimuli were the spoken words "bill", "dill", and "gill". The stimuli with conflicting transitions and spectral shape at onset were created by digitally filtering the onsets of the signals so that the onset spectrum was similar to that of one of the two other stimuli (e.g. the stimulus with /b/ transitions was given a rising, or /d/-like, spectral shape at onset). The stimuli with conflicting transition and abruptness of frequency change cues were created by digitally concatenating or removing waveform segments at signal onset. The duration of the burst and aspiration segments of "bill" and "dill" were approximately 9 msec in duration. To create "bill" and "dill" with non-abrupt frequency change following onset, three 9-msec segments were concatenated. The burst and aspiration segment of "gill" was 27 msec in duration. To create "gill" will an abrupt frequency change following onset, an 18-msec segment was removed from the signal following the initial 9-msec segment.

The test was a randomized sequence of eight tokens of each stimulus. A familiarization sequence consisted of five repetitions of the "bill", "dill," and "gill" stimuli with a normal complement of cues. The tests were conducted in a sound-attenuated booth. Signal presentation was by loudspeaker at 75 dB SPL.

Results

The results for stimuli constructed with conflicting formant transition and spectral tilt cues are shown in Table 1. For the normal-hearing subjects an inappropriate spectral tilt did not significantly alter identification responses [the difference in percent "d" responses to the stimulus with d-formants/d-tilt and to the stimulus with d-formants/b-tilt was not significant ($t=0.44$, $p=0.74$)]. Thus, formant transition cues in this vowel context appear to determine identification responses for normal listeners. For the implantees, spectral tilt had a far greater influence. For each patient, spectral tilt altered identification accuracy. For example, for Patient 1 the stimulus with b-transitions/b-tilt was identified as "b" on 62.5% of the trials and as "d" on 37.5% of the trials. In contrast, the stimulus with b-transitions/d/tilt was identified as "d" on 62.5% of the trials and as "g" on 37.5% of the trials. The stimulus was never identified as "b". A similar outcome was reported by Dorman et al. (1988) for another Ineraid patient. It appears, then, that the spectrum of the signal at onset plays a larger role in determining consonant identification for these implant patients than for normal-hearing listeners.

The results for stimuli constructed with conflicting formant transitions and abruptness of frequency change following signal onset are shown in Table 2. For the normal-hearing subjects variation in the abruptness dimension had no effect on the identification of "b" and "g". However, significantly more "d" responses were elicited by the stimulus with non-

TABLE 1
Percent Response as a Function of Stimulus Factors[a] and Hearing Status

Stimulus Factor		*Hearing Status*											
		Normal			*Patient 1*			*Patient 2*			*Patient 3*		
trans.	*tilt*	*b*	*d*	*g*	*b*	*d*	*g*	*b*	*d*	*g*	*b*	*d*	*g*
b	b	98	1	0	62	37	0	37	62	0	62	25	12
b	d	96	3	1	0	62	37	0	62	37	62	25	12
b	g	99	0	1	0	75	25	0	0	100	12	87	0
d	d	25	74	1	50	37	12	12	37	50	25	75	0
d	b	34	65	1	100	0	0	50	25	25	50	25	25
d	g	26	73	1	0	37	62	0	62	37	50	25	25
g	g	2	0	98	0	12	87	0	0	100	0	0	100
g	b	6	1	92	75	12	12	37	25	37	12	62	25
g	d	0	1	99	0	0	100	0	25	75	12	37	50

[a] Formant transitions and spectral tilt.

abrupt frequency change than the stimulus with abrupt frequency change ($t=2.75$, $p=0.013$). For the implantees, the abruptness of frequency change cue played a larger role in identification. When the non-abrupt spectral change for /g/ was made abrupt, all patients evidenced fewer /g/ responses. In the extreme instance, S3 dropped from 100% /g/ responses to 12.5% /g/ responses. When the abrupt onset for /b/ was lengthened, two of the three patients (1 and 3) evidenced a large reduction in the number of /b/ responses and a large increase in the number of /g/ responses.

TABLE 2
Percent Response as a Function of Stimulus Factors[a] and Hearing Status

Stimulus Factor		*Hearing Status*											
		Normal			*Patient 1*			*Patient 2*			*Patient 3*		
trans.	*abrupt.*	*b*	*d*	*g*	*b*	*d*	*g*	*b*	*d*	*g*	*b*	*d*	*g*
b	a	98	1	0	62	37	0	37	62	0	62	25	12
b	na	97	1	2	12	50	37	37	50	12	0	25	75
d	a	25	74	1	50	37	12	12	37	50	62	37	0
d	na	13	81	5	50	0	50	0	75	25	25	75	0
g	a	1	1	96	0	50	50	12	37	50	50	37	12
g	na	2	0	98	0	12	87	0	0	100	0	0	100

[a] Formant transitions and abruptness of frequency change following onset.

Discussion

Overall, we find that spectral tilt at signal onset and the abruptness of frequency change following signal onset affect the identification responses of implantees more than the identification responses of normal-hearing listeners. It is reasonable to assume that the crude quantization of frequencies in the F2/F3 region makes formant tracking a very difficult endeavour for implantees. For this reason, the spectrum at signal onset may play a more important role for implantees than for normal-hearing listeners. In similar fashion, the temporal cue of abruptness of frequency change following onset may play a more important role for implantees than for normal-hearing subjects.

EXPERIMENT 2
The Nature of Acoustic/Phonetic Categories

In the experiments described in this section we used the technique of generating a series of stimuli that varied along a small number of acoustic dimensions, in order to assess the ability of implant patients to use details of temporal and frequency cues for the purpose of phonetic categorization. We chose two continua for study based on the consonant and vowel identification ability of patients in previous experiments. Our data on consonant identification suggested that the voicing characteristic of stop consonants was well recognized. Therefore, we constructed a series of synthetic stimuli that varied in voice-onset time (VOT) to determine whether the acoustic/phonetic boundary between voiced and voiceless stops was positioned normally. Our data on vowel identification suggested that low-frequency F1s were well resolved. Therefore, we constructed a series of stimuli in which F1 and F2 co-varied in 20-Hz steps, to determine whether the acoustic/phonetic boundary between /ɪ/ (the vowel in "bit") and /ɛ/ (the vowel in "bet") was positioned normally.

Method

Subjects. Ten normal-hearing undergraduates and six implantees served as subjects. The implantees ranged in age from 24 to 61 years. For five patients the etiology of deafness was unknown. For another the etiology was Meniere's Disease. The consonant identification scores (16 consonants in "vCv" environment) ranged from 52 to 81% correct. The vowel identification scores (12 synthetic vowels in "bVt" environment) ranged from 22 to 79% correct. The word recognition scores of the implantees ranged from 48 to 100% correct.

Stimuli. To create the VOT continuum, the syllable /ga/ was synthesized using the Kewley-Port implementation of the Klatt algorithm (Klatt, 1980). The interval between the release burst and the onset of voicing in the first formant was varied over the range −10 msec (voicing occurred before the burst) to +70 msec (voicing was delayed 70 msec). For the stimuli in which voicing onset lagged the burst, aspiration excited the upper two formants for the duration of the voice onset time. The stimuli with short intervals between burst and onset of voicing were intended to be heard as /ga/. The stimuli with long intervals were intended to be heard as /ka/.

To create a continuum in which the frequency of steady-state formants varied, the vowel /ɪ/ was first synthesized. The frequency of F1 was 420 Hz, and the frequency of F2 was 1780 Hz. F3–F5 were fixed at 2570 Hz, 3300 Hz, and 3850 Hz, respectively. Stimulus duration was 150 msecs with a 25-msec rise–fall time. Nine stimuli were created by covarying F1 and F2, in 20-Hz steps, over the range 420–580 Hz and 1780–1620 Hz, respectively. The stimuli with low F1 and high F2 were intended to be heard as /ɪ/. The stimuli with high F1 and low F2 were intended to be heard as /ɛ/.

Procedure. Each test was presented as a forced-choice identification test with the alternatives listed in orthographic form at the top of the printed test sheet. The test sequence for each continuum consisted of eight tokens of each stimulus presented in random order. Each test sequence was preceded by a familiarization sequence in which the extreme stimuli from the continuum were presented as stimulus pairs. Eight repetitions of the pairs were presented. All tests were conducted in a sound-attenuated booth. Signal presentation level was 75 dB SPL. The stimuli were presented through a loudspeaker.

Results

The mean identification responses of the normal-hearing listeners (±1 *SD*) are shown as dotted functions in Figures 4 and 5. The identification functions of the implantees are shown as solid functions.

As shown in Figure 4, the mean VOT boundary (i.e. the location of 50% identification responses) for normal-hearing listeners was 42 msec, with a range of 34 to 50 msec. The VOT boundaries for Patients 1, 2, 3, and 6 were within the normal range. One patient (4) evidenced a shorter VOT boundary than normal (30 msec). Patient 5 showed consistent labelling of voiced signals, but inconsistent labelling of most of the signals that would normally have been heard as voiceless.

As shown in Figure 5, the mean boundary along the /ɪ/ – /ɛ/ continuum for normal-hearing listeners occurred at Stimulus 5 with a range of 4.0 to 6.5. Three patients (1, 2, 5) evidenced normal boundaries. For two patients (3, 4), the boundary was slightly beyond the normal range. The remaining patient (5) evidenced a normal boundary when the ascending portion of the labelling function was fit with a straight line, but was clearly unsure of the category affiliation of Stimuli 4–7. Patient 2 also evidence a shallow identification function. We infer that for these two patients the phonetic identity of the stimuli in the middle range of the continuum was unclear.

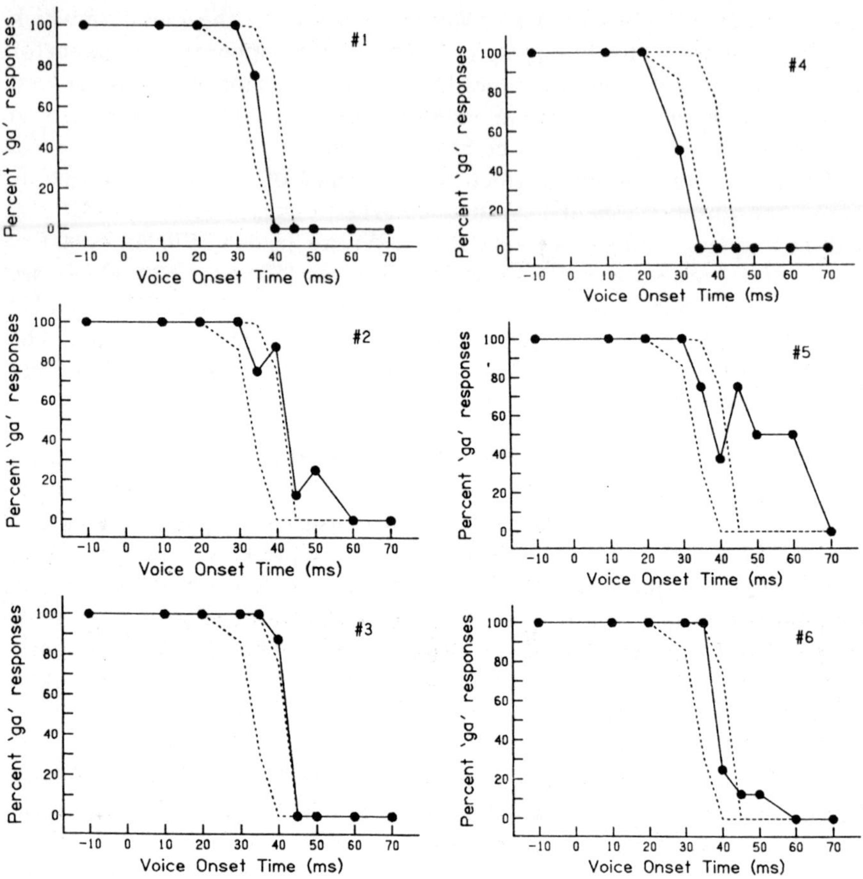

FIG. 4. Percent "ga" responses to stimuli that varied in VOT. Dotted functions indicate normal performance ± 1 *SD*.

Discussion

Two patients evidenced normal categorization, in terms of acoustic/phonetic boundaries and in slope of the identification function, of both continua. Two others evidenced boundaries only slightly outside the limits of normal. This outcome suggests that at least some implantees can appreciate the spectral/temporal detail available in the auditory representation of speech signals.

More patients were able to label the signals from the VOT continuum in a normal manner than signals from the /ɪ/-/ɛ/ continuum. This outcome probably reflects the greater number of acoustic cues available to the patients for the voicing contrast (see our discussion of cues to voicing, above).

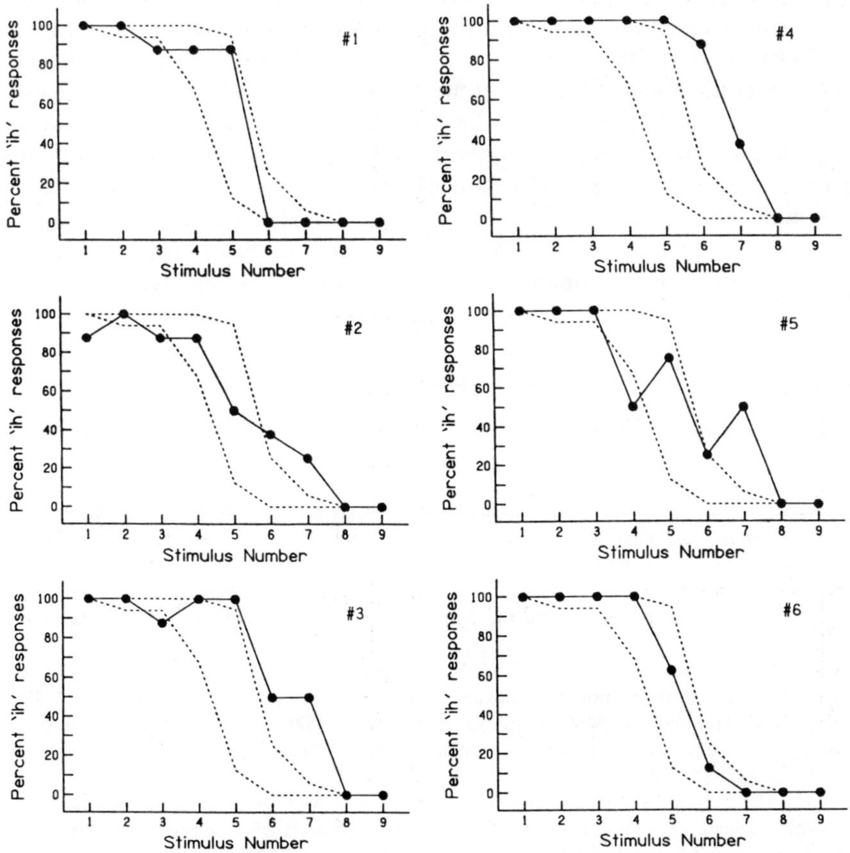

FIG. 5. Percent /ɪ/ responses to stimuli that co-varied in F1 and F2 frequency. Dotted functions indicate normal performance ±1 *SD*.

GENERAL DISCUSSION

Our aim in this report was to describe the information that enables patients who are "good" users of a multichannel cochlear implant to identify vowels and consonants. The experiments on vowel recognition suggest (1) that F1 is relatively well resolved, and (2) that at least large differences in F2 are resolved. The relatively good resolution of F1 is due, most probably, to rate coding of F1, although, as we noted previously, the present data do not rule out the possibility of F1 coding by the relative distribution of current among electrodes. The poorer resolution of F2 is due, most probably, to the limited amount for information available about place of stimulation for frequencies above 1 kHz.

The results of our experiments on consonant recognition indicate that the best patients extract most of the amplitude envelope information (including periodicity/aperiodicity) from the acoustic signal. This information allows accurate identification of consonant manner and voicing. For consonants, as for vowels, spectral information is limited. We suspect that rate coding adds to the identification of manner and voicing by providing information about the onset frequency of F1 (Dorman et al., 1988) and, in the case of the semivowels, about the onset frequency of some F2s. Place coding provides at least some information about the onset spectra of stop consonants. The identification of stop consonant place of articulation is assisted further by the characteristic spectral/temporal cues that follow signal onset.

REFERENCES

Blumstein, S., Issacs, E., & Mertus, J. (1982). The role of gross spectral shape as a perceptual cue to place of articulation in initial stop consonants. *Journal of the Acoustical Society of America, 72*, 43–50.

Dankowski, K. & McCandless, G. (1990). *Relationship between electrical and acoustical dynamic range and measures of speech discrimination.* Paper presented at the Second International Cochlear Implant Symposium, Iowa City, Iowa.

Dorman, M.F., Dankowski, K., Smith, L., & McCandless, G. (1989a). Identification of synthetic vowels by patients using the Symbion multichannel cochlear implant. *Ear and Hearing, 10*, 40–43.

Dorman, M.F., Dankowski, K., Smith, L., & McCandless, G. (1989b). Word recognition by 50 patients fitted with the Symbion multichannel cochlear implant. *Ear and Hearing, 10*, 44–49.

Dorman, M.F., Hannley, M., McCandless, G., & Smith, L. (1988). Acoustic/phonetic categorization with the Symbion multichannel cochlear implant. *Journal of the Acoustical Society of America, 84*, 501–510.

Dorman, M.F., Soli, S., Dankowski, K., Smith, L., McCandless, G., & Parkin, J. (1990). Acoustic cues for consonant identification by patients who use the Ineraid cochlear implant. *Journal of the Acoustical Society of America, 88*, 2074–2079.

Dubno, J. & Dorman, M.F. (1987). Effects of spectral flattening on vowel identification. *Journal of the Acoustical Society of America, 82*, 1503–1511.

Dynes, S. (1989). *Temporal discharge patterns in the electrically stimulated auditory nerve in cat.* Masters Thesis, Department of Physics, Massachusetts Institute of Technology.

Eddington, D. (1980). Speech discrimination in deaf subjects with cochlear implants. *Journal of the Acoustical Society of America, 68*, 885–891.

Gantz, B., Tyler, R., Knutson, J., Woodworth, G., Abbas, P., McCabe, B., Hinrichs, J., Tye-Murray, N., Lansing, C., Kuk, F., & Brown, C. (1988). Evaluation of five different cochlear implant designs: Audiologic assessment and predictors of performance. *Laryngoscope, 98*, 1100–1106.

Greenwood, D. (1990). A cochlear frequency position function for several species—29 years later. *Journal of the Acoustical Society of America, 87*, 2592–2605.

Hartmann, R. & Klinke, R. (1990). Response characteristics of nerve fibers to patterned electrical stimulation. In J.M. Miller & F.A. Spelman (Eds.), *Cochlear implants: Models for the electrically stimulated ear* (pp. 135–159). New York: Springer-Verlag.

Hochmair, E. & Hochmair-Desoyer, I. (1983). Percepts elicited by different speech-coding strategies. In C.W. Parkins & S.W. Anderson (Eds.), *Cochlear prostheses* (pp. 268–279). New York: New York Academy of Sciences.

Hochmair-Desoyer, I., Hochmair, E., Burian, K., & Stiglbrunner, H. (1983). Percepts from the Vienna cochlear prosthesis. In C.W. Parkins & S.W. Anderson (Eds.), *Cochlear prostheses* (pp. 295–306). New York: New York Academy of Sciences.

Hochmair-Desoyer, I., Hochmair, E., & Stiglbrunner, H. (1985). Psychoacoustic temporal processing and speech understanding in cochlear implant subjects. In R.A. Schindler & M.M. Merzenich (Eds.), *Cochlear implants* (pp. 291–303). New York: Raven Press.

Kewley-Port, D. (1983). Time varying features as correlates of place of articulation in stop consonants. *Journal of the Acoustical Society of America, 73*, 322–335.

Klatt, D. (1980). Software for a cascade/parallel formant synthesizer. *Journal of the Acoustical Society of America, 67*, 971–995.

Liberman, A.M., Delattre, P., Cooper, F., & Gerstman, L. (1954). The role of consonant-vowel transitions in the perception of the stop and nasal consonants. *Psychological Monographs, 68* (8, Whole No. 379), 1–13.

Lindholm, J., Dorman, M.F., Taylor, B.E., & Hannley, M. (1988). Stimulus factors influencing the identification of voiced stop consonants by normal-hearing and hearing-impaired adults. *Journal of the Acoustical Society of America, 83*, 1608–1614.

Rosen, S. (1989). Temporal information in speech and its relevance for cochlear implants. In B. Fraysee & N. Cochard (Eds.), *Cochlear implant: Acquisitions and controversies* (pp. 3–26). Basel: Cochlear AG.

Shannon, R. (1986). Temporal processing in cochlear implants. In M.J. Collins, T.A. Glattke, & L.A. Harker (Eds.), *Sensorineural hearing loss. The Reger conference* (pp. 349–367). Iowa City, IA: University of Iowa Press.

Smith, L. (1988). Clinical evaluation of pitch perception from a monopolar cochlear implant. *Biomedical Sciences Instrumentation, 24*, 153–159.

Soli, S. (1990). Perceptual evaluation of a neurally based encoding strategy for cochlear implants. In J.M. Miller & F.A. Spelman (Eds.), *Cochlear implants* (pp. 378–404). New York: Springer-Verlag.

Summerfield, A.Q. (1985). Speech-processing alternatives for electrical auditory stimulation. In R.A. Schindler & M.M. Merzenich (Eds.), *Cochlear implants* (pp. 195–222). New York: Raven Press.

Townshend, B., Cotter, N., Van Campernolle, D., & White, R.L. (1987). Pitch perception by cochlear implant patients. *Journal of the Acoustical Society of America, 87*, 106–115.

Tye-Murray, N. & Tyler, R. (1989). Auditory consonant and word recognition skills of cochlear implant users. *Ear and Hearing, 10*, 292–298.

Tyler, R.S., Moore, B.C.J., & Kuk, F.K. (1989a). Performance of some of the better cochlear-implant patients. *Journal of Speech and Hearing Research, 32*, 887–911.

Tyler, R.S., Tye-Murray, N., & Otto, S. (1989b). The recognition of vowels differing in a single formant by cochlear-implant patients. *Journal of the Acoustical Society of America, 86*, 2107–2112.

Van Tassel, D., Soli, S., Kirby, V., & Widin, G. (1987). Speech waveform envelope cues for consonant recognition. *Journal of the Acoustical Society of America, 82*, 1152–1161.

Revised manuscript received 23 October 1990

THE QUARTERLY JOURNAL OF EXPERIMENTAL PSYCHOLOGY, 1991, *43A* (3) 603–620

Formant Transition Duration and Amplitude Rise Time as Cues to the Stop/Glide Distinction

Margaret A. Walsh and Randy L. Diehl
University of Texas at Austin, Austin, Texas, U.S.A.

There is some disagreement in the literature about the relative contribution of formant transition duration and amplitude rise time in signalling the contrast between stops and glides. In this study, listeners identified sets of /bɑ/ and /wɑ/ stimuli in which transition duration and rise time varied orthogonally. Both variables affected labelling performance in the expected direction (i.e. the proportion of /b/ responses increased with shorter transition durations and shorter rise times). However, transition duration served as the primary cue to the stop/glide distinction, whereas rise time played a secondary, contrast-enhancing role. A qualitatively similar pattern of results was obtained when listeners made abrupt-onset/gradual-onset judgements of single sine-wave stimuli that modelled the rise times, frequency trajectories, and durations of the first formant in the /bɑ/-/wɑ/ stimuli. The similarities between the speech and non-speech conditions suggest that significant auditory commonalities underlie performance in the two cases.

Like other phonological contrasts, the distinction between stops and glides has multiple acoustic correlates. Stops (e.g. /b/ as in *boy* and /g/ as in *girl*) are produced with a complete articulatory closure followed, in non-final positions, by a rapid opening of the vocal tract. During closure, there is a buildup of oral air pressure such that articulatory release causes a transient burst of energy. This is followed by a relatively brief period of formant transitions and a relatively abrupt rise in amplitude envelope corresponding to the rapid opening movement. In contrast, glides (e.g. /w/ as in *wall* and /j/ as in *yell*) are produced with incomplete oral closure and a slower opening movement, resulting in the absence of an initial burst and in longer formant transition

---

Requests for reprints should be sent to Randy L. Diehl, the University of Texas at Austin, Austin, TX, U.S.A.

This research was supported by N.I.H. Grant NS25207 to the second author. We thank Quentin Summerfield and two anonymous reviewers for helpful comments on an earlier version of the paper.

durations and amplitude rise times (Mack & Blumstein, 1983; Miller & Baer, 1983; Walsh, 1989).

The earliest perceptual studies of the stop/glide distinction focused on the effects of manipulating certain frequency-time properties of formant transitions in synthetic speech stimuli. Liberman, Delattre, Gerstman, and Cooper (1956) found that the distinction between initial /b/ and /w/ and between initial /g/ and /j/ can be reliably signalled by varying formant transition duration and slope (while maintaining constant transition onset and offset frequencies). This result has since been replicated in many other studies (e.g. Cooper, Ebert, & Cole, 1976; Diehl, 1976; Miller & Liberman, 1979; O'Connor, Gerstman, Liberman, Delattre, & Cooper, 1957; Pisoni, Carrell, & Gans, 1983).

A problem for interpreting the results of these studies is that variation in frequency-time properties of formant transitions was virtually always confounded with variation in amplitude envelope properties. Either by design or because of inherent interactions between formant frequency and overall amplitude during synthesis, amplitude rise time tended to vary directly with transition duration. There is some uncertainty, therefore, whether the observed perceptual effects resulted from changes in frequency-time cues, envelope cues, or both.

In fact, several studies have challenged the primary role traditionally assigned to frequency-time cues in signalling the stop/glide contrast. Mack and Blumstein (1983) measured both amplitude and frequency characteristics near the consonantal release of stops and glides. Although the frequency-time properties (e.g. formant transition durations) of both manner classes varied considerably as a function of the following vowel, a measure of relative amplitude change was found to be rather stable across vowel contexts and to distinguish quite reliably between stops (/b/, /d/, and /g/) and glides (/w/ and /j/).

In a test of the perceptual role of the amplitude correlate described by Mack and Blumstein (1983), Shinn and Blumstein (1984) found that the amplitude envelope signalled the distinction between /b/-initial and /w/-initial syllables, even in the presence of conflicting formant frequency information. In their study they first synthesized a /bɑ/-/wɑ/ and a /bi/-/wi/ series by varying both frequency-time and amplitude envelope characteristics of the stimuli. Next, they created modified versions of each series by imposing either a stoplike or glidelike amplitude envelope on every stimulus item. In a forced-choice identification task, envelope cues generally overrode transition duration, slope, and frequency cues in specifying the stop/glide distinction for the various modified series.

The results of two other recent studies appear, however, to be at odds with the findings of Shinn and Blumstein (1984). Nittrouer and Studdert-Kennedy (1986) had listeners identify naturally produced tokens of /b/ and /w/ (in five following-vowel contexts) either in their original form or with modified amplitude envelopes. For the modified versions, the /b/ stimuli were given glidelike envelopes, whereas the /w/ stimuli were given stoplike envelopes. [The criteria for "stoplike" and "glidelike" envelopes were those established by Mack and Blumstein (1983) on the basis of their acoustical study of stops and glides.] The main finding was that envelope modification had virtually no effect on the labelling of /b/ stimuli and only a very small effect on the labelling of /w/ stimuli. Performance was almost entirely determined by the frequency-time properties of the stimulus items.

Moreover, in a study using synthetic speech stimuli in which frequency-time and envelope cues varied independently, Diehl and Walsh (1989) obtained results that were broadly compatible with those of Nittrouer and Studdert-Kennedy (1986). Variation in transition slope and duration (without concomitant changes in amplitude envelope) was sufficient to signal the stop/glide distinction. However, variation in rise time (with transition duration and slope fixed at values intermediate between the stop and glide categories) had only a modest effect on stop/glide labelling and did not reliably cue the distinction.

In view of the apparent discrepancies in the literature, one important aim of the present study was to try to clarify the individual and combined contributions of frequency-time cues and amplitude envelope cues in specifying the perceptual distinction between stops and glides. Diehl and Walsh (1989) studied the effects of transition-duration variation and rise-time variation in separate experiments, with the parameter in each experiment being overall stimulus length. Their design did not allow them to determine the extent to which the two variables might work together to signal the stop/glide contrast. It is possible, for example, that even the small effect of rise-time variation observed by Diehl and Walsh would be completely eliminated in the presence of the more robust signalling effect of transition-duration variation. In the present study, transition duration and rise time were varied orthogonally within the same experiments, providing a look at the effects of the two acoustic variables in combination. Specifically, in Experiment 1, transition, duration was the independent variable and rise time was the orthogonal parameter, whereas in Experiment 2 rise time was the independent variable and transition duration was the parameter.

Experiments 3 and 4 were motivated by another set of findings from Diehl and Walsh (1989). One goal of that study was to investigate the possible role of general auditory factors in the perception of stops and glides. For this purpose, Diehl and Walsh compared labelling performance on sets of stop and glide stimuli and on corresponding sets of non-speech stimuli consisting of single sine-wave patterns that modelled the first-formant trajectories and amplitude rise times of the speech tokens. (The sine-wave stimuli were categorized on the basis of perceived abruptness of onset.)

In most respects, listeners' performance on the speech and non-speech stimulus sets was closely parallel. Transition duration was an effective cue not only for the stop/glide distinction, but also for the non-speech distinction between abrupt and gradual onsets. Moreover, the locations of the category boundaries along the transition–duration dimension did not differ significantly between the two cases. When the stop/glide distinction was cued by tion of the stop/glide distinction and the perception of the abrupt-onset/ is, a longer following vowel shifted the stop/glide boundary towards longer values of transition duration, thus yielding more stop labelling responses (see Miller & Liberman, 1979, for an earlier demonstration of this effect). A very similar stimulus-length effect was also obtained for the corresponding sine-wave stimuli (see also Pisoni et al., 1983). As noted earlier, variation in amplitude rise time had only a small effect on stop/glide labelling, and the same was true for the sine-wave stimuli. There was one clear discrepancy between the speech and non-speech results: When the stop/glide distinction was signalled by rise-time variation alone, there was a stimulus-length effect, but no such effect was observed for the corresponding sine-wave stimuli. Despite this one difference, the overall results of Diehl and Walsh (1989) suggest that there are significant auditory commonalities between the perception of the stop/glide distinction and the perception of the abrupt-onset/gradual-onset distinction among auditory stimuli in general.

Here we explored further the extent to which perception of stops and glides is subserved by general auditory mechanisms. In Experiments 3 and 4 subjects identified single sine-wave analogs of the synthetic speech stimuli used in Experiments 1 and 2. The main question of interest was whether the individual and combined effects of variation in transition duration and rise time are similar across the speech and non-speech domains.

EXPERIMENT 1

In this experiment, formant transition duration and amplitude rise time were manipulated orthogonally to determine their individual and combined effects in signalling the stop/glide distinction.

Method

Stimuli. Two synthetic speech stimulus series were created using the parallel-resonance branch of the Klatt (1980) software synthesizer implemented on a PDP 11/34 computer. Each series ranged perceptually from /bɑ/ to /wɑ/ and varied in formant-transition duration from 20 msec to 120 msec, in 10-msec steps. The stimuli had five formants and included a variable-length steady-state vowel following the formant transitions. The transitions of the first three formants (F1, F2, and F3) rose linearly from their starting frequencies (250, 650, and 2000 Hz) to their steady-state values (750, 1200, and 2400 Hz). The frequencies of the fourth and fifth formants were fixed at 3300 and 3850 Hz, and the fundamental frequency (F0) was fixed at 100 Hz. Total stimulus duration was 300 msec.

The two stimulus series differed only in amplitude rise time, with values of 20 msec and 120 msec, respectively. The following steps were taken to control the rise time of each stimulus. First, to offset partially the effect of formant frequency on amplitude in the Klatt synthesizer, the nominal amplitude setting of the voicing source (AV) was reduced linearly from 68 dB to 60 dB over the duration of the formant transitions. This resulted in waveform periods that were more nearly uniform in peak amplitude. Next, each waveform period in the transition portion of a stimulus was scaled upwards or downwards so that the peak amplitude was identical to that of the steady-state portion of the stimulus. Finally, each stimulus waveform was multiplied by either a 20- or 120-msec negatively accelerated rise function (exponent equal to 0.3).

Procedure. Subjects in this and the other three experiments were introductory psychology students at the University of Texas, who participated in return for partial course credit. All subjects were native speakers of American English and reported having normal hearing. No subject served in more than one experiment.

The 12 subjects in the present experiment identified 15 randomized blocks of the 22 stimuli (11 transition durations × 2 rise times). The interstimulus interval was 2 sec, and the interblock interval was 3 sec. Subjects were asked to identify each stimulus item as either /bɑ/ or /wɑ/ by pressing a labelled response key. Between one and four subjects, assigned to separate response stations in a sound-proof chamber, served in each experimental session.

All stimuli were output at 10 kHz via a 14-bit D/A converter, low-pass filtered at 4.9 kHz, and presented to subjects over Beyer DT-100 earphones at a peak level of approximately 75 dB SPL. The same equipment and presentation levels were also used in the later experiments.

Results and Discussion

Results for both the short- and long-rise-time stimuli are shown in Figure 1. With rise time held constant within a series, transition duration was a robust cue for the stop/glide distinction. This replicates one of the main findings of Diehl and Walsh (1989) and is consistent with earlier claims about the perceptual significance of transition duration based on studies in which transition duration and rise times were systematically confounded. There was also an effect of amplitude envelope: the longer rise time shifted the stop/glide boundary towards smaller values of transition duration, resulting in a significantly greater overall percentage of /wɑ/ responses, $t(11)=3.13$, $p<0.025$, two-tailed. It appears that frequency-time and envelope properties

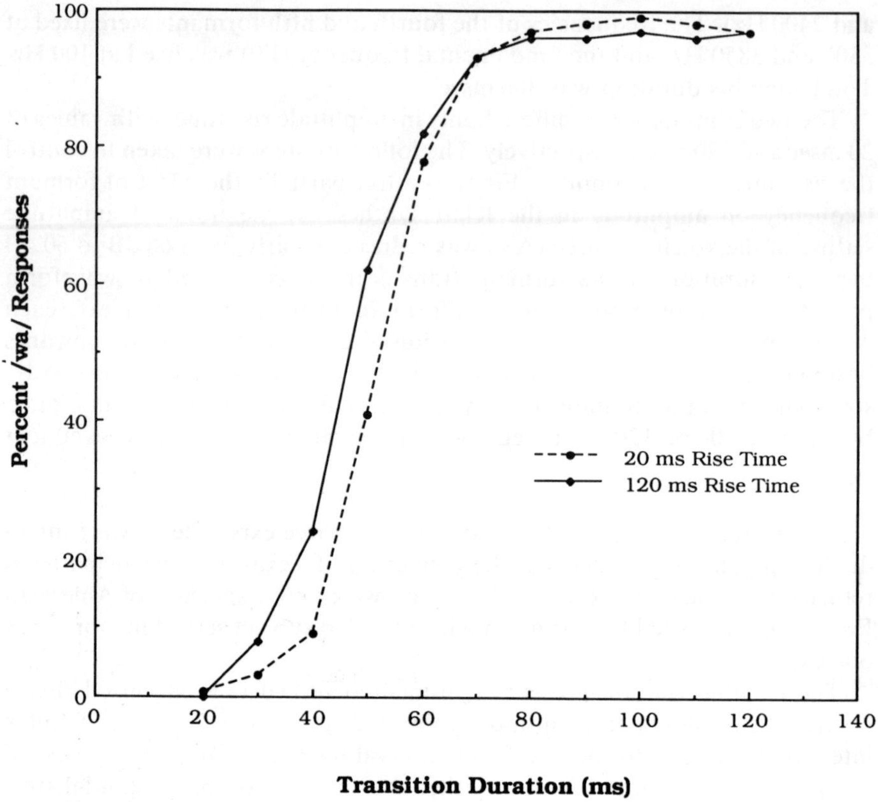

FIG. 1. Identification functions for the /bɑ/-/wɑ/ stimuli used in Experiment 1. The parameter is rise time.

both help to signal the distinction between stops and glides, with transition duration playing a major role and rise time playing at least a supporting role.

EXPERIMENT 2

In this experiment, rise time and transition duration were again manipulated orthogonally, but rise time now served as the independent variable and transition duration as the parameter. This design enabled us to evaluate whether variation in rise time alone is sufficient to distinguish stops and glides and, if so, whether transition duration plays an enhancing role in signalling the contrast (analogous to the enhancing role of rise time observed in Experiment 1).

Method

Stimuli. Two stimulus series were synthesized and edited to vary in rise time from 5 msec to 105 msec, in 10-msec steps. The amplitude envelope was controlled using the same type of procedure described in Experiment 1. In one series transition duration was fixed at 30 msec, whereas in the other series it was fixed at 50 msec.[1] Synthesis parameter values were otherwise the same as those used in Experiment 1.

Procedure. Pilot work indicated that when the two stimulus series were presented in a mixed format as in Experiment 1, listeners tended to disregard the rise-time cue and to identify the items as /ba/ or /wa/ mainly on the basis of the 20-msec difference in transition duration. Moreover, listeners found the task quite difficult. Accordingly, several changes were made in the testing procedure for the actual experiment. The two stimulus series were presented in a blocked format (with order counterbalanced across subjects) to encourage greater use of the rise-time cue in identifying the stimuli. Before identifying a given series, subjects were first trained, via feedback lights, to label the two series-endpoint stimuli as /ba/ or /wa/. Subjects responded to 20 randomized repetitions of each training stimulus. After training, subjects labelled 15 randomized blocks of the entire 11-stimulus series and were then trained and tested on the other series. Subjects were instructed to press a response key according to whether each item sounded more like the short-rise-time (5 msec) or the long-rise-time (105 msec) endpoint stimulus. Twelve subjects served in the experiment.

Results and Discussion

Figure 2 displays the results of Experiment 2. Although linear trend tests showed that variation in rise time had a reliable effect on the overall percentage of /wa/ responses—$F(1, 11) = 13.56$, $p < 0.005$, 30-msec formant transitions, and $F(1, 11) = 17.30$, $p < 0.005$, 50-msec formant transitions—relatively extreme rise-time values failed to yield a stimulus that was unambiguously /ba/- or /wa/-like. This essentially replicates the modest effect of rise-time variation observed by Diehl and Walsh (1989). Despite the relatively small change in transition duration across the two stimulus series,

[1] In pilot studies we discovered that extreme transition durations (e.g. 20 and 120 msec) completely overrode any effect of rise time, with virtually 100% of responses to the short-transition series resulting in /ba/ judgements, and virtually 100% of responses to the long-transition series resulting in /wa/ judgements. We chose 30- and 50-msec transition durations because these values straddled the stop/glide boundary as determined in Experiment 1.

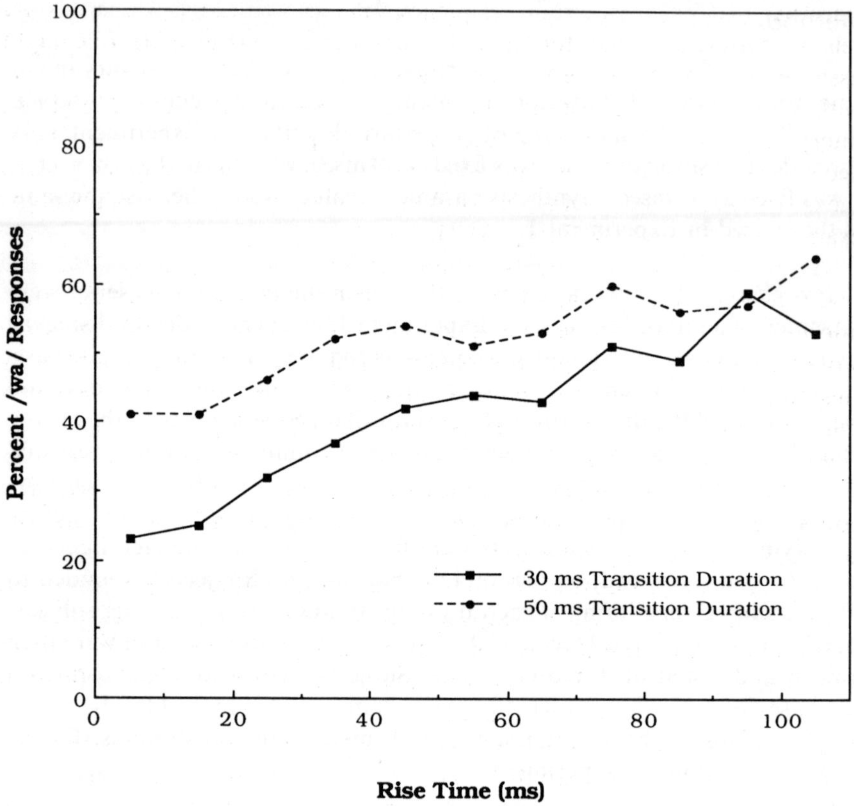

FIG. 2. Identification functions for the speech stimuli used in Experiment 2. The parameter is transition duration.

the longer transition duration produced a significant increase in the percentage of /wɑ/ responses [$t(11) = 5.84$, $p < 0.001$].

Together, the findings of Experiments 1 and 2 indicate that *both* transition duration and rise time contribute to the perceptual distinction between stops and glides. For listeners with normal hearing in quiet, transition duration appears to be the more important variable, acting as a primary cue to the distinction, whereas rise time is a secondary, contrast-enhancing cue. It is reasonable to conclude that the covariation between transition duration and rise time in naturally produced stops and glides yields greater perceptual distinctiveness than would be had by differences in either variable alone.

What is the basis of the mutually reinforcing character of transition duration and rise time in signalling the perceptual distinction between stops and glides? A rather obvious answer can be framed in terms of perceptual learning. Inasmuch as certain frequency-time and envelope properties are reliable correlates of the stop/glide distinction and are detectable, one might assume that, for language learners, these properties will acquire cue value with respect to the distinction. The results of Experiments 1 and 2 might be interpreted, then, to reflect the listeners' long experience with the correlated acoustic attributes of stops and glides. (That even infants can quickly learn the correlated attributes of arbitrarily defined categories has been shown, for example, by Younger & Cohen, 1983.)

As it stands, the perceptual-learning account in no way implies that the observed positive correlation between transition duration and rise time affords a more natural perceptual basis for the category distinction than would be afforded by, say, an inverse correlation between these variables. By this account, the relation of mutual enhancement between short transition durations and short rise times in perceptually specifying the category *stop consonant* arises simply from the fact that they happen to be correlated cues. From the standpoint of perceptual learning, the direction of the correlation could well be arbitrary (although it is clearly not arbitrary from the standpoint of speech production).

Alternatively, it is possible that the positive correlation between transition duration and rise time across stops and glides creates a category distinction that is auditorily natural or robust. For example, brief transition durations and short rise times may both contribute to a relatively broadband activation of frequency channels within a small time interval, which may be a principal auditory correlate of abrupt onsets in general. Unlike the perceptual-learning hypothesis, this account of the results of Experiments 1 and 2 makes no reference to linguistic experience. It is based rather on acoustic/auditory factors that are presumably common across speech and non-speech stimulus domains.

One way to test a general auditory account of this type is to invite listeners to categorize *nonspeech* stimulus sets in which frequency transition duration and amplitude rise time are varied orthogonally in the manner of the /bɑ/-/wɑ/ stimuli used in the first two experiments. Experiments 3 and 4 were designed accordingly.

EXPERIMENT 3

In this experiment, subjects performed two-category labelling of single-sine-wave stimuli that abstractly mimicked certain frequency-time and amplitude-envelope properties of the /bɑ/-/wɑ/ stimuli used in Experiment 1. The purpose was to investigate whether the stimulus effects observed in that experiment are unique to the perception of stops and glides or whether they characterize auditory perception of the more general category distinction between abrupt and gradual onsets.

Method

Stimuli. Using a waveform synthesis program implemented on a PDP 11/34 computer, we created two series of single-sine-wave stimuli as analogs of the short- and long-rise-time stop/glide series used in Experiment 1. Each sine-wave stimulus modelled the centre-frequency trajectory of the first formant of its corresponding speech stimulus. That is, there was an initial linear frequency transition from 250 to 750 Hz, after which the frequency remained constant at this terminal value. As was the case for the speech stimuli, the frequency transition duration varied in each series from 20 msec to 120 msec, in 10-msec steps. Total stimulus duration was 300 msec. For one stimulus series, there was an initial 20-msec rise in amplitude; for the other series, the initial rise extended 120 msec. The rise functions were negatively accelerated with an exponent of 0.3. Every item had a constant peak amplitude equal to that of the corresponding /bɑ/-/wɑ/ stimuli and a final decay time of 10 msec.

Procedure. Nine subjects participated in the experiment. Before identifying the full stimulus set, they were trained to label the four endpoint stimuli of the two series. Forty randomized blocks of the four stimuli were presented, and subjects were required to learn by means of feedback lights to press either of two response keys labelled "abrupt onset" and "gradual onset." These corresponded, respectively, to the endpoint stimuli with the short and long frequency transitions. (Thus, by the experimenter-defined category mappings, rise time was an irrelevant variable.) After training, subjects heard 15 randomized blocks of the full 22-item stimulus set (11 transition durations × 2 rise times). As in Experiment 1, the interstimulus interval was 2 sec, and the interblock interval was 3 sec. Subjects were instructed to "press the button corresponding to the training category that each stimulus sounds more like."

Results and Discussion

Figure 3 shows the mean percentage of times a given stimulus was judged as more similar to the "gradual-onset" training category (i.e. the category defined by the long frequency transitions.) For both rise-time conditions, variation in transition duration effectively signalled the distinction between abrupt and gradual onsets. This is perhaps not surprising given that the training categories were experimentally defined with respect to differences in transition duration. However, it is nonetheless noteworthy that the transition-duration variable yielded identification functions that were only slightly less steep in the region of the category boundary than those found for the corresponding stop/glide stimuli. What is clearly not an artifact of training is the effect of the envelope parameter: the long rise time produced a significant

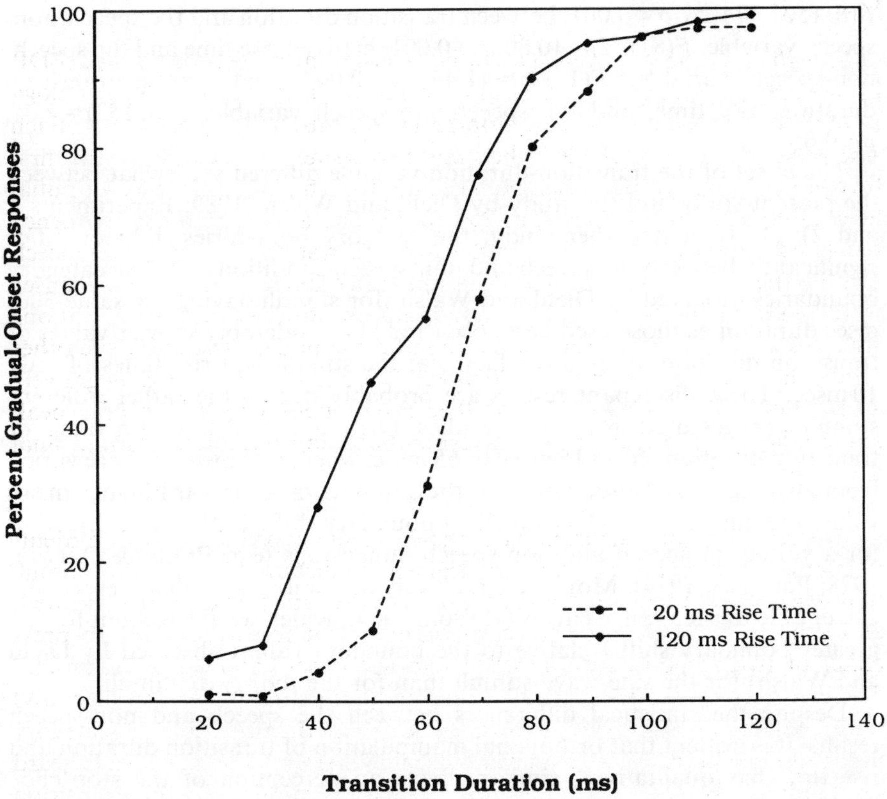

FIG. 3. Identification functions for the sine-wave stimuli used in Experiment 3. The parameter is rise time.

increase in the overall percentage of "gradual-onset" responses, $t(8) = 4.5$, $p < 0.002$. The boundary shift was in the same direction, but about twice as large, as that for the corresponding speech stimuli. Probit analyses located the transition-duration boundary values (i.e. the 50% identification cross-over points) for the short- and long-rise-time series at 54.9 msec and 48.1 msec for the speech stimuli and at 69.4 msec and 54.2 msec for the non-speech stimuli.

An 11 (levels of transition duration) × 2 (levels of rise time) × 2 (speech vs. non-speech) cross-experiment analysis of variance was performed on the percentages of /wɑ/ responses in Experiment 1 and gradual-onset responses in Experiment 3. There were significant main effects of transition duration, $F(8, 152) = 297.80$, $p < 0.001$; rise time, $F(1, 19) = 35.32$, $p < 0.001$; and the speech/non-speech variable, $F(1, 19) = 13.37$, $p < 0.002$. Also, there were significant interactions between transition duration and rise time,

$F(8, 152) = 15.26$, $p < 0.001$; between transition duration and the speech/non-speech variable, $F(8, 152) = 10.80$, $p < 0.001$; between rise time and the speech/non-speech variable, $F(1, 19) = 11.44$, $p < 0.004$; and among transition duration, rise time, and the speech/non-speech variable, $F(8, 152) = 2.04$, $p < 0.05$.

The effect of the transition-duration variable differed somewhat between the present study and the study by Diehl and Walsh (1989, Experiments 1 and 2): (1) In that earlier study, the category boundaries did not differ significantly between the speech and non-speech conditions. (2) The category boundaries observed by Diehl and Walsh (for stimuli having the same 300-msec duration as those used here) occurred at considerably shorter values of transition duration, despite the fact that the stimuli had rise times of only 10 msec. These discrepant results are probably due to the rather different stimulus ranges used in the two studies. Diehl and Walsh used a range of transition durations from 15 msec to 65 msec, whereas transitions here varied from 20 msec to 120 msec. Shifts in the stimulus range toward higher mean values are known to produce labelling boundary shifts in the same direction for a variety of speech and non-speech dimensions (e.g. Brady & Darwin, 1978; Parducci, 1974). Moreover, relatively unfamiliar stimuli are especially susceptible to such range effects (Helson, 1964), which would account for the greater boundary shift (relative to the boundary values observed by Diehl and Walsh) for the sine-wave stimuli than for the /ba/-/wa/ stimuli.

Despite the statistical differences between the speech and non-speech results, it is evident that orthogonal manipulation of transition duration and rise time has qualitatively similar effects on perception of the stop/glide distinction and perception of the non-speech distinction between abrupt and gradual onsets. It seems, therefore, that the results of Experiment 1 are not likely to be explained strictly in terms of perceivers' previous learning of the correlated attributes of stops and glides. If the natural correlation between transition duration and rise time enhances the contrast between stops and glides, it is apparently because of acoustic/auditory factors that are not unique to the perception of speech. One possibility, mentioned earlier, is that brief transition durations and rise times both contribute to a relatively broadband activation of auditory frequency channels within a small time interval, which may signal abrupt onsets in general. In the General Discussion, however, we describe some recent evidence from our laboratory that casts doubt on this "frequency dispersion" hypothesis.

EXPERIMENT 4

In the final experiment, listeners performed two-category identification of sine-wave analogs of the speech stimuli used in Experiment 2. A main question was whether the modest effect of rise-time variation in cueing the stop/glide distinction would also be observed for the labelling of abrupt and gradual onsets in non-speech stimuli.

Method

For each speech stimulus used in Experiment 2, we created a single-sine-wave pattern that modelled the centre-frequency trajectory, duration, and rise time of the first formant. Thus, rise times varied across both series from 5 msec to 105 msec, in 10-msec steps, and were negatively accelerated (exponent equal to 0.3); transition durations for the two series were set at 30 msec and 50 msec, respectively. The procedure, including training on series-endpoint stimuli and blocked presentation of the two transition-duration conditions, was identical to that of Experiment 2, except that the response keys corresponding to the short- and long-rise-time training categories were labelled "abrupt onset" and "gradual onset." Twelve subjects took part in the experiment.

Results and Discussion

Figure 4 shows the mean number of times subjects labelled items as being more similar to the long-rise-time ("gradual onset") training category. As was the case for the corresponding speech stimuli in Experiment 2, variation in rise time yielded significant linear trends in both transition-duration conditions—30-msec transitions, $F(1, 11) = 23.75$, $p < 0.001$; 50-msec transitions, $F(1, 11)$, 6.43, $p < 0.02$—but again the effects were relatively weak. Even the endpoint stimuli used in training were labelled inconsistently. Unlike Experiment 2, transition duration had no overall effect on labelling performance [$t(11)$, $p > 0.5$].

A 2 (levels of transition duration) × 11 (levels of rise time) × 2 (speech vs. non-speech) cross-experiment analysis of variance on the percentages of /wɑ/ responses in Experiment 2 and gradual-onset responses in this experiment showed significant main effects of transition duration, $F(1, 22) = 8.48$, $p < 0.01$, and rise time, $F(8, 176) = 16.39$, $p < 0.001$, but no significant main effect of the speech/non-speech variable [$F(1, 22) = 0.62$, $p = 0.44$]. There were also significant interactions between transient duration and rise time, $F(8, 176) = 3.80$, $p < 0.001$, and between transition duration and the speech/non-speech variable, $F(1, 22) = 4.72$, $p < 0.05$. However, there were no significant interactions between rise time and the speech/non-speech variable [$F(8, 176) = 1.56$, $p > 0.1$] nor among transition duration, rise time, and the speech/non-speech variable [$F(8, 176) = 0.62$, $p > 0.5$].

Thus, the main difference between the results of Experiments 2 and 4 was the absence of a reliable effect of the transition-duration parameter in the latter, non-speech experiment. One possible explanation for this difference derives from the observation that the abrupt-onset/gradual-onset category

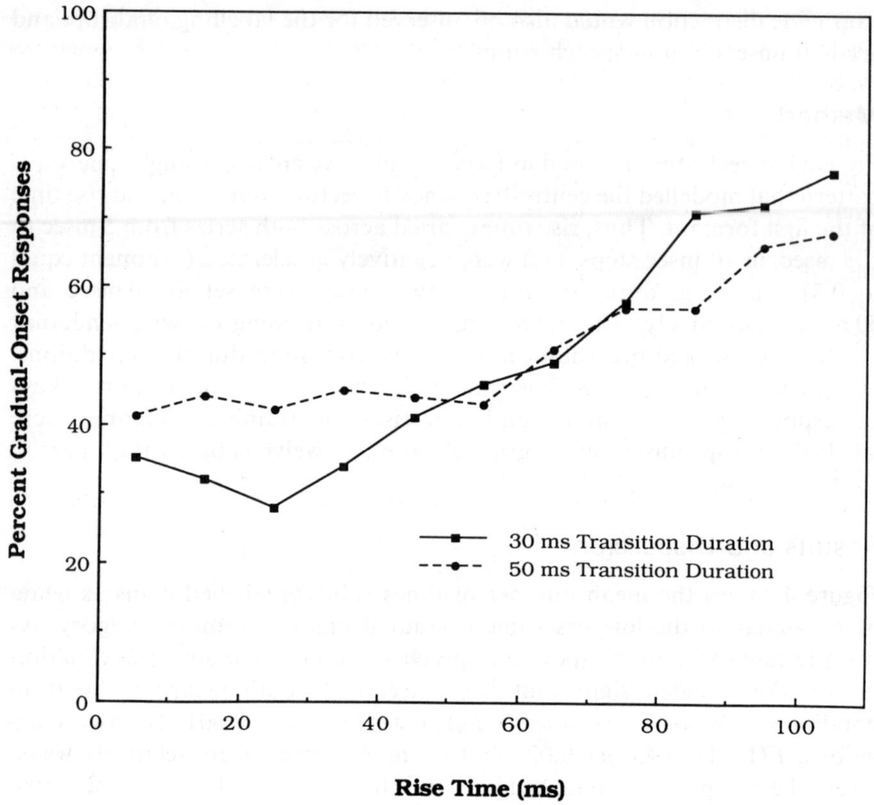

FIG. 4. Identification functions for the sine-wave stimuli used in Experiment 4. The parameter is transition duration.

boundary (Experiment 3) occurs *ceteris paribus* at a higher value of transition duration than does the stop/glide boundary (Experiment 1). In the speech case, the transition-duration value of 30 msec corresponds clearly to a perceived stop, whereas the 50-msec transition duration occurs near the stop/glide boundary (being within the glide category at least for longer values of rise time). However, in the non-speech case, the 30- and 50-msec values of transition duration are both within the abrupt-onset category (for the range of rise times used in the present study). This may help to account for the absence of a transition-duration effect in Experiment 4.

Despite training on the series-endpoint stimuli, listeners in the present experiment were unable to make reliable abruptness-of-onset judgements on the basis of rise-time variation alone. This failure indicates that the robust effect of transition duration observed in the previous experiment is not merely an artifact of the training procedure. It appears then, that the relative contributions of transition duration and rise time in signalling the stop/glide distinction in speech are approximately matched by their relative contributions in signalling the abrupt-onset/gradual-onset distinction among non-speech stimuli.

GENERAL DISCUSSION

Frequency-time cues and amplitude-envelope cues were independently manipulated to determine their effects in signalling the distinction between stops and glides (Experiments 1 and 2) and the distinction between abrupt and gradual onsets among analogous non-speech stimuli (Experiments 3 and 4). Consistent with results of Diehl and Walsh (1989), variation in transition duration effectively cued both the stop/glide and the abrupt-onset/gradual-onset contrasts, whereas comparable changes in rise time had only a modest effect on labelling performance in both the speech and non-speech conditions. Unlike the study by Diehl and Walsh (1989), transition duration and rise time were here varied within the same stimulus sets, allowing examination of the effects of the two variables in combination. Although transition duration clearly served as the primary cue (for listeners with normal hearing in quiet), rise time appeared to play a contrast-enhancing role in both the stop/glide and abrupt-onset/gradual-onset distinctions. That is, a brief rise time made the stimuli with shorter transitions appear more stoplike or more abrupt in onset, whereas a long rise time made the items with longer transitions seem more glidelike or more gradual in onset.

Despite some statistical differences between the effects observed in the speech and non-speech conditions, the qualitative similarities point to the likelihood that significant auditory commonalities underlie performance in the two cases. The perception of speech stops and glides may then be described as an instance of the perception of abrupt and gradual onsets in general (see Diehl & Walsh, 1989, for additional evidence on this point).

Earlier we suggested a frequency-dispersion account of the pattern of results observed in Experiments 1 and 3. Both rapid formant transitions and abrupt rise times may activate a relatively broad range of auditory frequency channels within a brief time interval, and such broadband activation may be a principal basis for the perception of abrupt onsets in general. This would account for the shift in location of the category boundaries along the transition-duration dimension produced by the parametric variation in rise time.

Recently, Bonvini, Walsh, and Diehl (1990) obtained evidence that calls into question the above hypothesis. Subjects labelled two series of synthetic speech stimuli that varied in transition duration and ranged perceptually from /bɑ/ to /wɑ/. The two series differed only in the frequency extent and slope of the formant transitions. Another group of subjects categorized single-sine-wave analogs of the speech stimuli as having either abrupt or gradual onsets. By the frequency-dispersion hypothesis, the series with the greater transition extents should have yielded more stop or abrupt-onset responses. A perceptual-learning account would make the opposite prediction in the case of the /bɑ/-/wɑ/ stimuli, because, in natural speech, glides typically have greater formant-transition extents than do the corresponding stops (Mack & Blumstein, 1983; Walsh, 1989). The results were mixed: in both the speech and non-speech conditions the effect of varying transition extent was inconsistent across subjects, yielding no significant overall shift in the category boundary. This appears to rule out the simple version of the frequency-dispersion hypothesis. Thus, at this point the auditory basis of the category boundary shifts observed in Experiments 1 and 3 remains unclear.

In the Introduction, we noted some discrepancies in the literature concerning the relative effectiveness of frequency-time and amplitude-envelope information in signalling the stop/glide distinction. Recall that Shinn and Blumstein (1984) reported evidence favouring a primary role for envelope cues, whereas Nittrouer and Studdert-Kennedy (1986) and Diehl and Walsh (1989) obtained results suggesting that frequency-time cues are more important. The present findings clearly support the latter position. These various studies differed in quite a number of ways, particularly with respect to stimulus design. The synthetic /bɑ/-/wɑ/ and /bi/-/wi/ stimuli used by Shinn and Blumstein had formant frequencies and timing characteristics that were adapted from the values of natural tokens of a male talker. By comparison, the stimuli used in the present study and in the study by Diehl and Walsh were rather stylized, having formant trajectories that did not closely model those typical of natural speech. One might conclude that our results are somehow attributable to the unnaturalness of our stimuli, and that the Shinn and Blumstein findings are a truer reflection of the relative importance of envelope and formant cues in natural speech.

Several facts, however, cast doubt on such a conclusion. First, when subjects in the Shinn and Blumstein (1984) study were allowed to perform free identification of the stimuli, the results were sufficiently variable to suggest that the stimulus parameters may not have been altogether natural. For example, the /bɑ/ endpoint stimulus from the series with appropriately interpolated amplitude envelopes was labelled as having an initial /v/ or /vw/ 30% of the time. (The segment /v/ shares with /w/ the feature value [+continuant], whereas /b/ is [-continuant].) Also, the /bi/ endpoint stimulus in the interpolated-amplitude series was labelled as beginning with /d/ 73% of the time. A second, more important reason to doubt the above conclusion is that our results are consistent with those of Nittrouer and Studdert-Kennedy (1986). As we noted, in their study the stimulus items included amplitude-modified versions of *naturally produced* /b/- and /w/-initial syllables. Moreover, the envelope modifications were based on criteria established by Mack and Blumstein (1983) and used by Shinn and Blumstein (1984). It appears unlikely, then, that the discrepancy between our results and those of Shinn and Blumstein can be ascribed to putative differences in stimulus naturalness.

We note that our results support Shinn and Blumstein's (1984) general view that envelope properties play a role in signalling the stop/glide contrast. We differ from them in our evaluation of the relative importance of those properties.

Finally, given the relatively modest effect of rise time in our experiments, it is useful to re-evaluate some results of earlier studies that appear to implicate rise time as a robust cue for the perceptual distinction between the affricate /ʧ/ as in *chop* and the fricative /ʃ/ as in *shop* (Cutting & Rosner, 1974; Gerstman, 1957; Howell & Rosen, 1983). In each of these studies, rise time was varied by removing successive portions of the initial frication segment such that rise time was directly related to frication duration. In a recent set of experiments, Walsh and Kluender (submitted) had listeners identity sets of /ʧɑ/-/ʃɑ/ stimuli (edited from natural tokens) in which rise time and frication duration were independently varied. Whereas variation in frication duration was sufficient to signal the contrast between affricates (short frication segments) and fricatives (long frication segments), rise time had only a small effect on identification performance. The pattern of results was, in fact, analogous to that of the stop/glide experiments in the present study. Rise-time variation across a range from 20 msec to 120 msec yielded a significant linear trend in labelling performance (with shorter rise times yielding more affricate labelling responses), but this range of variation was not sufficient to signal the distinction reliably. However, rise time did have an enhancing effect on the perception of the distinction, with short rise times shifting the affricate/fricative boundary towards greater values of frication duration.

Although waveform envelope properties appear to provide some information for consonant distinctions (see, e.g., Van Tassell, Soli, Kirby, & Widen, 1987), the role of rise time in speech perception may be much more limited than is generally believed.

REFERENCES

Bonvini, P.E., Walsh, M.A., & Diehl, R.L. (1990). *Effects of transition extent in signaling the /b/-/w/ distinction*. Unpublished raw data.

Brady, S.A. & Darwin, C.J. (1978). Range effect in the perception of voicing. *Journal of the Acoustical Society of America, 63*, 1556–1558.

Cooper, W.E., Ebert, R.R., & Cole, R.A. (1976). Perceptual analysis of stop consonants and glides. *Journal of Experimental Psychology: Human Perception and Performance, 2*, 92–104.

Cutting, J.E. & Rosner, B.S. (1974). Categories and boundaries in speech and music. *Perception & Psychophysics, 16*, 564–570.

Diehl, R.L. (1976). Feature analyzers for the phonetic dimension *stop* vs. *continuant*. *Perception & Psychophysics, 19*, 267–272.

Diehl, R.L. & Walsh, M.A. (1989). An auditory basis for the stimulus-length effect in the perception of stops and glides. *Journal of the Acoustical Society of America, 85*, 2154–2164.

Gerstman, L.J. (1957). *Perceptual dimensions for the friction portion of certain speech sounds*. Unpublished PhD dissertation, New York University.

Helson, H. (1964). *Adaptation-level theory*. New York: Academic Press.

Howell, P. & Rosen, S. (1983). Production and perception of rise time in the voiceless affricate/fricative distinction. *Journal of the Acoustical Society of America, 73*, 976–984.

Klatt, D. (1980). Software for a cascade/parallel formant synthesizer. *Journal of the Acoustical Society of America, 67*, 971–995.

Liberman, A.M., Delattre, P.C., Gerstman, L.J., & Cooper, F.S. (1956). Tempo of frequency change as a cue for distinguishing classes of speech sounds. *Journal of Experimental Psychology, 52*, 127–137.

Mack, M. & Blumstein, S.E. (1983). Further evidence of acoustic invariance in speech production. *Journal of the Acoustical Society of America, 73*, 1739–1750.

Miller, J.L. & Baer, T. (1983). Some effects of speaking rate on the production of /b/ and /w/. *Journal of the Acoustical Society of America, 73*, 1751–1755.

Miller, J.L. & Liberman, A.M. (1979). Some effects of later-occurring information on the perception of stop consonants and semi-vowels. *Perception & Psychophysics, 25*, 457–465.

Nittrouer, S. & Studdert-Kennedy, M. (1986). The stop-glide distinction: Acoustic analysis and perceptual effect of variation in syllable amplitude envelope for initial /b/ and /w/. *Journal of the Acoustical Society of America, 80*, 1026–1029.

O'Connor, J.O., Gerstman, L.J., Liberman, A.M., Delattre, P.C., & Cooper, F.S. (1957). Acoustic cues for the perception of initial /w, j, r, l/ in English. *Word, 13*, 24–43.

Parducci, A. (1974). Contextual effects: A range-frequency analysis. In E.C. Carterette & M.P. Friedman (Eds.), *Handbook of perception: Vol. II. Psychophysical judgment and measurement* (pp. 127–141). New York: Academic Press.

Pisoni, D.B., Carrell, T.D., & Gans, S.J. (1983). Perception of the duration of rapid spectrum changes in speech and nonspeech signals. *Perception & Psychophysics, 34*, 314–322.

Shinn, P. & Blumstein, S.E. (1984). On the role of the amplitude envelope for the perception of [b] and [w]. *Journal of the Acoustical Society of America, 75*, 1243–1252.

Van Tassell, D.J., Soli, S.D., Kirby, V.M., & Widen, G.P. (1987). Speech waveform envelope cues for consonant recognition. *Journal of the Acoustical Society of America, 82*, 1152–1161.

Walsh, M.A. (1989). *Acoustic measurements of stops and glides produced at varying speaking rates*. Unpublished raw data.

Walsh, M.A. & Kluender, K.R. (submitted). Amplitude rise time and the perception of the voiceless affricate/fricative distinction.

Younger, B.A. & Cohen, L.B. (1983). Infant perception of correlation among attributes. *Child Development, 54*, 858–867.

Revised manuscript received 30 November 1990

THE QUARTERLY JOURNAL OF EXPERIMENTAL PSYCHOLOGY, 1991, *43A* (3) 621–645

Single Band Amplitude Envelope Cues as an Aid to Speechreading

Ken W. Grant, Louis D. Braida, and Rebecca J. Renn

Research Laboratory of Electronics, Massachusetts Institute of Technology, Cambridge, Massachusets, U.S.A.

Amplitude envelopes derived from speech have been shown to facilitate speech-reading to varying degrees, depending on how the envelope signals were extracted and presented and on the amount of training given to the subjects. In this study, three parameters related to envelope extraction and presentation were examined using both easy and difficult sentence materials: (1) the bandwidth and centre frequency of the filtered speech signal used to obtain the envelope; (2) the bandwidth of the envelope signal determined by the lowpass filter cutoff frequency used to "smooth" the envelope fluctuations; and (3) the carrier signal used to convey the envelope cues. Results for normal hearing subjects following a brief visual and auditory-visual familiarization/training period showed that (1) the envelope derived from wideband speech does not provide the greatest benefit to speechreading when compared to envelopes derived from selected octave bands of speech; (2) as the bandwidth centred around the carrier frequency increased from 12.5 to 1600 Hz, auditory-visual (AV) performance obtained with difficult sentence materials improved, especially for envelopes derived from high-frequency speech energy; (3) envelope bandwidths below 25 Hz resulted in AV scores that were sometimes equal to or worse than speechreading alone; (4) for each filtering condition tested, there was at least one bandwidth and carrier condition that produced AV scores that were significantly greater than speech-reading alone; (5) low-frequency carriers were better than high-frequency or wideband carriers for envelopes derived from an octave band of speech centred at 500 Hz; and (6) low-frequency carriers were worse than high-frequency or wideband carriers for envelopes derived from an octave band centred at 3150 Hz. These results suggest that amplitude envelope cues can provide a substantial benefit to speechreading for both easy and difficult sentence materials, but that

---

Requests for reprints should be sent to Ken W. Grant, Army Audiology and Speech Center, Walter Reed Army Medical Center, Washington, DC 20307-5001, U.S.A.

The authors wish to thank Quentin Summerfield, Arthur Boothroyd, William Rabinowitz, and an anonymous reviewer for their helpful comments on earlier drafts of this manuscript. This research was supported by NIH grants DC 00010 and DC 00117 to Massachusetts Institute of Technology, Cambridge, Massachusetts.

---

frequency transposition of these signals to regions remote from their "natural" spectral locations may result in reduced performance.

Listeners with a severe-to-profound sensorineural-neural hearing loss often experience speech as "blurred" and "distorted" even after it has been amplified through an appropriately fitted hearing aid. Plomp (1978) has described this aspect of the hearing loss as a loss of acuity, and in particular as a loss of frequency discrimination (i.e. the ability to discriminate between two tones of different frequency) and frequency selectivity (i.e. the ability to resolve the sinusoidal components in a complex sound). Reduced frequency selectivity has been implicated as one of the factors making resolution of different spectral components of speech (e.g. formant frequencies, intonation patterns, etc.) more difficult (Hoekstra & Ritsma, 1977; Wightman, McGee, & Kramer, 1977; Scharf & Florentine, 1982; Moore & Glasberg, 1986; Rosen & Fourcin, 1986; Tyler, 1986). Under these circumstances, severely-to-profoundly impaired listeners tend to rely more heavily than do normal-hearing listeners on the temporal and amplitude variations in speech and on speechreading in order to comprehend spoken language (Erber, 1972b; Rosen & Fourcin, 1986; Van Tasell, Soli, Kirby & Widen, 1987: Rosen & Smith, 1988).

One way to compensate for impaired frequency selectivity is to preprocess the speech signal in a way that maximizes the salience of selected speech features known to be important for communication. For example, those features that complement speechreading may be emphasized, whereas at the same time other speech features that are redundant with speechreading may be disregarded. In doing so, less overall speech information is transmitted to the listener, but more information specific for enhancing speechreading may be received. Previous studies that have adopted this approach to signal simplification (Rosen, Fourcin, & Moore, 1981; Rosen & Fourcin, 1983; Moore et al., 1984; Breeuwer & Plomp, 1984, 1985, 1986; Grant, Ardell, Kuhl, & Sparks, 1985; Grant, 1987a, 1987b; Rosen, Walliker, Fourcin, & Ball, 1987) have shown that trained normal-hearing listeners and some hearing-impaired listeners can make substantial use of auditory sinewave analogs representing various speech features such as voicing-duration, amplitude-envelope, fundamental frequency (F0), and formant frequency cues when combined with speechreading.

An obvious question raised by these studies is whether simplified auditory signals of the type mentioned above can provide more benefit to speechreading than conventional amplification, and how much training is necessary to achieve this result. Results from Rosen and Fourcin (1983) and Grant (1987a) have shown that some severely-to-profoundly hearing-impaired subjects perform better on tasks focusing on the perception of intonation and stress with non-speech, sinewave analogs of F0 than they do with amplified speech. Results for other types of auditory signal amplification have not been directly compared to normal speech.

Training is one of the most important issues that continues to plague research on sensory substitution and aids to speechreading, especially when novel speech coding schemes are used. Unless one is convinced that subjects have been sufficiently trained (which is seldom possible given the time and motivation required to achieve performance asymptotes, even under a single condition), any conclusions comparing speech recognition results obtained with conventional amplification and coded speech signals or between two different coded speech signals should be considered preliminary until a much larger research effort addressing the learning issue is completed.

With this caveat in mind, the purpose of the present study was to investigate the potential benefit to speechreading when speech envelope cues are presented to normal-hearing subjects. We chose to evaluate normal hearing subjects in these initial studies in order to establish realistic performance expectations for future work with impaired listeners. Consistent with our long-term goal to develop an effective communication aid to speechreading for individuals who do not currently benefit from hearing aids, speech envelope signals (as opposed to formant frequency or fundamental frequency signals) were selected because (1) they have been shown to result in significant improvements to speech perception when presented in combination with speechreading, (2) are easily extracted from continuous speech, (3) have relatively narrow bandwidths and are therefore appropriate for listeners with very limited residual hearing, and (4) are easily transposed in frequency, so that they can be optimally matched to the individual's best region of hearing.

Background

Previous work on the benefit of presenting speech envelope cues as a supplement to speechreading has led to widely differing results, ranging from little or no benefit (Erber, 1972a; Risberg & Lubker, 1978) to substantial benefit (Risberg, 1974; Ardell, 1980; Grant et al., 1985; Breeuwer & Plomp, 1984, 1986). These studies are summarized in Table 1. One way to interpret differences in results among studies is in terms of the processing strategies employed during envelope extraction and presentation. Figure 1 shows a typical processing scheme that extracts and presents speech envelope signals (after Horii, House, & Hughes, 1971), with the shaded blocks indicating the three parameters under investigation in the present study. An additional variable not under consideration in this study is whether the rectifier used half-wave or full-wave rectification. All of the studies listed in Table 1, as well as the present study, used full-wave rectification.

1. The *pre-filter* determines the spectral region(s) of the speech signal from which the envelope is derived. Both wideband and narrowband pre-filters have been used. For example, in the studies by Breeuwer and Plomp (1984, 1986), $\frac{1}{3}$- and 1-octave pre-filters centred at 500, 1600, and 3160 Hz

TABLE 1

Survey of Selected Studies Evaluating the Contribution of Speechreading and Amplitude Envelopes to Speech Perception

Study	*Prefilter*	*Smoothing Filter*	*Carrier*	*Materials*	*Condition*	*Score*
Erber (1972a)	2000 Hz lowpass	20 Hz	500-Hz OBN	240 nouns	SA, S + AM	58–65 (PHI) 26–32 (adults) 41–49 (children)
Risberg (1974)	100–2700 Hz	30 Hz	120-Hz pulse train bandpass filtered at 500 Hz, 250-Hz bandwidth	15 familiar closed-set sentences	SA, S + AM, AM	40–72–19
Risberg & Lubker (1978)	100–2700 Hz	30 Hz	120-Hz pulse train bandpass filtered at 500 Hz, 250-Hz bandwidth	24 unknown questions	SA, S + AM	38–42

Ardell (1980)	300 Hz lowpass	100 Hz	225-Hz tone	connected discourse tracking	SA, S + AM	38–68
Breeuwer & Plomp (1984)	$\frac{1}{3}$ octaves and octaves at 500, 1600, and 3160 Hz	20 Hz	tone at centre frequency of the pre-filter	20 lists of 13 easy sentences	SA, S + AM	*$\frac{1}{3}$-oct** 500 23–55 1600 23–44 3160 23–44 *1-oct* 500 23–66 1600 23–46 3160 23–41
Breeuwer & Plomp (1986)	WB	20 Hz	250-Hz pulse train filtered from 160 to 400 Hz	10 lists of 13 easy sentences	SA, S + AM	17–46

* Scores are for six different pre-filter conditions.

Note: All scores in percent correct except Ardell (1980), which are in percent of normal tracking rate (i.e. 108 words per minute). SA = speechreading alone; OBN = octave band of noise; PHI = profoundly hearing-impaired; WB = wideband speech.

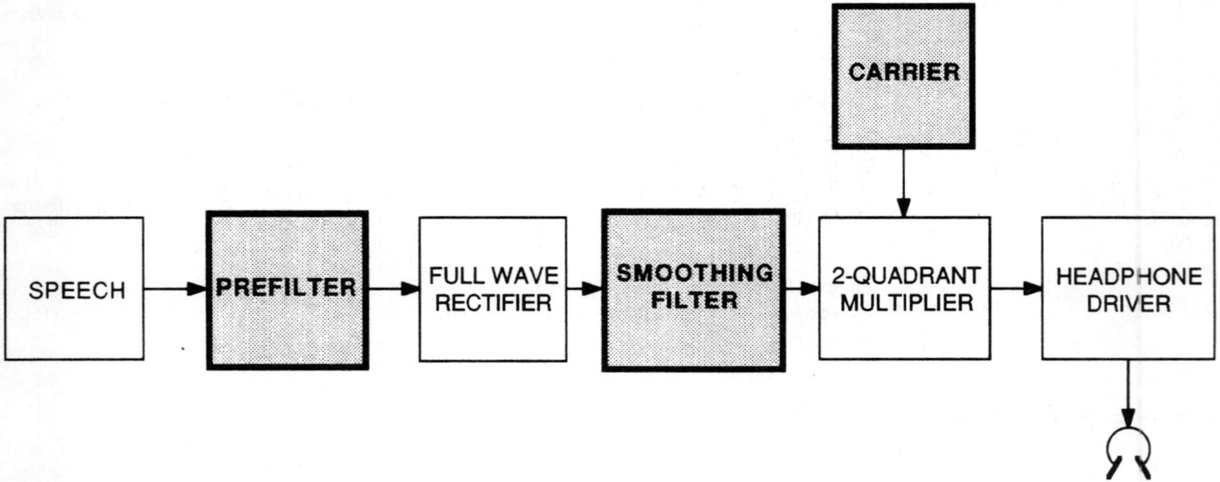

FIG. 1. Schematic showing the processing used to extract and present speech envelope cues. Shaded areas indicate the three parameters varied in Experiments 1 and 2. Pre-filter values were either wideband speech or octave bands at 500, 1600, and 3150 Hz. Smoothing filter values ranged from 12.5-Hz to 1600-Hz lowpass. Carrier signals included wideband noise as well as sinusoids at 200, 500, 1600, and 3150 Hz.

were tested. In addition, several two-band envelope combinations were also studied. For most of the conditions evaluated by Breeuwer and Plomp (1984), a tone carrier at the pre-filter centre frequency was used to convey the envelope cues to untrained normal-hearing listeners. The results obtained with sets of everyday sentences indicated that (1) AV performance with any of the envelope cues was significantly greater than speechreading alone, (2) the 500-Hz pre-filter was more effective in aiding speechreading than either the 1600- or 3160-Hz pre-filter (see Table 1), and (3) differences between $\frac{1}{3}$- and 1-octave pre-filter bandwidths were significant only for the 500-Hz pre-filter condition. In their later study (Breeuwer & Plomp, 1986), an envelope signal derived from the wideband speech signal was used to modulate a 250-Hz pulse train that was bandpass filtered from 160 to 400 Hz. While the results with this envelope cue were also significantly better than speechreading alone (see Table 1), it is not possible to compare the earlier results obtained with the narrowband pre-filters to that of the wideband pre-filter because different carriers and different subjects were employed. Thus, to our knowledge, no study has compared AV performance with the overall speech envelope (i.e. no pre-filter) to other speech envelopes within the same subject group.

2. The *smoothing filter* affects the envelope bandwidth, the degree to which the envelope can follow rapid fluctuations in speech energy, and the overall group delay of the system (i.e. the apparent asynchrony between auditory and visual speech elements). It is necessary to follow the full-wave rectifier with a lowpass filter because the effect of rectification on the filtered signal can be a substantial increase in bandwidth. The "smoothing" lowpass filter is used to select those components associated with the envelope of the bandpass signal. Previous studies investigating the relation between amplitude envelope cues and speechreading used smoothing filters with cutoff frequencies between 20 and 100 Hz. However, the effect on the reception of continuous speech of varying the smoothing filter has not been tested. In a related study, Van Tasell et al. (1987) studied the effect of smoothing filter on information transmission of auditorily presented /aCa/ syllables. Envelopes were derived from a 4-kHz lowpass prefilter, smoothed with a 20, 200, or 2000-Hz lowpass filter, and then multiplied with pink noise. Information transmitted (Miller & Nicely, 1955) increased from 22% to 29% to 35% for the three smoothing filters, respectively.

3. The *carrier* determines the spectral centre and timbre of the resulting amplitude-modulated signal and can be used to transpose the envelope information to any frequency region. Pure tones, complex tones, and noise carriers have been used to vary the quality and bandwidth of the resulting AM signal.

Schematized examples of speech envelopes derived either from the wide-band speech waveform or from an octave band centred at 500 or 3150 Hz are shown in Figure 2 for the sentence "Show the Enterprise's home port". The middle panel of this figure shows the original speech waveform. For each pre-filter, the result of using either a 100-Hz or 12.5-Hz smoothing filter is shown. A comparison of the original speech waveform to that of the wideband envelope with a 12.5-Hz smoothing filter shows an overall group delay of approximately 60 msec. In addition to the group delay imposed by the

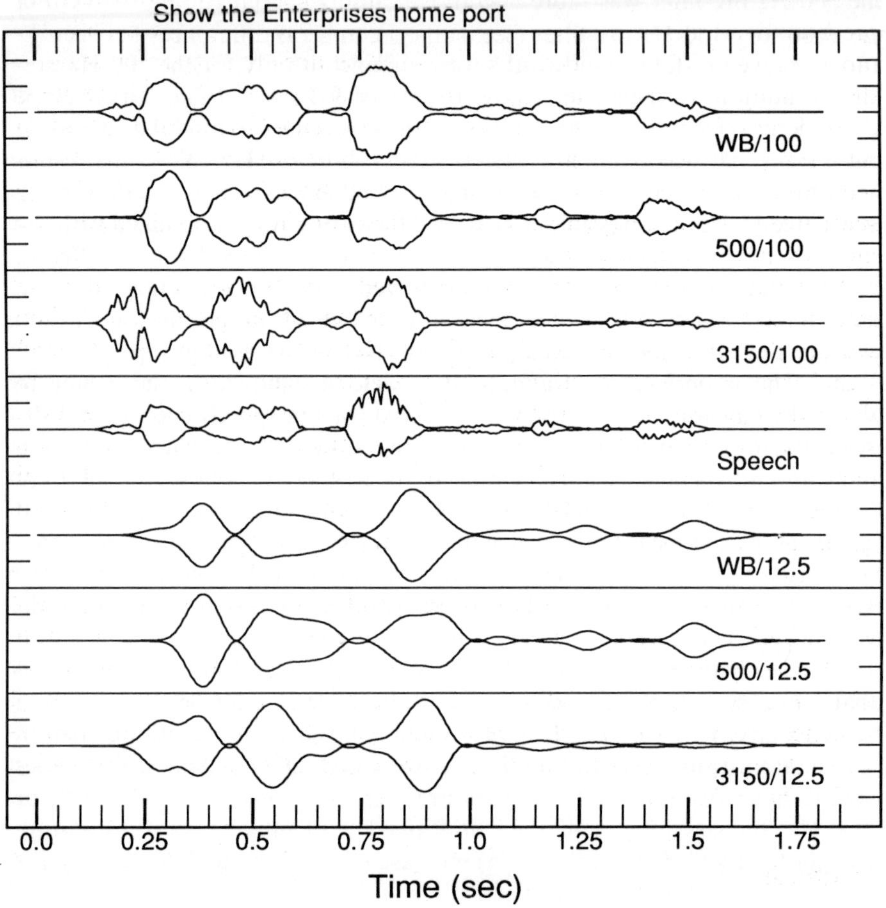

FIG. 2. Schematized envelope signals for the sentence "Show the Enterprise's home port" obtained with three different pre-filters (WB = wideband; 500 = octave band centred at 500 Hz; 3150 = octave band centred at 3150 Hz) and two different smoothing filters (100 = 100-Hz lowpass; 12.5 = 12.5 Hz lowpass). Also shown (middle panel) is the waveform envelope of the original unprocessed sentence. Envelopes were obtained by digitizing the sentence at 16-kHz sampling rate, pre-filtering the signal with an 8-pole Butterworth bandpass filter, full-wave rectifying the output of the bandpass filter, and then smoothing the result with an 8-pole Butterworth lowpass filter. To obtain the plots, the maximum and minimum values for non-overlapping 100-point segments were computed for each of the seven signals shown.

lowpass smoothing filter, a second type of "delay" that is directly related to the spectrum content of the speech signal and the pre-filter can be observed. For example, with a 500-Hz pre-filter and a 12.5-Hz smoothing filter, the onset of the envelope signal relative to the onset of the word "show" in the speech signal is delayed nearly 120 msec, because the initial /ʃ/ is not represented in the envelope signal. For the 3150-Hz pre-filter, the combined delay due to the 12.5-Hz smoothing filter and the interaction between the pre-filter and the spectrum content of the speech signal is substantially less (approximately 60 msec), because the envelope does reflect the presence of the initial fricative consonant. It is important to consider the magnitude of these delays because it can result in noticeable and perceptually disruptive AV asynchrony. According to McGrath and Summerfield (1985), delays on the order of 80 msec or more are likely to affect AV performance for average speechreaders, and delays as small as 40 msec can affect AV performance for more experienced speechreaders.

In addition to the different delays imposed by the combination of smoothing filter, pre-filter, and spectrum content of the speech signal, there are also deviations in the waveform shape relative to the unprocessed speech signal's envelope. Due to the common carrier frequency running throughout the envelope signal, many of these waveform perturbations are heard as extra syllables. For example, with a 3150-Hz pre-filter and 100-Hz smoothing filter, the word "show" appears to have three syllables. Note, that although the 500-Hz pre-filter/100-Hz smoothing filter envelope is missing the initial /ʃ/ in "show", it appears to convey the correct number of syllables.

In the present study, the pre-filter, carrier, and smoothing filter were systematically varied to cover a wide range of possible cases. Experiment 1 varied both pre-filter and carrier while holding smoothing filter constant at 100 Hz lowpass. Experiment 2 investigated a range of smoothing filters for three pre-filter/carrier conditions. For both experiments, two types of sentence materials were used—one with a high degree of contextual information (CUNY sentences) and one with a low degree of contextual information (IEEE–Harvard sentences).

Methods

Subjects. Ten subjects participated in this study: six in Experiment 1 and four in Experiment 2. All were native speakers of American English, and all had normal hearing and normal or corrected vision. None of the subjects had previously been employed in any speechreading experiments. Subjects were paid for their participation.

The subjects were first screened for speechreading ability using three lists (Lists A, C, and E) of the CID/NTID everyday sentence test (Davis & Silverman, 1978). Subjects viewed the sentence lists on a 19-in. colour monitor (SONY Model KV 2080R) from a distance of approximately 6 ft. Each list contained ten sentences, with five key words per sentence. A score of 20% key-word identification was required for participation in the study. Previous data with these same sentence materials (Grant, 1988) have shown that approximately 85% of normal-hearing subjects pass this screening level. For the ten subjects used in the present study, the average screening score was 36% correct, with a range of 21 to 60% correct.

Speech Materials. The speech materials used in this study consisted of both CUNY (Boothroyd, Hnaith-Chislm, & Hanin, 1985) and IEEE sentences (IEEE, 1969). IEEE sentences were videotaped using a three-tube colour camera (Ikegami ITC-730A), a tram Lavelier close-talk microphone, and a $\frac{3}{4}$-in. U-matic video recorder (JVC 8250). Overhead lighting was provided by a combination of soft and spot lights (Mole Richardson Studio Lighting) against a blue background. CUNY sentences were purchased on Laser Disc format. Sentences from the original recordings (CUNY and IEEE) were dubbed onto $\frac{1}{2}$-in. Hi-Fi VHS format (NEC 961U).

Instrumentation and Procedures. All envelope conditions were obtained by the method described by Horii et al. (1971). Pre-filtering was accomplished with a $\frac{1}{3}$-octave multifilter bank (GR Model 1925). Attenuation rates were locally very steep (approximately 80 dB/octave) for the first 40–50 dB and then became less steep. The smoothing filter was an 8-pole damped response lowpass filter (Krohn-Hite Model 3343R). At the cutoff frequency, the filter response was approximately 24 dB down. The 3-dB point was located at approximately one-third of the cutoff frequency. Envelope signals were presented binaurally over headphones (TDH-39) at a comfortable listening level.

Previous studies by Breeuwer and Plomp (1984, 1985, 1986) showed that untrained normal-hearing subjects can achieve a fairly large AV advantage over speechreading alone for everyday sentence materials when presented with a 500-Hz tone amplitude-modulated by the envelope from an octave band centred at 500 Hz (e.g. 66% S+AM vs. 23% SA, see Table 1). In our earlier work with similar signals (Grant, Renn & Yu, 1988) we had found that some listeners had great difficulty utilizing auditory envelope cues with speechreading, especially for difficult sentence materials such as the IEEE/Harvard lists. Therefore, in order to familiarize the subjects with speechreading alone and with speechreading with reduced auditory cues, all subjects were tested for 3 hr in a connected discourse tracking (CDT) procedure (DeFilippo & Scott, 1978). In this procedure, short passages of connected discourse are presented to subjects who are required to repeat verbatim what was read. If an error is made, the talker repeats the missed word or words until they are perceived correctly. In addition to simple repetition, the talker may use a variety of directed feedback options. Among the most common of these options are repeating previous portions of text as a review and reading ahead in the text as a preview to upcoming material. At the end of each session, the number of words correctly repeated is converted to a words-per-minute (WPM) score.

During the tracking evaluations, the subject and talker were seated in separate sound-treated rooms. The subject viewed the talker through a closed-circuit TV system consisting of a colour video camera (JVC Model S-62U) and a 19-in. colour monitor (Sony Model KV 2080R). Auditory signals were presented binaurally over headphones (TDH-39) at a comfortable listening level. The subject responded by speaking into a microphone connected to a speaker located in the talker's booth.

Three receptive conditions were evaluated using the tracking procedure: speechreading alone (SA), speechreading, plus lowpass filtered (300-Hz cutoff) speech (S + FIL300), and speechreading plus speech envelope (S + AM) cues (pre-filter = octave band at 500 Hz; smoothing filter = 100-Hz lowpass; carrier = 375 Hz)[1]. Each condition was evaluated for six 10-min sessions in randomized order. The speech materials used were the same for each subject and were at a fourth-grade reading level. The talker was a male speaker (KWG) with considerable practice with the CDT procedure.

Following familiarization/training, subjects were tested with two sets of sentence materials. CUNY sentences were presented in lists of 12 sentences each, and scoring was based on the total number of words correctly identified (102 words per list). IEEE sentences were presented in lists of ten sentences each, and scoring was based on the number of key words correctly identified (50 words per list).

Experimental Conditions. The first experiment reported below examined the effects of using different carrier signals to convey envelopes derived from different pre-filter regions of speech. For Experiment 1, the smoothing filter was fixed at 100-Hz lowpass. The second experiment examined the effect of smoothing filter for three different pre-filter/carrier configurations. In all, there were 19 different AV conditions in Experiment 1 and 18 different AV

---

[1] Note that with the exception of speechreading alone, the conditions evaluated with the tracking procedure were different from the test conditions evaluated in Experiments 1 and 2. This was done deliberately because of the large number of conditions evaluated in the two experiments and the time-intensive nature of the tracking procedures. Thus, the "training" conditions were used to familiarize the subjects with speechreading, with and without low-intelligibility auditory signals. A more formal training procedure, in which all of the training conditions were also used as test conditions, was incorporated into a later study, which tested both single-band and two-band envelope combinations as supplements to speechreading.

TABLE 2
Experimental Conditions

Pre-filter	*Smoothing Filter*	*Carrier*
*Experiment 1**		
		Wideband noise
Wideband speech		200 Hz tone
Octave band at 500 Hz	100 Hz	500 Hz tone
Octave band at 1600 Hz		1600 Hz tone
Octave band at 3150 Hz		3150 Hz tone
Experiment 2		
	12.5 Hz	
	25 Hz	
Octave band at 500 Hz	50 Hz	200-Hz tone
	100 Hz	
	200 Hz	
	12.5 Hz	
	25 Hz	
Octave band at 3150 Hz	50 Hz	200-Hz tone
	100 Hz	
	200 Hz	
	12.5 Hz	
	25 Hz	
	50 Hz	
Octave band at 3150 Hz	100 Hz	3150-Hz tone
	200 Hz	
	400 Hz	
	800 Hz	
	1600 Hz	

* All combinations were tested except the 1600-Hz pre-filter/3150-Hz carrier condition.

conditions in Experiment 2. The different AV conditions are shown in Table 2. In addition, speechreading alone measures were obtained for both subject groups. In Experiment 1, all possible combinations of pre-filter and carrier were tested, with the exception of the 1600-Hz pre-filter/3150-Hz carrier condition. Due to the limited number of sentence lists available, not all of the conditions could be tested without repeating lists, and this particular condition was eliminated because of its limited application for hearing-impaired listeners (i.e. transposing the envelope cues to a higher frequency region). In Experiment 2, the selection of smoothing filters was restricted on the low end so as not to allow the overall group delay due to processing to exceed 80 msec and on the high end so as not to exceed the carrier frequency or the lower edge of the pre-filter bandwidth. Testing with CUNY sentence materials was completed before testing began with the IEEE sentences. Subjects wrote their responses and were encouraged to guess if they were unsure of the sentence's content. Three different CUNY lists and three different IEEE lists were presented for each condition, and within a list each sentence was presented once for identification without feedback. At no time were any of the sentences repeated. Conditions for the two separate experiments were presented in random order, but all conditions were tested once before any condition was repeated.

Result

Experiment 1—Effects of Pre-filter and Carrier

The data from Experiment 1 were subjected to a three-factor (four pre-filters, five carriers) repeated measures (three lists) ANOVA with sentence type (CUNY or IEEE) treated separately.[2] For the CUNY sentence data, recall that one condition (1600-Hz pre-filter/3150-Hz carrier) was omitted due to the limited number of available sentence sets. Therefore, in order to run a balanced repeated measures ANOVA, the missing data cells were filled with the mean values obtained for each of the three repetitions, respectively.

The results of this analysis showed that pre-filter was a significant factor for both CUNY and IEEE sentences, $F(3, 100) = 10.8$, $p < 0.01$ and $F(3, 100) = 15.4$, $p < 0.01$, respectively, and that carrier was not a significant factor for either set of sentence materials. For IEEE sentences, carrier approached but did not reach significance [$F(4, 100) = 2.2$, $p = 0.07$]. The Pre-filter × Carrier interaction was not significant for either type of sentence materials. For CUNY sentences, and to a lesser extent with IEEE sentences, scores continued to improve with repeated evaluations, $F(2, 200) = 131.1$, $p < 0.01$, and $F(2, 200) = 8.3$, $p < 0.01$, respectively, indicating that the subjects had not yet reached asymptotic performance. This finding is consistent with that of Breeuwer and Plomp (1986) and Van Tasell et al. (1987), who also found that a subject's ability to use envelope cues effectively was quite variable and would probably be influenced by training. The amount and type of training necessary to stabilize the responses is not known.

Although the above analysis failed to reveal a significant Pre-filter × Carrier interaction, subjects frequently reported that the AM signals sounded more "natural" when the carrier frequency was near the pre-filter frequency. Subsequent post hoc analyses using two-tailed t-tests to compare all possible combinations of pre-filter/carrier conditions showed that there were signifi-

---

[2] Although a repeated measures design was used, recall that no sentence was ever presented more than once. Thus, the conditions were tested three times, each time with a different sentence list.

cant effects for carrier type when the data were averaged across repetitions. For the CUNY data, carrier was significant ($p<0.05$) for both the 500-Hz and 3150-Hz pre-filter conditions—that is, for these pre-filter conditions, significant differences were found among the different carriers tested. For the IEEE data, significant effects for the different carrier signals were found for all but the wideband pre-filter condition.

The main results from Experiment 1 are shown in Figure 3. For both sentence types, substantial AV advantages over speechreading alone were

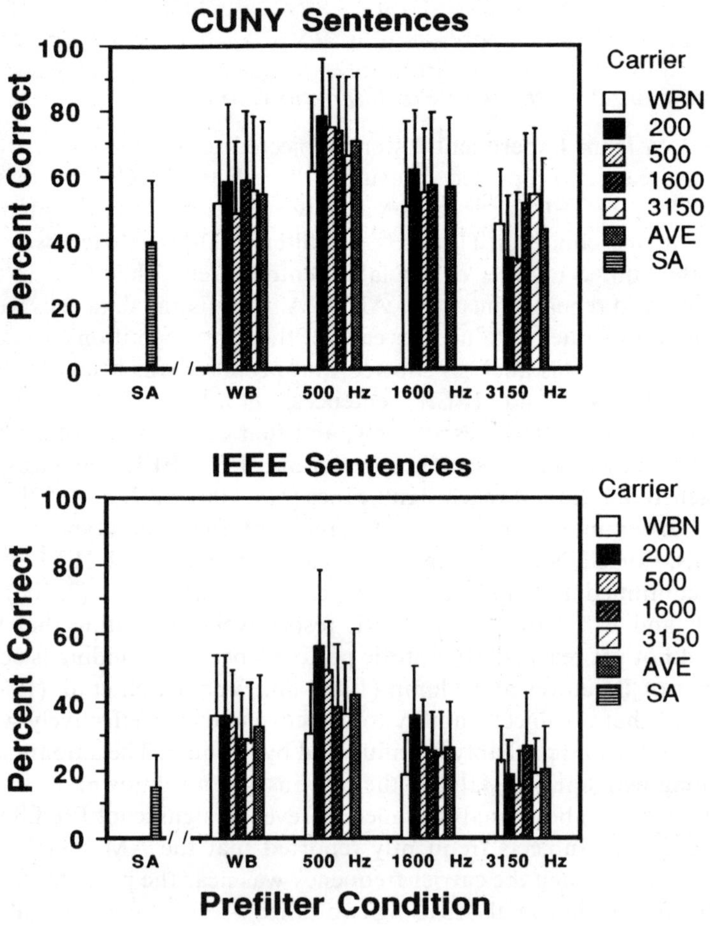

FIG. 3. Average AV results and standard deviations (error bars) for six normal-hearing subjects in Experiment 1. Pre-filters were either wideband speech or octave bands centred at the specified frequency. Smoothing filter was fixed at 100-Hz lowpass. Each bar represents a different carrier condition. Average scores for all carriers within a single pre-filter condition are also shown (AVE). WBN = wideband noise; SA = speechreading alone.

found for some of envelope signals tested. Although some of the envelope conditions failed to benefit speechreading, at least one carrier in each pre-filter group resulted in significant improvements over speechreading alone (significance was based on unpaired, two-tailed t-tests for means averaged across repetitions, $p < 0.05$). Specifically, for both sets of sentence materials, we found that (1) all carriers tested with the 500-Hz pre-filter condition resulted in AV scores that were significantly better than speechreading alone; (2) for the wideband and 1600-Hz pre-filter conditions, scores for the 200-Hz and 1600-Hz carrier conditions were significantly greater than speechreading alone; and (3) for the 3150-Hz pre-filter condition, the 1600-Hz carrier condition for IEEE sentences and the 3150-Hz carrier condition for CUNY sentences resulted in scores significantly greater than those for speechreading alone.

On average, envelopes obtained from the 500-Hz pre-filter condition provided more benefit to speechreading than the other pre-filter conditions, including wideband speech. Specifically, the average score for this pre-filter (across carrier and repetition) was significantly greater than the average score obtained with any other pre-filter condition, including wideband speech. In addition, the 500-Hz pre-filter/200-Hz carrier condition was better than any other condition tested, and the 200-Hz carrier produced the best results for all pre-filters except the 3150-Hz pre-filter condition where high-frequency carriers (and wideband noise) were better than low-frequency carriers. Results obtained with the wideband noise carrier were generally not as good as those obtained with tone carriers, except for the 3150-Hz pre-filter.

As mentioned previously, there were large individual differences among the subjects in their overall ability to speechread and in their ability to use auditory envelope cues with speechreading. Figure 4 shows the range of these differences with IEEE sentence scores obtained from the worst (SL) and best (CT) speechreader evaluated in Experiment 1. Note that in spite of the large skill differences in speechreading alone scores (5% vs. 29%), the patterns of relative performance between conditions were quite similar for each subject and similar to the average data shown in Figure 3.

Experiment 2—Effects of Smoothing Filter

In Experiment 2, three pre-filter/carrier conditions (500 Hz/200 Hz, 3150 Hz/200 Hz, and 3150 Hz/3150 Hz) were evaluated with different smoothing filters. Five different smoothing filters were used for the first two pre-filter/carrier conditions, and eight different smoothing filters were used for the 3150-Hz/3150-Hz condition. Due to the different number of smoothing filter conditions tested, a complete three-factor repeated measures ANOVA was not applicable. Instead, the data for each pre-filter/carrier condition were treated separately and analysed with a two-factor (smoothing

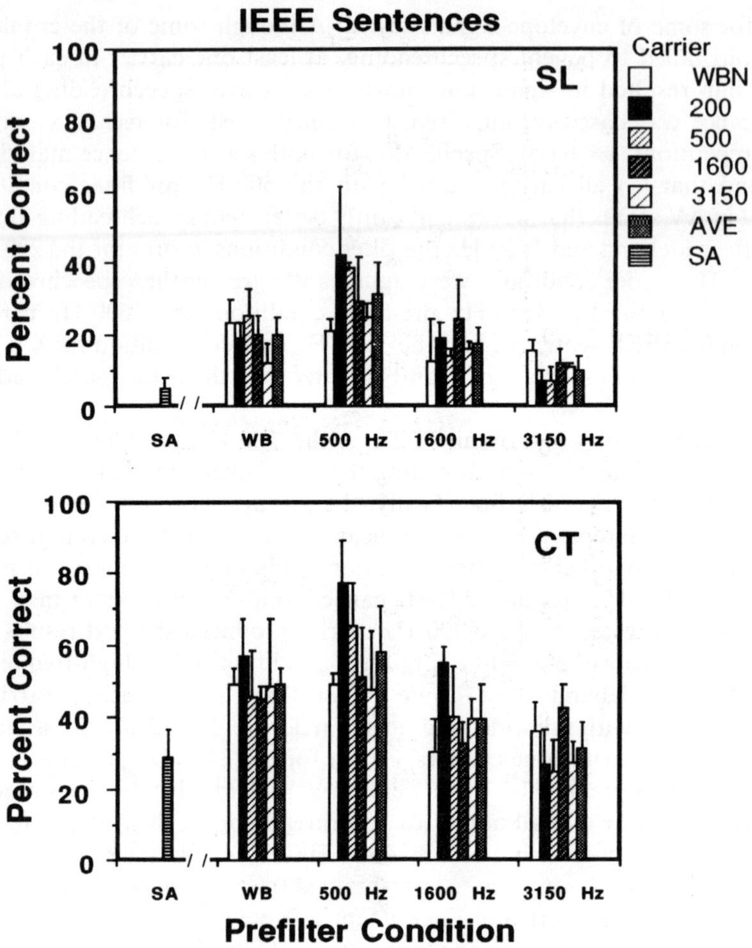

FIG. 4. Individual AV results and standard deviations (error bars) for the worst and best speechreader from Experiment 1. See Figure 3 for condition code.

filter, list) repeated measures ANOVA. This analysis indicated that smoothing filter was a significant factor only for the 3150-Hz/3150-Hz condition evaluated with IEEE sentences, $F(7, 24) = 10.9, p < 0.01$). Results for this prefilter/carrier condition obtained with CUNY sentences approached but did not reach significance, $F(7, 24) = 1.9$, $p = 0.07$.

The main results from Experiment 2 are shown in Figure 5. Note that several of the functions tend to rise and then level off as the centre frequency of the smoothing filter was increased. Post-hoc *t*-tests based on a comparison

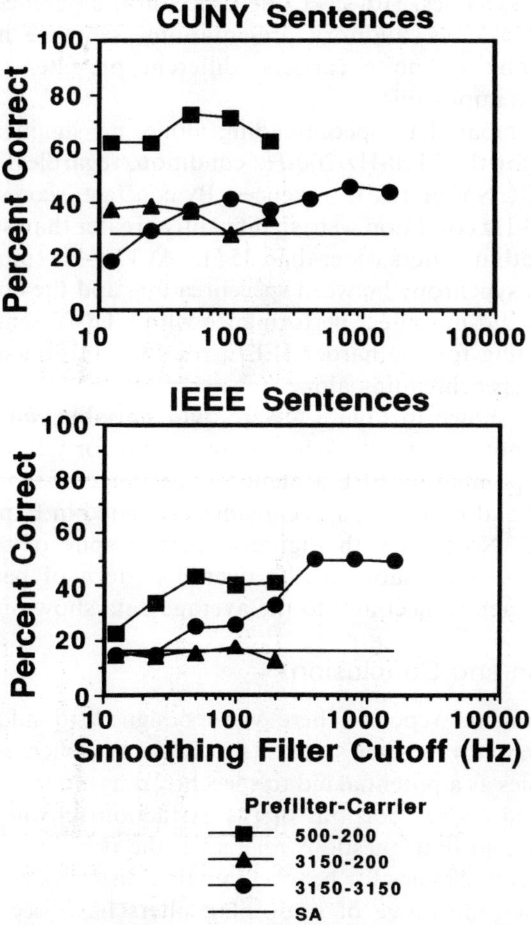

FIG. 5. Average AV results for three pre-filter/carrier conditions as a function of smoothing filter. Data are for four normal-hearing subjects in Experiment 2. Average standard deviations (not shown) across pre-filter/carrier conditions were 16% for CUNY sentences and 13% for IEEE sentences. SA = speechreading alone.

among means for all scores within a given pre-filter/smoothing filter condition showed that this rising trend was significant ($p < 0.05$) for the 3150-Hz/3150-Hz condition for both CUNY and IEEE sentences and for the 500-Hz/200-Hz condition for the IEEE sentences. This is in agreement with the results of Van Tasell et al. (1987), who found a significant increase in the amount of information transmitted when the smoothing filter was increased from 25 Hz to 200 Hz for auditory presentations of envelope cues derived from /aCa/ syllables. However, the procedural differences between the two studies (i.e. AV vs. auditory presentations, sentence materials vs. /aCa/ syllables, tone vs. noise carriers, different pre-filters, etc.) make direct comparisons impossible.

When compared to speechreading alone, no significant AV advantage was found for the 3150-Hz/200-Hz condition, regardless of smoothing filter for either CUNY or IEEE sentences. By contrast, scores obtained with the 500-Hz/200-Hz condition were significantly greater than speechreading alone for all smoothing filters wider than 25 Hz. At 12.5-Hz smoothing, there was a noticeable asynchrony between speechreading and the envelope signal. This asynchrony did not affect performance with CUNY sentence materials but was distracting for the harder IEEE, resulting in non-significant improvements over speechreading alone.

The data shown in Figure 5 were quite variable, with average standard deviations (not shown) of 16 percentage points for CUNY sentences and 13 percentage points for IEEE sentences. The range of scores obtained by the worst (AC) and best (GF) speechreader evaluated in Experiment 2 is shown in Figure 6. Note, as with Figure 4, that in spite of the large individual differences between subjects, the overall pattern of performance is quite similar for each subject and to the average data shown in Figure 5.

Discussion and Conclusion

The experiments reported here were designed to address many of the questions raised in earlier studies (see Table 1), which evaluated amplitude envelope cues as a potential aid to speechreading. In these earlier studies, the pre-filter and carrier portions of the extraction scheme were typically not independent, so that questions related to the possible effects of frequency-lowering envelope cues for hearing impaired listeners were left unanswered. Similarly, a wide range of smoothing filters have been used by different researchers, but the only study that formally addressed this aspect of the extraction scheme (e.g. Van Tasell et al., 1987) did not evaluate AV performance.

Based on the results of the present study, we are now in a position to come to the following conclusions:

1. Speech envelopes derived from wideband speech signals, regardless of the carrier frequency or carrier type (e.g. tone or noise), are not the best signals for aiding speechreading. Envelopes derived from low-frequency speech regions (e.g. from lowpass filtered speech or from octave bands of speech with centre frequencies around 500 Hz) provide more benefit to speechreaders for smoothing filters up to 200 Hz. For smoothing filters above 200 Hz, no direct comparisons across different pre-filter/carrier combinations have been made. This conclusion was suggested earlier by Ardell (1980) and Grant et al. (1985), based on the premise that envelope signals

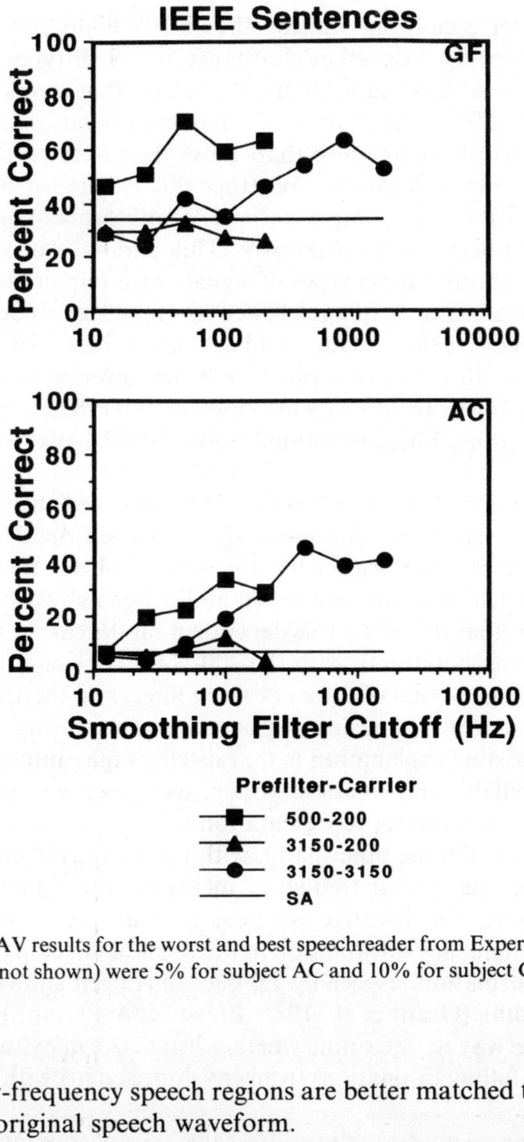

FIG. 6. Individual AV results for the worst and best speechreader from Experiment 2. Average standard deviations (not shown) were 5% for subject AC and 10% for subject GF. SA = speechreading alone.

derived from low-frequency speech regions are better matched to the syllabic structure of the original speech waveform.

2. Tone carriers are better than noise carriers for conveying envelope signals. This is probably true, because noise carriers have their own amplitude modulations that are independent of the speech signal's modulations.

3. For envelopes derived from the 3150-Hz pre-filter conditions, lowering the carrier from 3150 Hz to 500 Hz or 200 Hz significantly reduced performance for both types of sentence materials. On the other hand, lowering the envelopes derived from the wideband 1600-Hz or 500-Hz prefilter conditions did not affect performance. For envelopes derived from the

500-Hz pre-filter conditions, raising the carrier from 500 Hz or 200 Hz to 3150 Hz significantly reduced performance for both types of sentence materials. For normal hearing listeners, it appears that envelope cues that are greatly displaced from their "natural" frequency locations are more difficult to integrate with speechreading than those that were presented at or near their original spectral locations. Whether this is true for impaired listeners (presumably with less listening experience than normals) or for well-trained normal hearing listeners is not known. This finding is of some concern for possible application of these types of signals with impaired listeners because of the probable need to frequency-lower envelope signals derived from high-frequency speech regions. Our results suggest that, for normal hearing listeners at least, this may be a problem if the lowering is severe.

4. Similar to the results of Van Tasell et al. (1987), our results show an effect for smoothing filter reductions below 200 Hz, presumably because of the imposed signal delay, which reduced auditory-visual synchrony (e.g. especially for the 12.5-Hz smoothing condition), and the distortions in the envelope shape relative to the input speech waveform. Unfortunately, we were not able to separate these two sources of error due to limitations in our ability to re-synchronize the processed audio signals with the video signals. Note, however, that this effect was dependent on the carrier frequency for the 3150-Hz pre-filter condition, with the 200-Hz carrier offering no support to speechreading, regardless of the smoothing filter, and the 1600-Hz and 3150-Hz carriers offering increasing support with increasing smoothing filter cutoff. One possible explanation is that listeners may interpret the 3150/200 envelope as syllabic information, which, as shown earlier (see Figure 2), would lead to an incorrect representation of the number of syllables in the speech utterance. On the other hand, with the 3150/3150 envelope signal, as the smoothing filter cutoff frequency increases, the signal obtains a more noise-like timbre for fricative sounds, and at the same time contains fundamental frequency information in the form of envelope periodicity. This additional information, especially F0 cues, has been shown to significantly aid speechreading (Grant et al., 1985; Breeuwer & Plomp, 1986). Studies are currently underway to determine whether listeners can extract useful F0 cues (e.g. rising vs. falling intonation) from envelope signals with different degrees of smoothing.

Although we do not formally address the issue of training in this study, we feel that this is an important factor in a subject's ability to use envelope cues effectively while speechreading. In the present study, subjects were exposed to envelope cues through use of the Connected Discourse Tracking procedure. Admittedly, this exposure or training phase was very brief, lasting only three hours. Yet, in spite of the brevity of this exposure, we feel that without it the subject's scores would have been substantially lower. To illustrate this point with the 500-Hz pre-filter condition, we compared IEEE sentence identification performance of four subjects, two tested with no previous exposure and two tested after familiarization training using the tracking procedure. The two pairs of subjects were matched, as closely as was possible, according to their speechreading-alone scores. The first subject pair represented above-average speechreaders (approximately 20% correct), and the second subject pair represented below-average speechreaders (approximately 5% correct). The scores for both trained subjects were substantially higher than for the untrained subjects, indicating that the tracking procedure was effective in facilitating the subject's ability to combine speech envelope cues with speechreading. Unfortunately we were not able to demonstrate the effects of familiarization/training within the same subject because of the large number of different experimental conditions investigated and the limited number of sentence lists available.

Another factor that can influence the magnitude of the AV scores is the difficulty of the speech materials. For difficult sentence materials (e.g. IEEE sentences), average AV scores for the best envelope signals were only 58% correct. Although this level of performance was much better than that for speechreading alone, there is clearly room for improvement. We must remember, however, that simple envelope signals like those evaluated in this study convey very limited amounts of segmental information pertaining to consonants (Van Tasell et al., 1987) and virtually no segmental information pertaining to vowels. In the absence of additional auditory cues for segment identification, listeners presumably rely more heavily on their knowledge of the language and on the sentence context. With easier sentence materials having a greater degree of contextual information (e.g. CUNY sentences), the average AV scores would be expected to be higher, as was indeed the case in the present study (approximately 78%). This materials difference was evident in the studies by Risberg (1974) and Risberg and Lubker (1978), who used the same envelope signal with a closed-set of simple sentences and an open-set of unknown questions, respectively. With familiar sentences, the envelope signal provided an improvement over speechreading alone of approximately 32 percentage points. With unfamiliar sentences, the envelope signal provided only a small advantage over speechreading alone (approximately 4 percentage points). The fact that our subjects obtained a large AV advantage over speechreading alone with difficult sentence materials was probably due to the selection of pre-filter, carrier, and smoothing filter, as well as the initial training given to the subjects.

It is interesting to note that the beneficial value of the different speech envelopes does not correspond to the intelligibility of the filtered speech bands from which the envelopes originate. According to Articulation Theory (French & Steinberg, 1947; ANSI, 1969), a $\frac{1}{3}$-octave or 1-octave band of speech centred at 1600 Hz is more intelligible both auditorially and audiovisually than is either a $\frac{1}{3}$- or 1-octave band of speech centred at 3150 Hz or

500 Hz. For example, intelligibility scores obtained for $\frac{1}{3}$-octave bands at 500, 1600, and 3150 Hz and IEEE/Harvard sentence materials (Grant, 1988) were 0.9, 24.6, and 8.4% correct, respectively, for auditory-only presentations, and 41.5, 86.3, and 65.5% correct for auditory–visual presentations. Similar measures obtained for 1-octave bands at these same centre frequencies resulted in intelligibility scores of 20.6, 77.0, and 48.5% correct for auditory only presentations, and 79.8, 94.1, and 89.5% correct for auditory–visual presentations. From the data shown in Figure 3, IEEE/Harvard auditory–visual scores obtained with envelope cues derived from octave bands at 500, 1600, and 3150 Hz were 48.9, 25.3, and 18.8% correct, respectively, when sinusoidal carriers equal to the pre-filter centre frequency were used. Thus, low-frequency envelope cues appear to be more beneficial to speechreading than mid- or high-frequency envelope cues, and mid-frequency speech cues are more beneficial to speechreading than low- or high-frequency speech cues.

In comparison to other simple auditory signals, such as fundamental and formant frequency signals, envelope signals of the type used here and by Breeuwer and Plomp have been shown to provide similar improvements to speechreading after some initial training. For example, Breeuwer and Plomp (1984, 1986), showed that a two-band envelope signal, derived by combining the envelopes from an octave band at 500 Hz and an octave band at 3160 Hz, provided significantly more benefit to speechreading than did single band envelope signals, F0 signals, or formant frequency signals when (1) the AM carriers were sinusoids at the pre-filter centre frequencies (i.e. 500 Hz and 3160 Hz, respectively), and (2) the subjects were relatively untrained. Later experiments with trained subjects showed smaller differences in the aided speechreading scores among the different signals. In the present study, scores obtained by moderately trained subjects listening to CUNY sentences (the difficulty of which is comparable to that of the sentences used by Breeuwer and Plomp) under the best single band envelope condition (i.e. 500-Hz pre-filter/200-Hz carrier) was 78% correct. Pilot experiments with two-band envelope signals in our laboratory also show a small improvement over single-band scores when the carriers were at the centre frequency of the pre-filter bands (approximately 90% correct for CUNY sentences). One potential problem with the two-band envelope results is that the high-frequency envelope band may have to be frequency-lowered for hearing-impaired listeners with low-frequency residual hearing. As was shown in Figure 3 however, when the high pre-filter condition was lowered, scores tended to decrease. Thus, one of the challenges for future research in this area will be to find display configurations that allow for the possibility of presenting multiple envelope signals to listeners with a greatly reduced bandwidth of usable hearing.

Along with limitations in usable bandwidth, many severely-to-profoundly hearing-impaired listeners have limitations in usable dynamic range. The

AM signals used in the present study had a 30+ dB dynamic range, and it is therefore important to consider what might happen if the dynamic range of the signals were restricted or compressed. Unfortunately, there are no data that directly speak to this issue. In earlier studies by Grant et al. (1985) and Breeuwer and Plomp (1986), a fixed-frequency fixed-intensity signal gated on and off with the voiced portions of the speech signal was evaluated as an aid to speechreading. In the Grant et al. study, the voicing signal proved to be a significant aid to speechreading, but not as good as when the amplitude of the signal was allowed to vary. In the Breeuwer and Plomp (1986) study, listeners were not able to take advantage of the voicing signal when presented with speechreading. If we assume that speech envelope signals provide both suprasegmental cues for stress and rhythm (in terms of amplitude and duration variations across speech segments) and segmental cues for consonant manner of articulation (in terms of the rate of attack onset for each segment), then the small benefits provided by the voicing signal used by Grant et al. (1985) and Breeuwer and Plomp (1986) are easily explained.

In summary, we have shown that a number of different speech envelope signals can provide speechreaders with valuable cues to improve their speech identification performance. These signals are extremely simple relative to normal speech signals and may be useful for hearing-impaired listeners who have trouble extracting cues from speech. However, practical problems concerned with matching the bandwidth and dynamic range of the envelope signal to that of the listener's residual hearing still remain.

As a final note, it is evident from the above discussion that the term "speech envelope" is one that has to be carefully defined for each application. Clearly there is no one speech envelope, and different envelopes have different values as far as the speechreader is concerned. What is most commonly meant by the term "speech envelope" refers to the single band envelope derived from the wideband pre-filter condition. We have shown, however, that this may not be the best envelope signal to use if the intention is to aid speechreading. In this regard, it will be important for future studies to show that hearing-impaired listeners can also make use of envelope signals, and that they find these types of simplified auditory displays better than conventional amplification.

REFERENCES

ANSI (1969). *American National Standard methods for the calculation of the Articulation Index, ANSI S3.5–1969*. New York: American National Standards Institute.

Ardell, L.H. (1980) *The contribution of fundamental frequency and time-intensity cues to connected-discourse perception by speechreaders*. M.S. thesis, University of Washington, Seattle.

Boothroyd, A., Hnath-Chislm,T., & Hanin, L. (1985). A sentence test of speech perception: Reliability, set-equivalence, and short-term learning. *City University of New York, Report No. RCI10.*

Breeuwer, M. & Plomp, R. (1984). Speechreading supplemented with frequency-selective sound-pressure information. *Journal of the Acoustical Society of America*, *76*, 686–691.

Breeuwer, M. & Plomp, R. (1985). Speechreading supplemented with formant-frequency information from voiced speech. *Journal of the Acoustical Society of America*, *77*, 314–317(L).

Breeuwer, M. & Plomp, R. (1986). Speechreading supplemented with auditorily presented speech parameters. *Journal of the Acoustical Society of America*, *79*, 481–499.

Davis, H. & Silverman, S.R. (1978). *Hearing and deafness* (pp. 536–538). New York: Holt, Rinehart & Winston.

Davis, H., Stevens, S.S., Nichols, R.H. Jr., Hudgins, C.V., Marquis, R.J., Peterson, G.E., & Ross, D.A. (1947). *Hearing aids—An experimental study of design objectives*. Cambridge, MA: Harvard University Press.

DeFilippo, C.L. & Scott, B.L. (1978). A method for training and evaluating the reception of ongoing speech. *Journal of the Acoustical Society of America*, *63*, 1186–1192.

Erber, N.P. (1972a). Speech-envelope cues as an acoustic aid to lipreading for profoundly deaf children, *Journal of the Acoustical Society of America*, *51*, 1224–1227.

Erber, N.P. (1972b). Auditory, visual and auditory-visual recognition of consonants by children with normal and impaired hearing. *Journal of Speech and Hearing Research*, *15*, 413–422.

French, N.R. & Steinberg, J.C. (1947). Factors governing the intelligibility of speech sounds. *Journal of the Acoustical Society of America*, *19*, 90–119.

Grant, K.W. (1987a). Encoding voice pitch for profoundly hearing-impaired listeners. *Journal of the Acoustical Society of America*, *82*, 423–432.

Grant, K.W. (1987b). Identification of intonation contours by normally hearing and profoundly hearing-impaired listeners. *Journal of the Acoustical Society of America*, *82*, 1172–1178.

Grant, K.W. (1988). Further studies on the auditory-visual Articulation Index. *Journal of the Acoustical Society of America*, *83*, S86(A).

Grant, K.W., Ardell, L.H., Kuhl, P.K., & Sparks, D.W. (1985). The contribution of fundamental frequency, amplitude envelope, and voicing duration cues to speechreading in normal-hearing subjects. *Journal of the Acoustical Society of America*, *77*, 671–677.

Grant, K.W., Renn, R.J., & Yu, J.S. (1988). Amplitude envelopes and speechreading. *Journal of the Acoustical Society of America*, *84*, S45(A).

Hoekstra, A. & Ritsma, R.J. (1977). Perceptive hearing loss and frequency selectivity. In E.F. Evans & J.P. Wilson (Eds.), *Psychophysics and physiology of hearing* (pp. 263–271). London: Academic Press.

Horii, Y., House, A.S., & Hughes, G.W. (1971). A masking noise with speech-envelope characteristics for studying intelligibility. *Journal of the Acoustical Society of America*, *49*, 1849–1856.

IEEE (1969). IEEE recommended practice for speech quality measurements. New York: Institute of Electrical and Electronic Engineers.

McGrath, M. & Summerfield, Q. (1985). Intermodal-timing relations and audiovisual speech recognition by normal-hearing adults. *Journal of the Acoustical Society of America*, *77*, 678–685.

Miller, G.A. & Nicely, P.E. (1955). An analysis of perceptual confusions among some English consonants. *Journal of the Acoustical Society of America*, *27*, 338–352.

Moore, B.C.J., Douek, E., Fourcin, A.J., Rosen, S.M., Walliker, J.R., Howard, D.M., Abberton, E., & Frampton, S. (1984). Extra-cochlear stimulation with speech patterns: Experience of the EPI group (U.K.). In W.D. Keidel & P. Finkenzeller (Eds.), *Cochlear implants in clinical use* (pp. 148–162). Basel: Karger.

Moore, B.C.J. & Glasberg, B.R. (1986). The role of frequency selectivity in the perception of loudness, pitch and time. In B.C.J. Moore (Ed.) *Frequency selectivity in hearing* (pp. 251–308). London: Academic Press.

Plomp, R. (1978). Auditory handicap of hearing impairment and the limited benefit of hearing aids. *Journal of the Acoustical Society of America, 63*, 533–549.

Risberg, A. (1974). The importance of prosodic speech elements for the lipreader. In H.B. Nielson & E. Klamp (Eds.), *Visual and audio-visual perception of speech* (Sixth Danavox Symposium, *Scandinavian Audiology* (Suppl. 4), 153–164.

Risberg, A. & Lubker, J.L. (1978). Prosody and speechreading. *STL-QPSR, 4*, 1–16.

Rosen, S.M. & Fourcin, A.J. (1983). When less is more—Further work. In *Speech, Hearing and Language* (vol. I, pp. 3–27). London: University College, Dept. of Phonetics and Linguistics. 3–27.

Rosen, S.M. & Fourcin, A.J. (1986). Frequency selectivity and the perception of speech. In B.C.J. Moore (Ed.), *Frequency selectivity in hearing* (pp. 373–487). London: Academic Press.

Rosen, S.M., Fourcin, A.J., & Moore, B.C.J. (1981). Voice pitch as an aid to lipreading. *Nature, 291*, 5811, 150–152.

Rosen, S.M. & Smith, D.A.J. (1988). Temporally-based auditory sensations in the profoundly hearing-impaired listener. In H. Duifhius, J.W. Horst, & H.P. Wit (Eds.), *Basic Issues in Hearing* (pp. 431–449). London: Academic Press.

Rosen, S.M., Walliker, J.R., Fourcin, A.J., & Ball, V. (1987). A microprocessor-based acoustic hearing aid for the profoundly impaired listener. *Journal of Rehabilitation Research and Development, 24*, 239–260.

Scharf, B. & Florentine, M. (1982). Psychoacoustics of elementary sounds. In G.A. Studebaker & F.H. Bess (Eds.), *The Vanderbilt hearing-aid report* (pp. 3–15). Upper Darby, PA: Monographs in Contemporary Audiology.

Tyler, R.S. (1986). Frequency resolution in hearing-impaired listeners. In B.C.J. Moore (Ed.), *Frequency selectivity in hearing* (pp. 309–371). London: Academic Press.

Van Tasell, D.J., Soli, S.D., Kirby, V.M., & Widen, G.P. (1987). Speech waveform envelope cues for consonant recognition. *Journal of the Acoustical Society of America, 82*, 1152–1161.

Wightman, F.L., McGee, T., & Kramer, M. (1977). Factors influencing frequency selectivity in normal and hearing-impaired ears. In E.F. Evans & J.P. Wilson (Eds.), *Psychophysics and physiology of hearing* (pp. 296–306). New York: Academic Press.

Revised manuscript received 1 January 1991

THE QUARTERLY JOURNAL OF EXPERIMENTAL PSYCHOLOGY, 1991, *43A* (3) 647–677

Crossmodal Integration in the Identification of Consonant Segments

Louis D. Braida

Massachusetts Institute of Technology, Cambridge, Massachusetts, U.S.A.

Although speechreading can be facilitated by auditory or tactile supplements, the process that integrates cues across modalities is not well understood. This paper describes two "optimal processing" models for the types of integration that can be used in speechreading consonant segments and compares their predictions with those of the Fuzzy Logical Model of Perception (FLMP, Massaro, 1987). In "pre-labelling" integration, continuous sensory data is combined across modalities before response labels are assigned. In "post-labelling" integration, the responses that would be made under unimodal conditions are combined, and a joint response is derived from the pair. To describe pre-labelling integration, confusion matrices are characterized by a multidimensional decision model that allows performance to be described by a subject's sensitivity and bias in using continuous-valued cues. The cue space is characterized by the locations of stimulus and response centres. The distance between a pair of stimulus centres determines how well two stimuli can be distinguished in a given experiment. In the multimodal case, the cue space is assumed to be the product space of the cue spaces corresponding to the stimulation modes. Measurements of multimodal accuracy in five modern studies of consonant identification are more consistent with the predictions of the pre-labelling integration model than the FLMP or the post-labelling model.

In many situations speech reception is improved if the listener integrates cues derived from the visible actions of the talker's face with those derived from the acoustic signal. For example, speechreading is substantially facilitated by

---

Requests for reprints should be sent to Louis D. Braida, Research Laboratory of Electronics, Massachusetts Institute of Technology, Cambridge, MA 02139, U.S.A.

This work was supported by the N.I.H. (Grants R01-DC00117 and P01-DC00361). I am grateful for critical discussions with P.J. Blamey, M.M. Cohen, E.M. Eide, K.W. Grant, G.R. Lockhead, N.A. Macmillan, D.W. Massaro, R.M. Nosofsky, W.M. Rabinowitz, C.M. Reed, B.H. Repp, S.M. Rosen, Q. Summerfield, R.M. Uchanski, P.M. Zurek, and an anonymous reviewer. Data and background materials were generously provided by P.J. Blamey, D.A. Busacco, K.W. Grant, A.A. Montgomery, Q. Summerfield, S.D. Soli, and B.E. Walden.

the feeble auditory cues available to those with profound hearing impairments. Conversely, auditory communication in noisy environments is facilitated even by dimly perceived facial actions (e.g. Erber, 1979; Neely, 1956). At present, understanding of the process by which such cues are combined is fairly tentative. Although the standard method for computing the Articulation Index (ANSI, 1969) explicitly takes the availability of speechreading into account, the correction procedure is largely empirical and does not predict the benefit to speechreading provided by acoustic signals of negligible auditory intelligibility (e.g. Breeuwer & Plomp, 1985, 1986). Similarly, recent studies of audiovisual interaction at the segmental level using discrepant visual and auditory signals (e.g. McGurk & MacDonald, 1976a, 1976b) are often interpreted to mean that cues are combined in a highly selective fashion (e.g. with place of articulation derived through vision and manner of articulation derived through audition). But it is unclear whether the unexpected pattern of responses elicited by such discrepant stimuli reflects primarily the effects of resolution or those of response bias.

This paper is concerned with the integration process that occurs in multimodal speech reception. Although there are a variety of approaches to the study of multimodal integration (e.g. Massaro, 1987), we begin with the problem of predicting accuracy (percentage of correct responses) in consonant identification experiments in which the stimuli consist of short speech segments. Identification experiments are comparatively well understood (e.g. Bush, Galanter, & Luce, 1963; Durlach & Braida, 1969), and, as will be discussed, there are good theoretical reasons to focus on overall accuracy initially. In this paper we restrict attention to stimuli consisting of CV or VCV syllables distinguished by the consonant. When the visual display is supplemented by auditory or tactile displays, only supplements derived from the acoustic signal corresponding to the same utterance are considered. Although such experiments are widely used clinically to evaluate the performance of auditory prostheses, there is currently little understanding of how much improvement one should expect in the multimodal condition compared to the unimodal conditions. Quantitative prediction of multimodal accuracy requires both a precise description of unimodal cues and an explicit specification of the integration process in the multimodal case.

For purposes of this paper, five studies of consonant identification are particularly relevant (see Table 1), because they report confusion matrices for the visual (V), auditory (A), or tactile (T), and audiovisual (AV), tactile–visual (TV), or tactile–audiovisual (TAV) presentation conditions rather than simply overall measures of performance.

Binnie, Montgomery, and Jackson (1974) tested A, V, and AV identification of the 16 consonants /p, t, k, f, θ, s, ʃ, b, d, g, v, ð, z, ʒ, m, n/ in C-/ɑ/ context using ten normally hearing and sighted subjects. Speech materials were videotaped, with the auditory presentation partially masked by broadband noise at S/N = −18, −12, and −6 dB. Each subject received 20 presentations of each consonant in each condition.

Busacco (1988) measured A, V, and AV identification of the 20 consonants /p, t, k, f, θ, s, ʃ, b, d, g, v, ð, z, ʒ, m, n, l, r, w, j/ in C-/ɑ/ context using twenty middle-aged (MA) (mean 42.4 years) and twenty elderly (E) (mean 72.2 years) male subjects. Groups were roughly matched for hearing loss (roughly 57 dB in the 1–4 kHz range) and NU-6 word score (roughly 64% correct). Speech materials were videotaped, with acoustic stimulation restricted to the less sensitive ear of each subject. Each consonant syllable was presented 20 times to each subject in each condition.

Campbell (1974) tested A, V, and AV identification of the 6 Dutch consonants /p, t, s, b, d, z/ in C-/ɪ/ context. Speech materials were videotaped, with the auditory presentation partially masked by broadband noise at S/N = −15, −12, and −9 dB. Each of three normal-hearing subjects received 42 presentations of each consonant in each condition. Campbell also conducted supplementary identification and discrimination experiments with smaller stimulus sets. These will not be analysed in this paper.

Erber (1972) tested three groups (PD—profoundly deaf, SI—severely hearing-impaired, and NH—normal-hearing) of five children each on identification of the 8 consonants /b, d, g, p, t, k, m, n/ in /ɑ/-C-/ɑ/ context. Materials were videotaped. Each subject was presented each consonant 45 times in the A, V, and AV conditions.

Sparks and Grant (1979) tested two subjects on the identification of the 22 consonants /p, t, k, b, d, g, m, n, f, v, s, z, θ, ð, ʃ, ʒ, w, r, l, j, ʧ, ʤ/ in C-/ɑ/ context in conditions A, T, V, AV, TV, and TAV. Live voice presentation was used with the subjects alternating as sender and receiver. Auditory presentation employed 300-Hz lowpass filtering and tactile presentation employed the MESA tactile aid (Sparks, Kuhl, Edmonds, & Gray, 1978) to encode the acoustic signal. The number of presentations of each syllable to each subject varied from condition to condition: T–15, V–32, A–35, AV–60, TV–60, and TAV–60.

The studies considered are typical of identification experiments in that each stimulus was presented roughly an equal number of times, and the subjects were informed of the composition of the stimulus set and forced to choose a response from the closed response set known to them. The major limitations of these studies include the fact that data have been pooled across subjects rather than reported on an individual basis and that none of the studies characterizes the physical properties of the speech stimuli used, so that it is difficult to relate results across studies. Despite these drawbacks the data from the studies listed in Table 1 are suitable for testing models of integration. In each study the same set of subjects was tested in each condition. The effect of pooling is partially compensated for by the large number of presentations in the resulting confusion matrices. Consequently

TABLE 1
Observed and Predicted Accuracy for Studies of Multimodal Consonant Identification

		Percentage Correct Consonant Identification Scores					
		Observed Scores			*Predicted (T)AV Score*		
Study		*V*	*A/T*	*(T)AV*	*FLMP*	*Post.-L.*	*Pre.-L.*
Binnie et al.	S/N = −18 dB	43.2	6.3	47.7	42.3	47.7	49.1
	S/N = −12 dB	43.2	33.6	83.5	81.0	75.7	80.3
	S/N = −6 dB	43.2	53.4	88.6	91.3	86.4	89.6
Busacco	E	42.8	49.5	84.9	82.4	75.3	83.8
	MA	47.8	45.8	85.4	82.3	75.6	83.5
Campbell	S/N = −15 dB	44.9	54.0	88.4	90.9	85.4	89.1
	S/N = −12 dB	44.9	65.5	92.1	95.9	88.2	92.6
	S/N = −9 dB	44.9	77.7	94.7	97.1	93.3	96.5
Erber	PD	45.2	21.1	60.5	57.0	55.6	58.6
	SI	49.2	50.4	88.0	90.1	79.5	83.6
	NH	31.6	99.7	99.8	100.0	99.7	99.9
Sparks & Grant	AV	60.2	43.8	95.3	99.0	94.8	97.7
	TV	60.2	33.2	81.3	82.3	76.5	80.7
	TAV	60.2		97.5	99.7	97.2	99.1

Each row corresponds to a fixed set of conditions for a given subject group. Predicted scores for the multimodal condition were computed by fitting the FLMP, and pre- and post-labelling integration models to the unimodal data. See text for details.

the reliability of percentage correct scores (estimated using the conventional Bernoulli-trials assumption) corresponds to a standard deviation on the order of 0.4–1.2 percentage points. (Both Dowell et al. (1982) and Danhauer et al. (1990) report data from individual subjects who receive electrocochlear stimulation. These data are not considered in this paper because the small number of stimulus presentations makes precise analysis problematic.)

As the data in Table 1 indicate, although identification accuracy in the V condition does not vary greatly across studies, both accuracy in the A condition and the improvement obtained in the multimodal presentation conditions varies substantially from study to study. Both Boothroyd (1975) and Blamey (personal communication) have shown that fewer errors generally arise in the multimodal case than would be expected if a multimodal error required independent simultaneous errors for each modality separately. For example, in the Binnie et al. (1974) study, the visual error rate was 56.8%, and the auditory (S/N = −12 dB) error rate was 66.4%, but the multimodal error rate was only 16.5%, far lower than the 37.7% one would expect based on independent errors. Although the independent errors assumption is known to underestimate accuracy in other multimodal cases (e.g. Pollack, 1964), this result is significant. It is not found in all studies of audiovisual speech reception. For example, Massaro (1987) argues that the rate of occurrence of errors in the Sumby and Pollack (1954) study of audiovisual word recognition can be satisfactorily accounted for by the independent errors assumption.

At a more refined level of analysis concerned with confusions between specific pairs of consonants, many of the improvements afforded by multimodal presentation are readily interpretable, at least in qualitative terms. For example, in auditory presentation conditions that include additive broadband noise or severe lowpass filtering, Miller and Nicely (1955) found that consonants differing in place of articulation are relatively difficult to distinguish, but those differing in voicing or nasality are relatively easy to distinguish. By contrast, in visual presentation conditions consonants that differ in place of articulation are relatively easy to distinguish, but those that differ in terms of voicing or nasality are relatively difficult to distinguish (e.g. Owens & Blazek, 1985). In the audiovisual condition it should thus be possible to distinguish simultaneously between consonants that differ in either voicing or nasality or place of articulation. These observations elucidate the failure of the independent errors model to account for multimodal accuracy. Overall error rates are inadequate to predict multimodal identification accuracy from performance in the unimodal conditions. The pattern of unimodal perceptual confusions must also be specified. The error that occurs when the consonant /b/ elicits the response "g" in the A condition is of little consequence for the AV condition. Its effects can be resolved by visual cues. If, however, the same stimulus elicits the response "p", the consequences are serious. Visual cues provide little discrimination for consonant voicing. This notion has been analysed by Walden, Prosek, and Worthington (1974) in a test of the hypothesis that auditory signals improve the speechreading of consonants to the extent that the pattern of auditory confusions differs from that of visual confusions. They developed a measure of confusion redundancy derived from A and V confusion matrices that had moderate ability ($r = -0.70$) to predict the AV consonant recognition scores of listeners with hearing impairments.

The balance of this paper focuses on the problem of predicting multimodal identification accuracy based on integrating unimodal data. The properties of the unimodal data are inferred from the pattern of confusions observed in unimodal presentation conditions. Although the problem of predicting residual error patterns in the multimodal condition is considered briefly, detailed prediction of these patterns is beyond the scope of this paper.

Three models of integration are considered: the Fuzzy Logical Model of Perception (FLMP, Massaro, 1987) and two "optimum processing" models. Although these three models differ in complexity and formulation, each makes quantitative predictions for performance in experiments with multimodal stimuli based solely on performance in experiments with unimodal stimuli. The FLMP has been previously described and applied to a wide variety of experiments in audiovisual speech perception, but the two optimum processing models are relatively new. In the "pre-labelling" integration model, continuous-valued cues are combined across sensory systems to produce a vector of cues that is mapped into an identification response. For example, visual observation of the rate of lip opening might be combined with auditorily estimated "attack" characteristics and these combined with visual and auditory estimates of duration to produce a four-dimensional vector that characterizes the speech sound. In "post-labelling" integration each sensory system produces a discrete symbolic label, and the identification judgement is based on a vector of discrete labels. For example, in audiovisual reception of noisy speech, the auditory label might correspond to the consonant /p/ and the visual label to the consonant /d/, but the resulting pair of labels—for example, (P,D)—could specify that the response should correspond to the consonant /t/. In general, the identification accuracy associated with pre-labelling integration should never be inferior to that for post-labelling integration, but the size of the difference is not known. By formulating the pre-labelling and post-labelling models to achieve the greatest identification accuracy consistent with observed unimodal performance, it should be possible to derive quantitative estimates of this difference.

Section 1 describes the FLMP predictions for multimodal accuracy and evaluates its predictions. Section 2 describes a general class of post-labelling models and demonstrates that such models cannot satisfactorily account for multimodal accuracy. Section 3 describes a model (Braida, 1988) of consonant identification that interprets confusion matrices in terms of a subject's sensitivity and bias in using continuous-valued cues. Section 4 describes how pre-labelling sensitivity in multimodal presentation conditions is related to that in the corresponding unimodal conditions. Section 5 applies the pre-labelling model to data on consonant confusions and discusses how well it predicts overall accuracy in the multimodal presentation condition. Section 6 reviews the main results obtained in the previous sections and outlines some future research suggested by these results.

1. Fuzzy Logical Model of Perception

In the FLMP, the response to each stimulus is determined, in a probabilistic fashion, by the "feature value" of that stimulus for each of the possible responses. Feature values are not observed directly, but instead are inferred from response patterns. In unimodal (e.g. auditory) presentations, the conditional probability that response $\mathcal{R}_j$ is given when the stimulus is $\mathcal{S}_i$, $P_A(\mathcal{R}_j|\mathcal{S}_i)$ is taken as the feature value for response $\mathcal{R}_j$ associated with $\mathcal{S}_i$ in the auditory mode. In multimodal conditions, the feature value is assumed to be proportional to the product of the feature values for the corresponding unimodal conditions (Massaro & Cohen, personal communication). Thus, $P_{AV}(\mathcal{R}_j|\mathcal{S}_i)$, the probability that response $\mathcal{R}_j$ is given to stimulus $\mathcal{S}_i$ in the AV condition, is

$$P_{AV}(\mathcal{R}_j|\mathcal{S}_i)=\frac{P_A(\mathcal{R}_j|\mathcal{S}_i)P_V(\mathcal{R}_j|\mathcal{S}_i)}{\sum_{k=1}^{N} P_A(\mathcal{R}_k|\mathcal{S}_i)P_V(\mathcal{R}_k|\mathcal{S}_i)} \quad (1)$$

(The denominator term in Equation 1 normalizes the feature values for the N responses to conditional probabilities.)

As can be seen in Table 1, the FLMP makes reasonably accurate predictions of multimodal scores. Averaged over all studies FLMP predictions neither under- nor overestimate observed accuracy. However, there is a tendency to overestimate predicted multimodal scores when auditory performance is relatively good, and to underestimate them when auditory performance is poor. The predicted scores fail a simple χ^2 test (ignoring the Erber NH data and the Sparks and Grant TAV data, for which performance is very close to perfect, $\chi^2(12)=60.34$, $p<0.01$; including the two data sets does not alter this conclusion).

Some insight into the failure of the FLMP is provided by the data of Binnie et al. (1974) (at −18 dB S/N), for which the prediction was relatively poor. Here the score in the A condition was only slightly above chance, and the predicted AV score is somewhat below that in the V condition. If performance in the A condition had corresponded to unbiased random guessing, the predicted AV score would have equalled the observed V score.

Apparently the FLMP does not properly account for the effect that structured errors in one modality can have on multimodal accuracy. Consider the extreme case in which responses correspond to random guessing in one modality. If responses in the other modality are completely incorrect but perfectly consistent and different from stimulus to stimulus, the FLMP predicts there will be no correct responses in the multimodal condition. By contrast, the "optimum processor" models discussed in the following sections predict perfect accuracy under such conditions. Each of these models assumes that the probabilistic events that occur in a multimodal condition can be described as the joint occurrence of events that occur in unimodal conditions. These optimum processor models thus attribute accuracy in the multimodal condition to the joint consistency of unimodal percepts, rather than to the accuracy of unimodal responses.

2. Post-labelling Integration

In post-labelling integration the subject is assumed to make separate identification judgements about the stimulus based on the cues available in each modality, and to combine these judgements to determine the response to the multimodal stimulus. In the AV condition, for example, presentation of stimulus $\mathcal{S}_i$ generates a pair of labels (A_m, V_n) corresponding, respectively, to the auditory and visual judgements. The labels correspond to the responses that would be given in unimodal experiments. The collection of label pairs is assumed to be divided into mutually exclusive and collectively exhaustive sets. In particular, all labels belonging to the set Σ_j elicit response $\mathcal{R}_j$, so that

$$P_{AV}(\mathcal{R}_j|\mathcal{S}_j) = \sum_{m,n \in \Sigma j} P^*_{AV}(A_m, V_n|\mathcal{S}_i) \tag{2}$$

where $P^*_{AV}(A_m, V_n|\mathcal{S}_i)$ is the probability that stimulus $\mathcal{S}_i$ gives rise to the label pair (A_m, V_n), and $P_{AV}(\mathcal{R}_j|\mathcal{S}_i)$ is the probability that response $\mathcal{R}_j$ is given to this stimulus.

To relate multimodal identification to unimodal identification, we assume that the label produced for each modality is independent of the labels in the other modalities. Labelling judgements for each modality are thus assumed to be made by the same processes that operate in unimodal presentation conditions.

$$P^*_{AV}(A_m, V_n|\mathcal{S}_i) = P^*_A(A_m|\mathcal{S}_i) \times P^*_V(V_n|\mathcal{S}_i) \tag{3}$$

In particular, we assume that the probability of assigning labels is described by the confusion matrices observed in the unimodal presentation conditions. For example, in the A condition

$$P^*_A(A_m|\mathcal{S}_i) = P_A(\mathcal{R}_m|\mathcal{S}_i) \tag{4}$$

and in the V condition

$$P^*_V(V_n|\mathscr{S}_i)=P_V(\mathscr{R}_n|\mathscr{S}_i) \tag{5}$$

where $P_A(\mathscr{R}_m|\mathscr{S}_i)$ and $P_V(\mathscr{R}_n|\mathscr{S}_i)$ determine the frequencies observed in the auditory and visual unimodal confusion matrices.

There are many possible rules (or equivalently many possible choices of the Σ_j sets) that the subject can use to map the label pair (A_m, V_n) into a response. When the a priori stimulus presentation probabilities of the stimuli are equal, it is well known (e.g. van Trees, 1968) that no rule leads to greater identification accuracy (probability of responding correctly) than the *maximum likelihood* rule: for each (A_m, V_n) the response should be the identity of the stimulus for which $P^*_{AV}(A_m, V_n|\mathscr{S}_i)$ is greatest.

Let Θ_j denote the set of (m, n) for which $P^*_{AV}(A_m, V_n|\mathscr{S}_j)>P^*_{AV}(A_m, V_n|\mathscr{S}_i)$ for all $i\neq j$. Then, combining the above assumptions, the conditional response probabilities for the maximum likelihood rule are specified by

$$P_{AV}(\mathscr{R}_j|\mathscr{S}_i)=\sum_{m,n\in\Theta j} P_A(\mathscr{R}_m|\mathscr{S}_i)\times P_V(\mathscr{R}_n|\mathscr{S}_i) \tag{6}$$

If there is a set of (A_m, V_n) for which

$$P^*_{AV}(A_m, V_n|\mathscr{S}_i)=P^*_{AV}(A_m, V_n|\mathscr{S}_j)>P^*_{AV}(A_m, V_n|\mathscr{S}_k) \tag{7}$$

for all $k\neq i,j$, then these (A_m, V_n) may be mapped arbitrarily (on a deterministic or probabilistic basis) to either $\mathscr{R}_i$ or $\mathscr{R}_j$ without affecting identification accuracy. If there is no such set, the mapping that leads to greatest identification accuracy is unique.

The maximum likelihood assignment of label pairs for Erber's (1972) SI group is shown in Table 2. Clearly auditory labels corresponding to voiced consonants specify the response as a voiced consonant (and vice versa), but the same is not true for nasal auditory labels. Visual labels do not always specify the place of articulation of the consonant given as the response. The visual label N dominates the auditory labels D and T, specifying an "N" response, even though the nasal distinction is usually well conveyed auditorily to the hearing-impaired. Additional evidence of the distinctiveness of the visual N in Erber's (1972) experiments is discussed later.

Predictions of identification accuracy when post-labelling integration is used with the maximum likelihood rule are included in Table 1. These predictions were computed by using the conditional response frequencies in the A and V confusion matrices to estimate $P_A(\mathscr{R}_m|\mathscr{S}_i)$ and $P_V(\mathscr{R}_n|\mathscr{S}_i)$. Although the predictions are accurate in some cases, they systematically underestimate the multimodal accuracy in all cases. In several instances the underestimation is sizeable, especially compared to the estimated reliability of the data. For example, the underestimate for the Erber (1972) study with SI subjects is more than 10 times the binomial estimate of the standard

TABLE 2
Maximum Likelihood Assignment of A and V Labels for Erber's (1972) SI Group

Auditory Label	*Maximum Likelihood Label Assignment* — *Visual Label* B	D	G	P	T	K	M	N
B	B	D	G	B	D	G	B	N
D	B	D	G	B	D	G	B	N
G	B	D	G	B	D	G	B	G
P	P	T	K	P	T	K	P	N
T	P	T	K	P	T	K	P	N
K	P	T	K	P	T	K	P	T
M	M	N	M	M	N	M	M	N
N	N	N	G	M	N	G	M	N

Each row corresponds to an auditory label and each column to a visual label. Each cell entry specifies the AV response for a label pair. The responses shown in the table lead to the highest identification accuracy possible with post-labelling integration.

deviation of the percentage correct responses. Given the tendency to underestimate multimodal accuracy, it is not surprising that the predictions of the post-labelling model fail the χ^2 test [$\chi^2(12)=261.9$, $p<0.01$]. Note that in contrast to the FLMP, which showed no general bias towards underestimation of overall accuracy, the multimodal predictions of the post-labelling model never fall below the accuracy observed in the more accurate component modality.

The frequent underestimation of accuracy by the maximum likelihood rule makes it unlikely that post-labelling integration of unimodal cues can provide a general description of multimodal consonant identification. This is hardly surprising. In the context of signal detection, post-labelling integration leads to performance that is inferior to pre-labelling integration when both hits and false alarms are accounted for (e.g. Green & Swets, 1966). Part of this failure may also result from the use of inappropriate response strategies in the unimodal conditions. In difficult reception conditions, the available responses are often used with frequencies that differ substantially from the corresponding stimulus presentation frequencies. For example, in the V condition in the Binnie et al. study, the response "ma" was used 112 times, whereas the response "fa" was used 290 times. This unbalanced use of responses often makes it difficult to interpret the unimodal confusion matrices.

In subsequent sections we describe a method of predicting multimodal accuracy based on pre-labelling integration. Unimodal sensory data is assumed to be represented in continuous valued cues that are combined optimally before labels are assigned. The statistical properties of the cues are inferred from unimodal confusion matrices using a new type of multidimensional scaling. In essence, this technique derives estimates of a subject's ability to use the cues to resolve stimuli that is independent of response biases.

3. Model for Consonant Identification

In most consonant identification experiments, the confusions between stimuli cannot be attributed to the use of a single cue that can be characterized by a conventional scalar (one-dimensional) decision model. In this section we describe a generalization of the scalar model (Braida, 1988) that can be used to analyse performance in such experiments. This model is both a multidimensional extension of the theory of signal detection (e.g. Green & Swets, 1966; Durlach & Braida, 1969; Macmillan, Goldberg, & Braida, 1988), and also a new form of multidimensional scaling (e.g. Borg & Lingoes, 1987). Each presentation of one of the N possible stimuli (consonants) $\mathscr{S}_i$ is assumed to generate a D-dimensional vector of cues $\vec{X} = \langle x_1, x_2, \ldots, x_D \rangle$ described by the conditional probability density

$$p(\vec{X} \mid \mathscr{S}_i) = \prod_{k=1}^{D} p(x_k \mid \mathscr{S}_i) = \prod_{k=1}^{D} \frac{1}{\sqrt{2\pi}} \exp\left[-\frac{(x_k - s_{ik})^2}{2}\right] \tag{8}$$

Equivalently, the cue vector $\vec{X}$ may be thought of as displaced from the *stimulus centre* $\vec{S}_i = \langle s_{i1}, s_{i2}, \ldots, s_{iD} \rangle$ by an additive noise vector whose components are independent Gaussian random variables with zero means and common unit variance.

Corresponding to each response there is also a *response centre* or *prototype* $\vec{R}_i = \langle r_{i1}, r_{i2}, \ldots, r_{iD} \rangle$. (It is *not* necessarily true that $\vec{R}_i = \vec{S}_i$). The subject is assumed to respond $\mathscr{R}_k$ if and only if the distance from the observed vector of cues $\vec{X}$ to $\vec{R}_k$ is smaller than the distance to any other prototype, i.e., $\|\vec{X} - \vec{R}_k\| < \|\vec{X} - \vec{R}_j\|$ for all $j \neq k$. For any two vectors $\vec{Y}$ and $\vec{Z}$, the distance $\|\vec{Y} - \vec{Z}\|$ is defined in terms of the vector components y_k and z_k as

$$\|\vec{Y} - \vec{Z}\| = \sqrt{\sum_{k=1}^{D} (y_k - z_k)^2} \tag{9}$$

In effect, this rule partitions the D-dimensional space of cue vectors into N compact "response regions" that are bounded by hyperplanes (see Figure 1). All the points in each region are closer to the prototype in that region than to any other prototype. The probability that $\mathscr{R}_j$ is the response when the stimulus is $\mathscr{S}_i$ is the probability that the vector of cues $\vec{X}$ is closer to $\vec{R}_j$ than to any other prototype when $\mathscr{S}_i$ is presented. As the density $p(\vec{X} \mid \mathscr{S}_i)$ weights the relative likelihood of occurrence of cue vectors in these conditions,

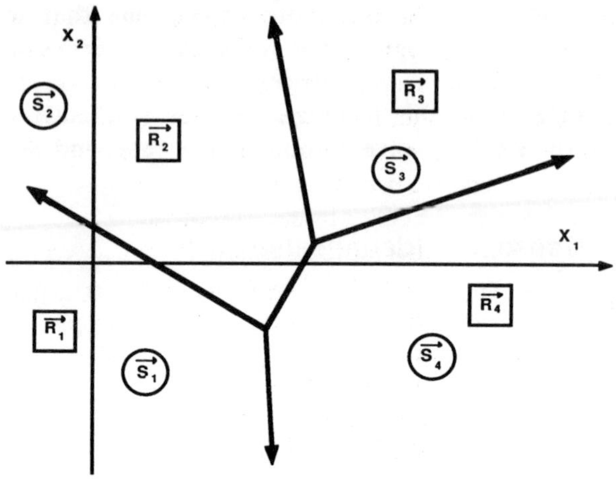

FIG. 1. Two-dimensional cue space for an identification experiment with four stimuli. Location of the stimulus centres (circles) relative to response prototypes (squares) is arbitrary in this figure. Response regions are bounded by line segments (extended bold lines), each of which coincides with a segment of the perpendicular bisector of a line connecting two response prototypes. All the points in a given response region are closer to the prototype in that region than to any other prototype. In general $P(\mathscr{R}_j|\mathscr{S}_i)$ is computed by integrating the multidimensional Gaussian density with mean $\vec{S}_i$ over the response region that contains $\vec{R}_j$.

$P(\mathscr{R}_j|\mathscr{S}_i)$ is determined by integrating the density with mean $\vec{S}_i$ over the response region containing $\vec{R}_j$.

Thus, the decision process in an identification experiment reflects the subject's comparison of cue vectors with prototypes. Errors result from the assumed noisiness of the cue vector, and the distribution of error responses reflects the relative locations of stimulus and response centres. The boundaries of the response regions are analogous to the decision criteria of signal detection theory. The locations of the prototypes, which determine these boundaries, are assumed to be at least partially under the control of the subject reflecting the effects of instructions and payoffs. By contrast, a subject's *sensitivity* $d'(i,j)$ in distinguishing stimulus $\mathscr{S}_i$ from stimulus $\mathscr{S}_j$, given in the multidimensional case by the expression

$$d'(i,j) = \|\vec{S}_i - \vec{S}_j\| = \sqrt{\sum_{k=1}^{D} (s_{ik} - s_{jk})^2} \tag{10}$$

is assumed to be determined by the physical characteristics of the stimuli and the properties of the subject's sensory system.

As discussed above, given the set of $\vec{S}_i$ and the set of $\vec{R}_j$, it is possible to predict the confusion matrix by numerical integration. The inverse problem of estimating the set of $\vec{S}_i$ and $\vec{R}_j$ that are most consistent with a given confusion matrix has yet to be solved completely. Braida (1988) described one procedure for estimating values of these parameters (i.e. the coordinates of the set of $\vec{S}_i$ and $\vec{R}_j$) corresponding to a given confusion matrix for a specified value of D. In this method, initial estimates of the stimulus centres are obtained by non-metric multidimensional scaling (KYST, Kruskal & Wish, 1978), and the response centres are initially aligned with the stimulus centres. Subsequent estimates of both sets of centres are obtained iteratively by attempting to improve the match (as specified by a χ^2-like measure) between the predicted matrix and the observed matrix.

Figure 2 illustrates how well the identification model can describe the cell entries in the corresponding confusion matrix. Matrices for Erber's (1972) SI group in the A and V conditions were fit using cue spaces of dimension $D=2$ and $D=3$. In these cases the addition of an extra dimension improves the quality of the fit modestly, reducing the rms error by roughly one-third. For larger matrices the improvement is usually greater. Most of the unimodal conditions considered in this paper are fit with $D=3$. However, the matrices reported by Campbell (1974), which are characterized by both a small number of consonants and a small number of presentations of each consonant, are fit with $D=2$, and the matrices reported by Busacco (1988), which are characterized by both a large number of consonants and large number of presentations of each consonant, are fit with $D=4$. For illustrative purposes, two-dimensional fits to Erber's (1972) data are included to permit visualization of results, but these are not used in predictions of multimodal accuracy.

To evaluate the quality of estimated parameter values (i.e. derived from the coordinates of the set of $\vec{S}_i$ and $\vec{R}_j$), the estimation procedure was applied to data derived from an *exact* numerical simulation of the model, i.e., matrices corresponding to the decision model with known stimulus and response centre locations. To do this, nominal model parameters (with $D=3$) were derived from the confusion matrices for the SI and PD groups in Erber's (1972) A and V conditions. These nominal parameters were used to create new confusion matrices using Monte Carlo simulation techniques consistent with the assumptions of the decision model. Each stimulus was presented 225 times in a given simulation, and each of Erber's conditions was simulated 40 times. For each simulation, new model parameters were estimated. These parameters were compared to the nominal parameters in terms of the bias and standard deviation of estimates of interstimulus sensitivity (Figure 3). The variability of the estimates reflects both the variability inherent in the Monte Carlo simulation process and additional variability in the parameter estimation process (which itself uses Monte Carlo techniques for numerical integration). For reference purposes, the standard deviation of estimates of d' (predicted by an analysis developed by Gourevitch & Galanter, 1967) for the two-stimulus scalar case with the same number of presentations of each stimulus is plotted as a solid line. Clearly the variability of parameter

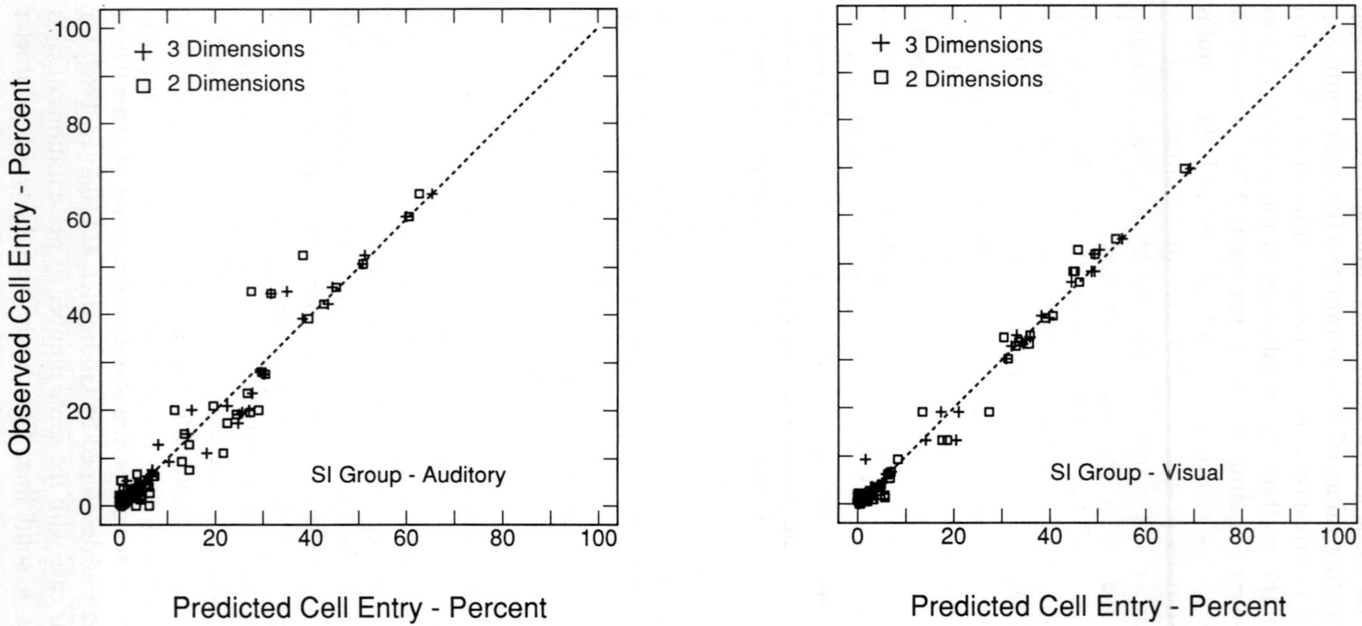

FIG. 2. Predicted and observed confusion matrix entries for Erber's (1972) SI group under A (left panel) and V (right panel) conditions. In each panel the abscissa is the matrix entry predicted by the identification model (expressed as a percentage), and the ordinate is the observed matrix entry. Predictions for both two- and three-dimensional cue spaces are shown.

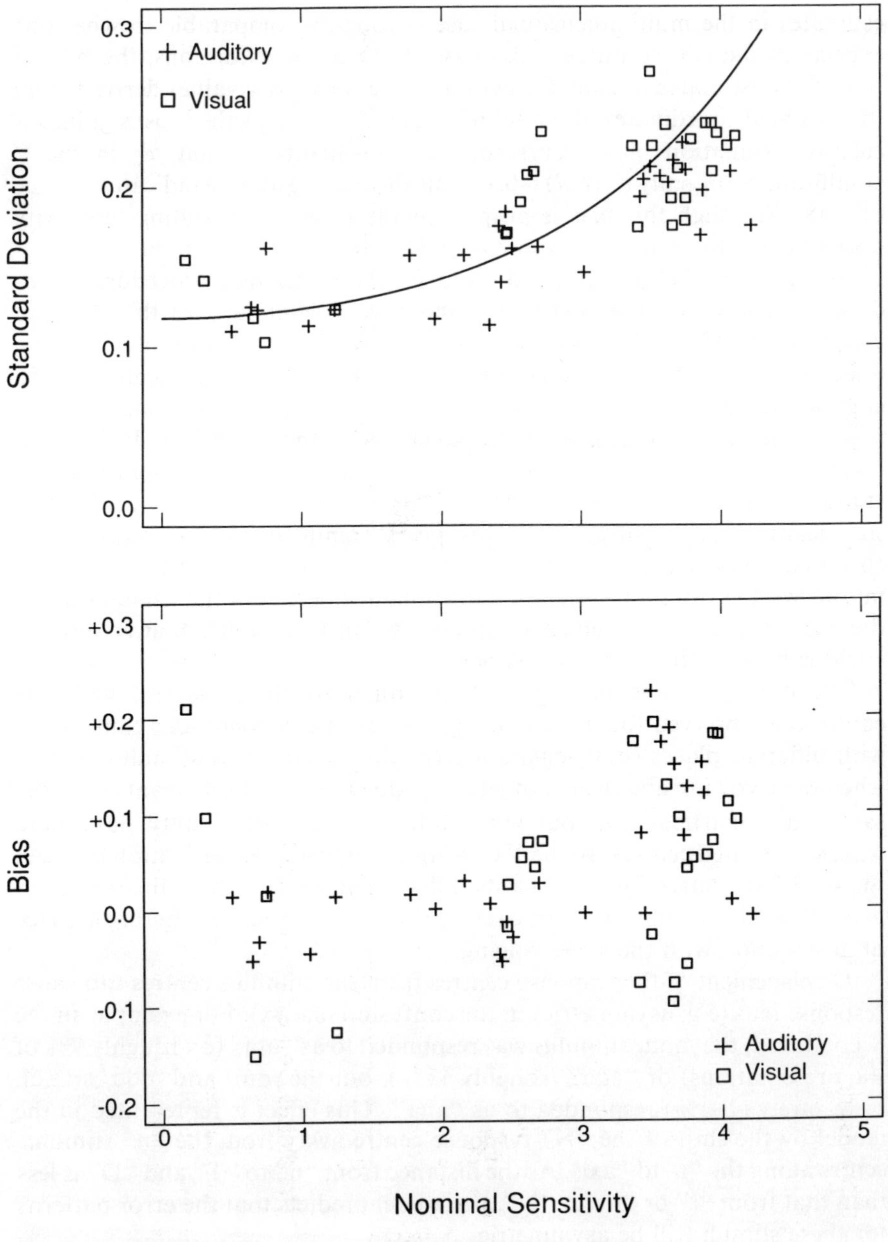

FIG. 3. Standard deviation (upper panel) and bias (lower panel) of estimates of interstimulus sensitivity for three-dimensional models corresponding to Erber's (1972) SI group A and V confusion matrices. The solid line in the upper panel corresponds to the Gourevitch and Galanter (1967) approximation to the standard deviation of sensitivity estimates in the two-stimulus scalar case.

estimates in the multidimensional case is roughly comparable to what one expects in the two-stimulus scalar case. With a few exceptions, the bias of sensitivity estimates is a small fraction of the sensitivity values derived from the assumed coordinates of the set of $\vec{S}_i$ and $\vec{R}_j$. Perhaps the most significant case of estimation bias occurs for the consonants /t/ and /d/ in the V condition. Nominally $d'_V(t, d) = 0.17$, but the mean estimate indicates a value of 0.38. Although this bias is proportionally large, the resulting sensitivity does not permit reliable discrimination between these consonants.

To visualize the cue spaces derived by the estimation procedures, two-dimensional fits to Erber's (1972) A and V confusion data for the SI group are plotted in Figure 4. Unlike traditional multidimensional scaling, the scale units in the panels of this figure are not arbitrary. One common unit, corresponding to the standard deviation of the Gaussian components of the additive noise vector, applies to all panels. Note that model predictions are insensitive to the absolute location and orientation of the configuration of stimulus and response centres. Only the relative locations of the centres are significant. Consequently, there is no special significance associated with the coordinate systems used in these panels. Association of particular orientations with various physical and perceptual properties of the stimuli used in the experiments (e.g. Clements, Braida, & Durlach, 1982; Soli & Arabie, 1979) is beyond the scope of this paper.

The configurations of Figure 4 are qualitatively consistent with the confusions observed for this subject group. In the A condition, consonants with different places of articulation have closely clustered stimulus centres when their voicing and degree of nasality are the same. Consonants with the same place of articulation, but which differ in voicing or nasality, have more widely separated centres. In the V condition, there is little separation between the stimulus centres for consonants differing in voicing when their place of articulation is the same, but large separation for consonants differing in place of articulation with the same voicing.

Displacement of the response centres from the stimulus centres can cause response bias (e.g. asymmetries in the confusion matrix). For example, in the V condition, the /ɑnɑ/ stimulus was responded to as "ata" (on roughly 9% of the presentations) or "ada" (roughly 13%), but the /ɑtɑ/ and /ɑdɑ/ stimuli were rarely (1–2%) responded to as "ana". This effect is represented in the model by the shift of the "N" response centre away from the "n" stimulus centre along the "n–td" axis. As the distance from "n" to "T" and "D" is less than that from "t" or "d" to "N", the model predicts that the error patterns for these stimuli will be asymmetric.

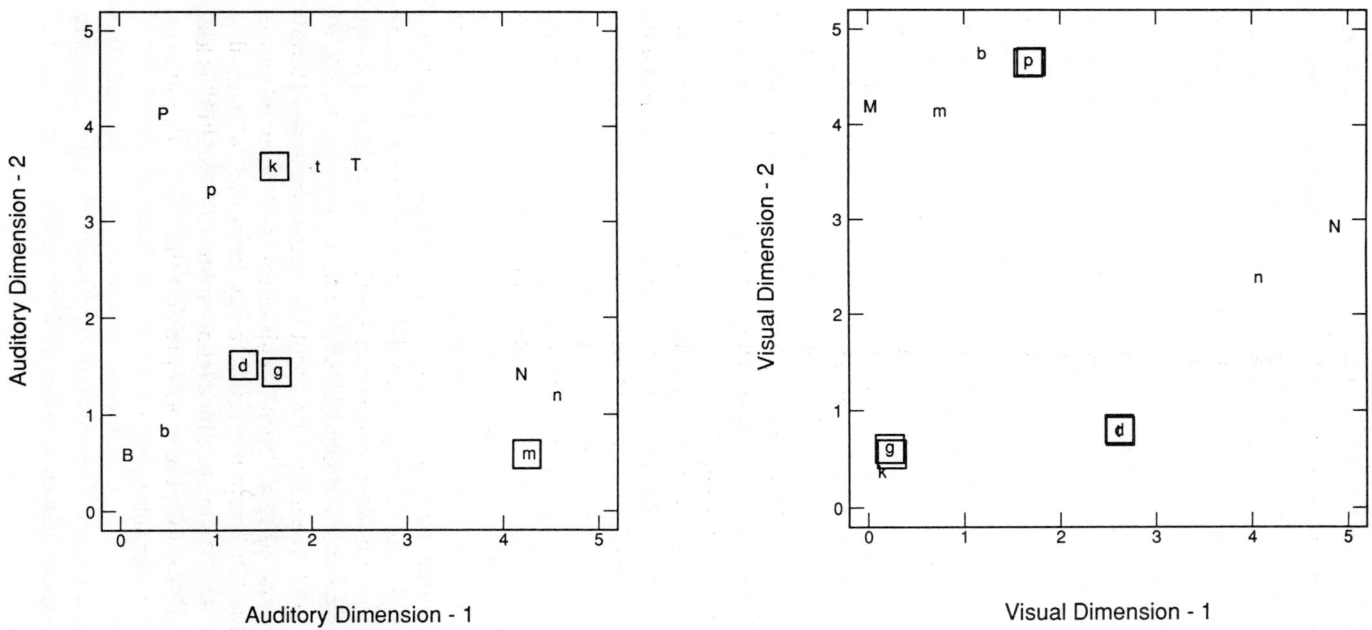

FIG. 4. Two-dimensional cue spaces for Erber's (1972) SI group. Lower-case letters mark stimulus centres, upper-case letters mark response centres. The squares in the left panel (auditory space) indicate nearly coincident stimulus and response centres, i.e. (d,D), (g,G), (k,K), and (m,M). Similarly, in the right panel (visual space) stimulus centres "t" and "d" are nearly coincident with each other and with response centres "T" and "D". Response centres "K" and "G" are nearly coincident with stimulus centre "g", and response centres "B" and "P" with stimulus centre "P". The common scale unit in the two panels corresponds to the standard deviation of components of the two-dimensional Gaussian cue densities.

4. Combining Cues from Different Modalities

In the multimodal presentation condition, we assume that cues are combined optimally and that there is no perceptual interference (e.g. masking or distraction) across modalities. We model the integration of cues by assuming that the cue densities in the multimodal condition are the "Cartesian products" of the densities corresponding to the separate modalities. This space is constructed from the orthogonal composition of the cue spaces corresponding to each of the stimulus modalities. A subset of the coordinates of each point in the product space corresponds to the coordinates of each of the subspaces for these modalities. Consider, for example, a multimodal AV condition. If the cue space corresponding to the A condition has dimension D_A with each stimulus represented by an auditory centre $\vec{A}_i = \langle a_{i1}, a_{i2}, \ldots, a_{iD_A} \rangle$, whereas that for the V condition has dimension D_V with each stimulus represented by a visual centre $\vec{V}_i = \langle v_{i1}, v_{i2}, \ldots, v_{iD_V} \rangle$, then in the AV condition the cue space has dimension $D_{AV} = D_A + D_V$ and each stimulus centre $\vec{S}_i$ has the coordinates

$$\vec{S}_i = \langle s_{i1}, s_{i2}, \ldots, s_{iD_{AV}} \rangle = \langle a_{i1}, \ldots, a_{iD_A}, v_{i1}, \ldots, v_{iD_V} \rangle \tag{11}$$

Locations of the stimulus centres in the combined cue space for three hypothetical identification experiments involving the consonants /p, t, k, b, d, g/ are shown in Figure 5. For simplicity, the figure assumes that confusions in the A and V conditions can satisfactorily be accounted for in one-dimensional cue spaces. The cue space in the AV condition is therefore predicted to be two-dimensional. This model for the combined condition predicts that there is a simple relation between a subject's sensitivity in distinguishing $\mathscr{S}_i$ from $\mathscr{S}_j$ in the multimodal condition, $d'_{AV}(i,j)$, and the corresponding unimodal sensitivities $d'_A(i,j)$ and $d'_V(i,j)$:

$$d'_{AV}(i,j) = \sqrt{d'_A(i,j)^2 + d'_V(i,j)^2} \tag{12}$$

It is well known that this Pythagorean relation satisfies the following inequalities:

$$d'_{AV}(i,j) \geqslant \max\,[d'_A(i,j),\, d'_V(i,j)] \tag{13}$$

and

$$d'_{AV}(i,j) \leqslant d'_A(i,j) + d'_V(i,j) \tag{14}$$

The geometric properties of the multimodal cue space thus capture the common observation that consonants can be distinguished in the AV condition if they can be distinguished in either or both of the A or V conditions. The model for the multimodal condition goes beyond this qualitative observation, however. The separation between stimulus centres in the Cartesian-product space places significant constraints on multimodal accuracy.

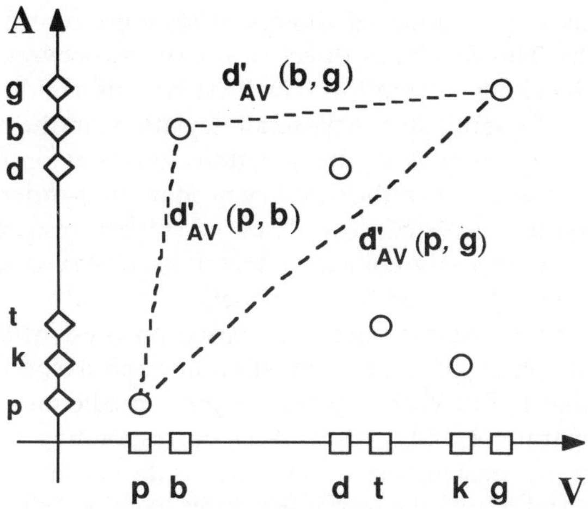

FIG. 5. Hypothetical cue spaces for /p, t, k, b, d, g/ identification experiments. Confusions in the A and V conditions are each assumed to be adequately described by scalar cues (*A* and *V*). Stimulus centres for the *A* (diamonds) and *V* (squares) scalar variables are shown on axes scaled to have a common unit, corresponding to the standard deviation of the cues. Stimulus centres in the AV condition are points in the *A*–*V* plane. As the *A* and *V* coordinates in the AV condition are assumed to be the same as the scalar coordinates in the A and V conditions, distances between points in the plane are just the Pythagorean sums of the *A* and *V* distances for the same stimulus pair. In all conditions the distance between a pair of points is the subject's sensitivity for distinguishing between the corresponding consonants.

5. Predicted Multimodal Accuracy

According to the assumptions stated in Section 4, the configurations derived from the unimodal confusion matrices determine the predicted stimulus centres for the multimodal configurations. Predicting accuracy in the multimodal condition requires a specification of the response centres as well. Unfortunately, the model presented in Section 4 does not predict the locations of the prototypes in the multimodal case, as response bias is logically unconstrained by sensitivity. The locations of response centres used in an experiment (relative to fixed stimulus centres) can be estimated iteratively. However, we have chosen to compute accuracy in the special case in which the bimodal response centres coincide with the bimodal stimulus centres, i.e.,

$$\vec{R}_i = \vec{S}_i = \langle a_{i1}, \ldots, a_{iD_A}, v_{i1}, \ldots, v_{iD_V} \rangle \quad (15)$$

The coincident centre condition has two special properties: (1) When the a priori stimulus presentation probabilities are equal, as they usually are in consonant identification experiments, it leads to the maximum value of identification accuracy among all choices of response centre locations (e.g. van Trees, 1968). This facilitates direct comparisons between the models of pre- and post-labelling integration. (2) Because this condition leads to a maximum value of overall accuracy, small deviations in the response centre locations from the stimulus centre locations produce only second-order changes in overall accuracy (although they produce first-order changes in the conditional response probabilities). Thus, if subjects use response centre locations that are close to the coincident locations, observed accuracy should be very close to that predicted by the model.

Predictions of identification accuracy based on pre-labelling integration under the assumption of coincident stimulus and response centres are included in Table 1. For each experiment these predictions were made by determining separate A and V cue spaces corresponding to the A and V confusion matrices, constructing an AV space as the Cartesian product of the A and V spaces and setting the response centres to coincide with the stimulus centres. The proportion of correct responses was then determined by integrating each stimulus density within its own response region and averaging the results across stimuli (consistent with the equal presentation probability assumption). Clearly the scores predicted by the pre-labelling model are both higher than those predicted by the post-labelling model and closer to observed values. This increase in predicted scores is unlikely to arise from poor descriptions of unimodal confusion matrices: on average, unimodal scores, predicted by the models of Section 3, with parameters used to predict multimodal scores, are about 1.2 percentage points less than observed, with an rms error of 1.7 points. This probably accounts for some of the underprediction of multimodal scores (roughly 0.5 percentage points averaged over studies). Note, however, that underestimation does not occur for all experiments, as for the post-labelling model. Moreover, predicted multimodal scores do not fail the χ^2 test [$\chi^2(12) = 17.09$, $p > 0.1$].

There is a second test of the model that is logically independent of the locations of the response centres in the multimodal condition. Interstimulus sensitivities predicted by Equation 12 based on models derived from A and V matrices can be compared with sensitivities corrresponding to a model of the AV matrix derived by the techniques described in Section 4. To the extent that these two sets of sensitivities are in agreement, the AV cue space is the orthogonal product of the A and V spaces. Although the value of this comparison is strongly model-dependent, the predicted and estimated sensitivities derive from completely separate sets of data, and the comparison is logically independent of assumptions about the locations of the response centres. The comparison for Erber's (1972) SI and PD group data is shown in Figure 6. As can be seen, there is good agreement between the two estimates of sensitivity for the conditions represented, although the larger values of sensitivity estimated for the AV matrix exceed the predictions of the

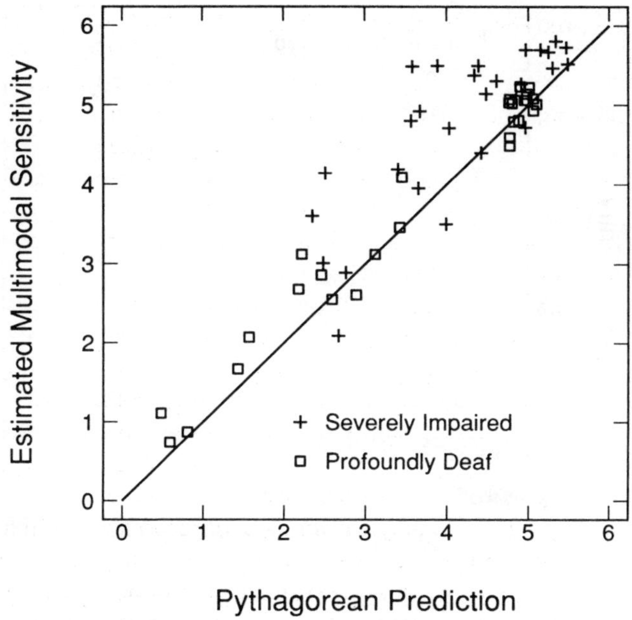

FIG. 6. Estimated and predicted values of interstimulus sensitivity for Erber's (1972) SI and PD groups in the AV condition. For each group, the identification model was used to derive a six-dimensional *AV* cue space corresponding to the AV confusion matrix. Estimated sensitivities are distances between stimulus centres in this space. Predicted values of sensitivity were obtained by applying Equation 12 to estimates of distances between stimulus centres in separate three-dimensional *A* and *V* cue spaces derived from A and V confusion matrices.

Pythagorean rule. Simulation studies (Braida, 1988) suggest that this is at least partially the result of a small overestimation of sensitivity in the higher-dimensional (e.g. *AV*) cue spaces. In any case, the practical consequences of this underestimation are likely to be small, because few confusions are expected when $d' > 4$.

Although the primary focus of this paper is on overall accuracy, it is also important that the pattern of response errors associated with the model be at least roughly consistent with those observed in the multimodal conditions. As discussed in Section 4, the error pattern predicted by the model depends on the location of the response centres relative to the stimulus centres, and we as yet have no theory that predicts response centre locations. Figure 7 compares the set of confusion matrix entries in the AV condition observed by Erber (1972) with that predicted by the model under the assumption of coincident stimulus and response centres. There is reasonably good agreement between the two patterns. Presumably this agreement could be substan-

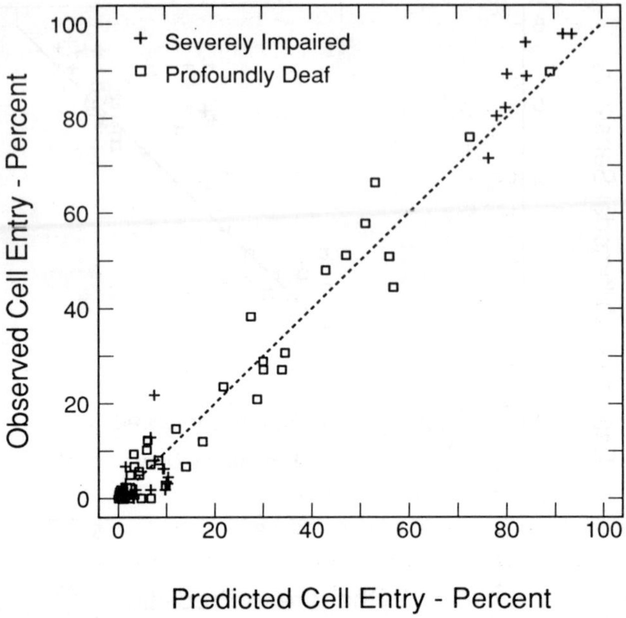

FIG. 7. Predicted and observed confusion matrix entries for the SI and PD groups in Erber's (1972) AV condition. For each group predicted entries were obtained by deriving three-dimensional *A* and *V* cue spaces corresponding to the A and V matrices, constructing a six-dimensional *AV* cue space as the Cartesian product of the A and V spaces, and setting response centres coincident with stimulus centres. Each predicted conditional response probability $P_{AV}(\mathscr{R}_j|\mathscr{S}_i)$ was then computed by integrating the density for $\mathscr{S}_i$ over the response region for $\mathscr{R}_j$ in the six-dimensional *AV* space.

tially improved if the correct locations of the response centres were used. Massaro (1987) has proposed use of an "rms" measure to describe the deviation between predicted and observed confusion matrices. As with overall accuracy, the pre-labelling model yields on average the smallest deviations, 17% smaller than those of the FLMP and 27% smaller than those of the post-labelling model.

DISCUSSION

Abstractly there need be little relation between multimodal performance and unimodal performance. On the one hand, unimodal cues could be integrated imperfectly (for example, as the result of perceptual interference), leading to lower than expected multimodal accuracy. On the other hand, in the multimodal case subjects could make use of intermodal cues that are unavailable in unimodal conditions, leading to higher than expected scores and unanticipated patterns of perceptual confusions. Such cues might arise if acoustic events were compared to visual events. For example, intermodal cues could result from estimating the loudness of segments relative to the degree of lip opening, or from estimating the duration of events bounded by the onset of audible sound and the subsequent visible closure of the lips. Accounts of multimodal integration that are equivalent to the post-labelling model must invoke such cues to account for higher than predicted multimodal accuracy. However, the success of the FLMP, and particularly the pre-labelling model, in accounting for audiovisual performance suggests that the contribution of intermodal cues is likely to be small in segment identification tasks.

The good predictions of identification accuracy based on the FLMP and the pre-labelling model of integration support the notion that there is little interference between the cues that originate in distinct modalities and, moreover, that subjects integrate these cues efficiently. Although precise estimates of efficiency await refinement of the estimation techniques used to establish parameters for the pre-labelling model, a finding of high efficiency would not be surprising. Subjects with usable visual and auditory abilities are likely to integrate auditory and visual cues routinely when communication is degraded (e.g. by noise, reverberation, poor articulation, hearing impairment, etc.). When tested on tasks of audiovisual speech reception, they are already highly practised in integration. Measures of integration efficiency for audiovisual speech stimuli are likely to be superior to those for less familiar stimuli.

The distinction between the pre-labelling and post-labelling models is common in the modelling of perceptual integration. Although predicted post-labelling integration accuracy was generally smaller than observed multimodal accuracy, the size of the discrepancy differed from study to study and in certain cases was probably negligible. On the other hand, the occurrence of substantial deficits in many cases indicates that subjects do adopt a pre-labelling integration strategy under certain conditions.

Only small differences between observed accuracy and that predicted by the post-labelling integration model were found in the −6 dB S/N condition in the Binnie et al. (1974) study, in the −9 and −15 dB conditions in the Campbell (1974) study, and in the AV condition in the Sparks and Grant (1979) study. In each of these cases the pre-labelling model overestimated performance. These two observations are consistent if suboptimal response regions are used in the AV condition.

The upper panel in Figure 8 illustrates response regions in a hypothetical two-dimensional AV cue space as well as those in the corresponding one-dimensional A and V cue spaces. In the one-dimensional spaces, the response regions are intervals along the scalar decision axes. In the two-dimensional space, the decision regions are compact regions in the plane. For the case

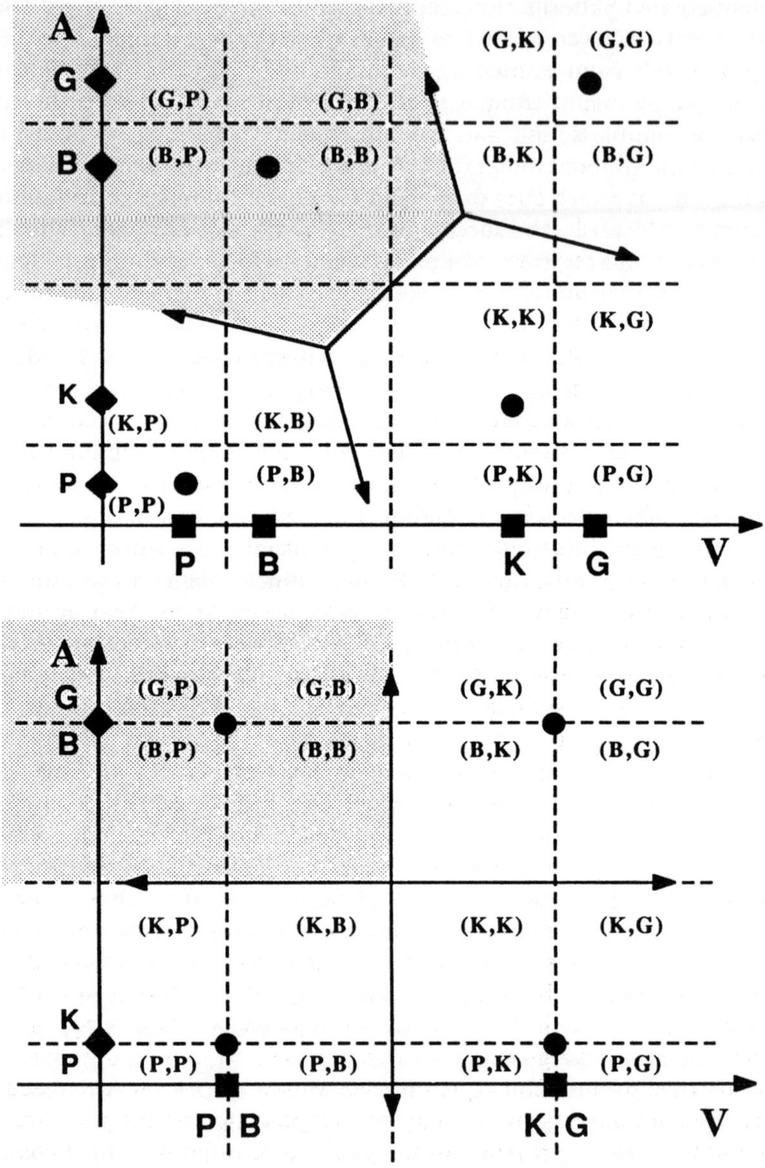

FIG. 8. Hypothetical cue spaces for /p, b, k, g/ identification experiments. Only response centres and response regions are shown; stimulus centres are not specified. As in Figure 5, confusions in the A and V conditions are described by scalar cues. In each panel, boundaries of two-dimensional *AV* response regions are marked by solid lines, and the response region for the "B" response is shaded. Dashed lines form rectangles corresponding to (A,V) label pairs in the post-labelling model. See text for details.

shown, the two-dimensional response centres are the Cartesian products of the one-dimensional centres.

It is possible to interpret the relation between pre- and post-labelling integration in this space. Each (A,V) label pair considered in the post-labelling model corresponds in the pre-labelling model to a rectangular region in the two-dimensional space (bounded by dashed lines), because such a region corresponds to the simultaneous occurrence of a specified A label and a specified V label in unimodal experiments. As seen in the upper panel, no two-dimensional response region corresponds to any grouping of rectangular regions. If the two-dimensional response centres coincide with the two-dimensional stimulus centres (which are themselves the Cartesian products of the one-dimensional stimulus centres), then the two-dimensional response regions lead to the highest identification accuracy. Any set of response regions constructed from collections of the rectangular regions must result in lower identification accuracy. Optimal decisions in the AV condition cannot be made by combining judgements made separately about the *A* and *V* cue vector components under such conditions.

The lower panel illustrates the same relation when pairs of the one-dimensional response centres become arbitrarily close to one another. Although there is no change in the one-dimensional decision regions or the label-pair rectangles, the two-dimensional response centres now describe rectangular response regions in the *AV* space. Each of these rectangular response regions corresponds precisely to a collection of the rectangular response regions constructed from the *A* and *V* response centres. Decisions in the AV experiment can be made as well by combining labelling judgements made separately for the *A* and *V* cue vector components. In terms of the analysis proposed by Ashby and Townsend (1986), such response centres enforce decisional separability: responses are based on the separate, as opposed to joint, properties of the components of the cue vector. However, such a strategy leads to inferior accuracy unless the stimulus centres coincide with the response centres. In the case illustrated this would correspond to an inability to discriminate between the pairs /p, k/ and /b, g/ in the A condition and a simultaneous inability to distinguish between /p, b/ and /k, g/ in the V condition. Such indistinguishability is not evident in the experiments considered in this paper. Consequently, when AV responses are based on decisional separability, accuracy may be well predicted by the post-labelling model, but the resulting performance is likely to be inferior to what could be achieved using a pre-labelling integration strategy.

The FLMP makes reasonably good predictions for multimodal accuracy, particularly given the ease with which these predictions can be computed. As noted above, the FLMP tends to underestimate the contribution of the acoustic signal when auditory accuracy is poor and overestimate it when accuracy is good. The usefulness of FLMP predictions is probably strongly dependent on the response biases of the subject, as consistent unimodal responses make little contribution to multimodal performance unless responses agree across modalities. Although the FLMP has been applied to a wide variety of studies of audiovisual speech reception, its predictions of multimodal accuracy derived from unimodal performance have not been analysed extensively. More typically, the adequacy of this model is evaluated by determining how well a common set of estimated auditory and visual feature values (i.e. $\hat{P}_A(\mathscr{R}_j|\mathscr{S}_i)$ and $\hat{P}_V(\mathscr{R}_j|\mathscr{S}_i)$) predict the set of observed $P_A(\mathscr{R}_j|\mathscr{S}_i)$, $P_V(\mathscr{R}_j|\mathscr{S}_i)$, and $P_{AV}(\mathscr{R}_j|\mathscr{S}_i)$. Such comparisons may yield more favourable evaluations of the FLMP's fits to observed confusion matrices.

To the extent that observed performance data reject the adequacy of post-labelling integration, many conventional descriptions of audiovisual speech reception must be revised. Strategies that group unimodal responses into "features" that are combined to determine the multimodal response are likely to underestimate accuracy in most cases. Such strategies are a class of techniques for labelling separately in each modality. To the extent that models of such strategies accurately account for unimodal confusions, they generally cannot predict identification accuracy superior to the maximum likelihood grouping of labels used in the post-labelling model, let alone to pre-labelling integration. In this respect it is interesting to note that in attempting to account for his own data, Campbell (1974) proposed a decision process for consonant identification that consists of a sequence of decisions based on linguistic features, with feature accuracy in the AV condition equal to that of the more accurate (A or V) modality. Although his estimates of feature accuracy describe unimodal accuracy reasonably well, they nevertheless tend to underestimate bimodal accuracy. For similar reasons the use of "viseme" groupings to describe visual stimuli is likely to underestimate the potential for multimodal integration of the pre-labelling type. Some current accounts of audiovisual speech perception are more consistent with the assumptions of the pre-labelling model. In particular, Summerfield (1987, 1989) reviews a variety of independent evidence that support the notion that audiovisual integration occurs before phonetic or lexical categorization takes place.

Additional research is needed to provide more incisive tests of the pre-labelling integration models described in Sections 3 and 4. The model of unimodal sensitivity needs to be evaluated in greater detail, on data from individual subjects. These evaluations should test the notion that model sensitivity is independent of those changes in response centre locations that can be affected by changes in presentation probabilities and payoffs (e.g. Chase, Bugnacki, Braida, & Durlach, 1982; Lippmann, Braida, & Durlach, 1976), as well as determine the extent to which the model provides a statistically adequate description of confusion matrices. This will entail the development of more robust techniques for estimating model parameters.

In a similar vein, the pre-labelling integration model needs to be tested over a larger range of stimuli. Except for the Campbell (1974) study, the consonants in the studies analysed were produced in the context of the vowel /ɑ/. According to the results of Owens and Blazek (1985), this is a particularly congenial environment for speechreading. The model needs to be tested and applied to consonant identification experiments that use more taxing vowel environments. The model should also be applied to identification experiments in which the stimuli are distinguished by the value of a vowel component. Available data on audiovisual vowel identification is sparse. The one study that published the confusion matrices needed for a test of the model (Hack & Erber, 1982) employed too few stimulus presentations per condition for a satisfactory test.

Models of audiovisual integration can also be extended to make predictions for the identification of stimuli with discrepant auditory and visual components (e.g. McGurk & MacDonald, 1976a, 1976b). To make and test predictions, unimodal and bimodal confusion matrices (including discrepant stimuli) are required. The predictions of the post-labelling model can be derived directly from these confusion matrices. To derive predictions for the pre-labelling model, both unimodal stimulus centres and bimodal response centres must be estimated. The model predicts that the stimulus centre corresponding to a discrepant combination of A and V stimuli is the Cartesian product of the *A* and *V* centres determined in the unimodal experiments. To predict the responses evoked by a discrepant stimulus, the probability density corresponding to this centre must be integrated over the response regions corresponding to the response centre locations for the non-discrepant stimuli. Unfortunately, the sets of matrices needed to make and test these predictions are not available. In a similar vein it is interesting to note that Repp (1976) attempted to account for the perceptual fusion of dichotically presented auditory syllables with a model that bears some similarities to pre-labelling integration. In Repp's "prototype" model, dichotic stimuli are mapped into separate auditory spaces, the resulting "multicategorical vectors" are combined, and the combination is mapped to a phonetic response category by comparison with prototypes. In contrast to the Cartesian-product integration process assumed in the pre-labelling model, however, Repp assumes that combination consists of averaging sense data either before or after multicategorical processing. As with discrepant audiovisual stimuli, it should be possible to apply the post- and pre-labelling models to the phenomenon of dichotic fusions, but the necessary matrices are not available.

To those accustomed to describe consonant identification with reference to the reception of various phonetic, articulatory, and acoustic features of speech sounds, it is perhaps surprising that a satisfactory account of multimodal accuracy can be developed in the abstract, without reference to such features. It is important to note, however, that multidimensional scaling analyses of unimodal confusion matrices often derive spaces (e.g. Figure 4) that can be interpreted, at least qualitatively, in terms of the acoustic–phonetic properties of speech. The extent to which the relevant detail in confusion matrices can be accounted for by linguistic features is not well understood. It is also important to ask whether features specified for clearly heard speech can account for audiovisual speech reception. Under degraded auditory reception conditions the perceptual effectiveness of feature differences is likely to be reduced non-uniformly. For example, as shown in Figure 4, the auditory $d'_A(b, p)$ is somewhat larger than $d'_A(k, g)$, even though each pair of consonants differs only in the voicing feature. Similarly, the visual distinctiveness of feature differences is often not specified by linguistic or articulatory constraints and consequently might be expected to vary from speaker to speaker. For example, in the visual space shown in Figure 4, $d'_V(t, n) \gg d'_V(b, m)$. (Although not shown in this figure, the PD subject group also showed good accuracy for the /d/–/n/ and /t/–/n/ distinctions.) Apparently the speaker in this study nasalized sounds in a manner that had greater visual consequences for dental than labial consonants. It seems plausible that those experienced in audiovisual communication would develop strategies that make use of all consistent perceptual differences in specific situations.

Although this paper focused on evidence for pre-labelling integration of cues from different sensory systems, the same analysis can logically be applied to the integration of cues from different channels in the same sensory system—for example, from low- and high-frequency bands of filtered speech. The amount of relevant data available on such integration is small (e.g. Miller & Nicely, 1955) but seems consistent with the finding for audiovisual consonant identification. Post-labelling integration is inadequate to describe the accuracy observed when bands are combined; pre-labelling integration provides a more satisfactory explanation.

The use of the pre-labelling model to relate identification scores derived from different presentation conditions is similar to the use of Articulation Theory to predict the effect of filtering on intelligibility. There are, however, substantial differences. The approach described in this paper is restricted to small closed sets of speech segments, but it can derive theoretical predictions for accuracy on combination conditions. Articulation Theory (e.g. ANSI, 1969) predicts intelligibility scores based on two sets of distilled empirical observations. One set is relevant to the computation of the Articulation Index, which is assumed to be independent of the type of speech material but dependent on presentation condition. The other set is relevant to the relation between Articulation Index values and intelligibility scores, which is assumed to be independent of presentation condition but dependent on the type of speech material. The computation of the Articulation Index might be placed on a firmer foundation by the use of explicit integration models. (Models for integration appropriate for vowels and models that relate syllable identification to consonant and vowel identification would also be required.) In a similar vein, explicit modelling of the integration process should provide new insights into the effectiveness of speechreading supplements whose unimodal intelligibility is practically negligible, such as those derived from fundamental frequency or the amplitude envelopes of filtered bands of speech. Although such signals provide little intelligibility for sentences or large sets of words, they can be used to identify consonants at levels well above chance. Unfortunately, the necessary triads of confusion matrices for these signals are not available.

There would appear to be several practical applications of these theoretical results. For example, many users of hearing aids, cochlear implants, and tactile aids often derive substantial communication benefit only when the prosthesis is used together with speechreading. The design of such prostheses is thus a matter of specifying the input to one modality when the performance of the device is ultimately evaluated on both unimodal and multimodal performance. Optimizing prosthesis design is likely to proceed most efficiently if intermodal integration is explicitly taken into account. This approach has long been advocated by Fourcin and his colleagues (e.g. Fourcin et al., 1979). To the extent that this integration can be modelled, it should be possible to apply these analytical techniques in reverse fashion: given a "target" level of performance for the audiovisual condition and a specified confusion matrix for the visual condition, determine an auditory confusion matrix consistent with the target level of accuracy. The prosthesis design problem can then be confined to achieving a specified auditory confusion matrix.

When multimodal reception is unsatisfactory, a prosthesis designer is forced to apportion the failing among the subject's poor use of visual cues, inability to use cues provided by the prosthesis, or difficulty in integrating these two sets of cues. The analytical techniques described in this paper provide a rational basis for this analysis. In addition, they can provide the clinician with insight into specific causes of poor accuracy that may be correctable through practice and training. Poorly chosen response centres produce inferior performance by inducing response bias. This can be identified in a given condition by using the pre-labelling model to analyse the confusion matrix, then predicting the confusion matrix that would be observed if response centres coincided with stimulus centres. On the other hand, if multimodal accuracy is lower than that predicted by the post-labelling model, it should be possible to improve scores with conventional training techniques. The potential for further improving accuracy by facilitating pre-labelling integration also should be considered. The development of appropriate training strategies for this case remains a challenge for the future.

REFERENCES

ANSI (1969). *American National Standard methods for the calculation of the Articulation Index, ANSI S3.5-1969.* New York: American National Standards Institute.

Ashby, F.G. & Townsend, J.T. (1986). Varieties of perceptual independence. *Psychological Review, 93,* 154–179.

Binnie, C.A., Montgomery, A.A., & Jackson, P.L. (1974). Auditory and visual contributions to the perception of selected English consonants for normally hearing and hearing-impaired listeners. *Video and Audio-visual Perceptions of Speech, Scandinavian Audiology* (Suppl *4*), 182–209.

Blamey, P.J. (1986). *Combining auditory and visual information in speech perception.* Personal communication.

Blamey, P.J., Cowan, R.S.C., Alcantara, J.I., Whitford, L.A., & Clark, G.M. (1988). Speech perception using combinations of auditory, visual, and tactile information. *Journal of Rehabilitation Research and Development, 26* (1), 15–24.

Boothroyd, A. (1975) *Interaction of speechreading and limited hearing.* S.A.R.P. No. 22, presented at the 1975 meeting of the American Speech and Hearing Association.

Borg, I. & Lingoes, J. (1987). *Multidimensional similarity structure analysis.* New York: Springer-Verlag.

Braida, L.D. (1988). Development of a model for multidimensional identification experiments. *Journal of the Acoustical Society of America, 84,* S142.

Breeuwer, M. & Plomp, R. (1985). Speechreading supplemented with formant frequency information from voiced speech. *Journal of the Acoustical Society of America, 77,* 314–317.

Breeuwer, M. & Plomp, R. (1986). Speechreading supplemented with auditorily presented speech parameters. *Journal of the Acoustical Society of America, 79,* 481–499.

Busacco, D.A. (1988). *The effect of age on the benefit derived from visual cues in auditory–visual speech recognition by the hearing impaired.* Ph.D. diss., Columbia University, New York.

Bush, R.R., Galanter, E., & Luce, R.D. (1963). Characterization and classification of choice experiments. In R.D. Luce, R.R. Bush, & E. Galanter (Eds.), *Handbook of mathematical psychology* (pp. 77–102). New York: John Wiley.

Campbell, H.W. (1974). *Phoneme recognition by ear and by eye: A distinctive feature analysis.* Ph.D. diss., University of Nijmegen, The Netherlands.

Chase, S., Bugnacki, P., Braida, L.D., & Durlach, N.I. (1982). Intensity perception. XII. Effect of presentation probability on absolute identification. *Journal of the Acoustical Society of America, 73,* 279–284.

Clements, M.A., Braida, L.D., & Durlach, N.I. (1982). Quantitative methods for the comparative evaluation of artificial tactile speech displays. IEEE Frontiers in Health Care, 1982. *Proc. 4th Conf. IEEE Eng. in Med. and Bio. Sci.* (pp. 362–367).

Danhauer, J.L., Ghadialy, F.B., Beck, D.L., Lucks, L.E., & Cudahy, E.A. (1990). Audio-visual consonant recognition with the 3M/House cochlear implant. *Journal of Rehabilitation Research and Development, 27* (3), 247–254.

Dowell, R.C., Martin, L.F.A., Tong, Y.C., Clark, G.M., Seligman, P.M., & Patrick, J.F. (1982). A 12-consonant confusion study on a multiple-channel cochlear implant patient. *Journal of Speech and Hearing Research, 25,* 509–516.

Durlach, N.I. & Braida, L.D. (1969). Intensity perception. I. Preliminary theory of intensity resolution. *Journal of the Acoustical Society of America, 46,* 372–383.

Erber, N.P. (1972). Auditory, visual, and auditory–visual recognition of consonants by children with normal and impaired hearing. *Journal of Speech and Hearing Research, 14,* 413–422.

Erber, N.P. (1979). Auditory–visual perception of speech with reduced optical clarity. *Journal of Speech and Hearing Research, 22,* 212–223.

Fourcin, A.J., Rosen, S.M., Moore, B.C.J., Douek, E.E., Clarke, G.P., Dodson, H., &

Bannister, L.H. (1979). External electrical stimulation of the cochlea: clinical, psychophysical, speech perceptual, and histological findings. *British Journal of Audiology*, *13*, 85–107.

Gourevitch, V. & Galanter, E. (1967). A significance test for one parameter isosensitivity functions. *Psychometrika*, *32*, 25–33.

Green, D.M. & Swets, J.A. (1966). *Signal detection theory and psychophysics*. New York: John Wiley.

Hack, Z.C. & Erber, N.P. (1982). Auditory, visual, and auditory–visual perception of vowels by hearing-impaired children. *Journal of Speech and Hearing Research*, *25*, 100–107.

Kruskal, J.B. & Wish, M. (1978). *Multidimensional scaling*. Beverly Hills, CA: Sage Publications.

Lippmann, R.P., Braida, L.D., & Durlach, N.I. (1976). Intensity perception. V. Effect of payoff matrix on absolute identification. *Journal of the Acoustical Society of America*, *59*, 129–134.

Macmillan, N.A., Goldberg, R.F., & Braida, L.D. (1988). Vowel and consonant resolution: Basic sensitivity and context memory. *Journal of the Acoustical Society of America*, *84*, 1262–1280.

Massaro, D.W. (1987). *Speech perception by ear and eye: A paradigm for psychological inquiry*. Hillsdale, NJ: Lawrence Erlbaum Associates, Inc.

McGurk, H. & MacDonald, J. (1976a). Visual influences on speech perception processes. *Perception and Psychophysics*, *24*, 253–257.

McGurk, H. & MacDonald, J. (1976b). Hearing lips and seeing voices. *Nature*, *264*, 746–748.

Miller, G.A. & Nicely, P. (1955). An analysis of perceptual confusions among some English consonants. *Journal of the Acoustical Society of America*, *27*, 328–352.

Neely, K.K. (1956). Effect of visual factors on the intelligibility of speech. *Journal of the Acoustical Society of America*, *28*, 1275–1277.

Owens, E. & Blazek, B. (1985). Visemes observed by hearing-impaired and normal-hearing adult viewers. *Journal of Speech and Hearing Research*, *28*, 381–393.

Pollack, I. (1964). Interaction between auditory and visual information sources in word identification. *Language and Speech*, *7*, 1–12.

Repp, B.H. (1976). Identification of dichotic fusions. *Journal of the Acoustical Society of America*, *60*, 456–469.

Soli, S.D. & Arabie, P. (1979). Auditory versus phonetic accounts of observed confusions between consonant phonemes. *Journal of the Acoustical Society of America*, *66*, 46–59.

Sparks, D.W. & Grant, K.W. (1979). Consonant recognition with the MESA. *Journal of the Acoustical Society of America*, *65*, S137.

Sparks, D., Kuhl, P., Edmonds, A., & Gray, G. (1978). Investigating the MESA (Multipoint Electrotactile Speech Aid): The transmission of segmental features of speech. *Journal of the Acoustical Society of America*, *63*, 246–257.

Sumby, W.H. & Pollack, I. (1954). Visual contribution to speech intelligibility in noise. *Journal of the Acoustical Society of America*, *26*, 212–215.

Summerfield, Q. (1987). Some preliminaries to a comprehensive account of audio-visual speech perception. In B. Dodd & R. Campbell (Eds.), *Hearing by eye: The psychology of lip-reading* (pp. 3–52). Hillsdale, NJ: Lawrence Erlbaum Associates, Inc.

Summerfield, Q. (1989). Visual perception of phonetic gestures. In I.G. Mattingly (Ed.), *Modularity and the motor theory of speech perception*. Hillsdale, NJ: Lawrence Erlbaum Associates, Inc.

van Trees, H.L. (1968). *Detection, estimation, and modulation theory*. New York: John Wiley.

Walden, B.E., Prosek, R.A., & Worthington, D.W. (1974). Predicting audiovisual consonant recognition performance of hearing-impaired adults. *Journal of Speech and Hearing Research*, *17*, 270–278.

Revised manuscript received 1 January 1991

THE QUARTERLY JOURNAL OF EXPERIMENTAL PSYCHOLOGY, 1991, *43A* (3) 679–699

A Further Examination of Attentional Effects in the Phonemic Restoration Illusion

Arthur G. Samuel

Yale University, New Haven, Connecticut, U.S.A.

Models of how listeners understand speech must specify the types of representations that are computed, the nature of the flow of information, and the control structures that modify performance. Three experiments are reported that focus on the control processes in speech perception. Subjects in the experiments tried to discriminate stimuli in which a phoneme had been replaced with white noise from stimuli in which white noise was merely superimposed on a phoneme. In the first two experiments, subjects practiced the discrimination for thousands of trials but did not improve, suggesting that they have poor access to low-level representations of the speech signal. In the third experiment, each (auditory) stimulus was preceded by a visual cue that could potentially be used to focus attention in order to enhance performance. Only subjects who received information about *both* the identity of the impending word and the identity of the critical phoneme showed enhanced discrimination. Other cues, including syllabic plus phonemic information, were ineffective. The results indicate that attentional control of processing is difficult but possible, and that lexical representations play a central role in the allocation of attention.

A description of the operation of an information processing system must include a characterization of the forms of representation used, the nature of the information flow, and the mechanisms that control processing. In the domain of speech perception, there is a large literature devoted to the representational issue, with evidence adduced for acoustic features (e.g. Sawusch, 1977), phonemes (e.g. Norris and Cutler, 1988), demisyllables (e.g. Fujimura, 1976), syllables (e.g. Massaro, 1975), and words (e.g. Samuel, 1986). There is also a substantial literature that focuses on the question of information flow. Research in this area is concerned with whether the information develops in a strictly "bottom-up" or "autonomous" way (e.g. Cutler & Norris, 1979; Cutler, Mehler, Norris, & Segui, 1987; Massaro,

Requests for reprints should be sent to Arthur G. Samuel, Department of Psychology, State University of New York, Stony Brook, NY 11794, U.S.A.

1989), or whether higher-level knowledge can influence the operation of lower-level analyses (e.g. Elman and McClelland, 1984, 1988; Marslen-Wilson & Welsh, 1978; McClelland & Elman, 1986). There are also partially interactive models in which top-down influences are allowed, but only among a subset of the levels in the system (e.g. Connine & Clifton, 1987; Samuel, 1981a, 1986; Tanenhaus & Lucas, 1987).

The literature dealing with control processes in speech perception is considerably sparser than the literatures on representation and information flow (see Nusbaum & Schwab, 1986). However, control issues are playing a growing role in assessing models of speech perception. For example, in Cutler and Norris's (1979) autonomous model, decisions in experimental tasks (such as phoneme monitoring) can be based on information encoded at either a phonemic or a lexical level. Control processes are invoked in the model to account for observed differences in performance across testing conditions: Task parameters such as word length, secondary tasks, and stimulus quality can bias attentional allocation towards either lexical or phonemic representations (Cutler et al., 1987). In fact, proponents of the autonomous model have argued that the model's inclusion of this control structure allows it to account for some empirical findings better than interactive models without such control processes (e.g. the TRACE model of McClelland and Elman, 1986).

To date, proponents of fully interactive models have not chosen to include control processes in their models, perhaps because these models already have many parameters and therefore great predictive power. However, Samuel and Ressler (1986) have provided an initial description of the use of control processes within a partially interactive framework, and such processes could be incorporated by interactive theories more generally. The present study extends Samuel and Ressler's examination of how listeners direct attention to different levels of representation of the speech signal.

Samuel and Ressler (1986) used the phonemic restoration illusion as a means to investigate attentional control in speech perception. The illusion occurs when listeners are presented with an utterance in which part of the speech signal is deleted (typically one phoneme) and replaced by an extraneous noise. Listeners report that the utterance sounds intact, despite the fact that objectively it is not (Warren, 1970). Samuel and Ressler suggested that the illusion might be at least partially attributable to a failure to attend to the low level (roughly, phonemic) needed to judge whether a phoneme is present. Under normal conditions, listeners would have little incentive to attend to such low levels because their goal is to understand the words of an utterance. Basing judgements on the lexical level in a restoration experiment, however, would produce the observed failures in performance. Samuel and Ressler noted that this analysis was similar to analyses that have been offered for visual illusions such as the Mueller–Lyer effect: Accurate perception of component parts (e.g. horizontal lines) may be undermined by predominant attention to the global pattern.

The present study, like Samuel and Ressler's study, examines whether the strength of the phonemic restoration illusion can be reduced with two techniques that have been used to reduce global dominance in visual illusions: training (e.g. Judd, 1902; Lewis, 1908) and cueing (Coren & Girgus, 1972; Dewar, 1967). The strength of restoration is assessed using Samuel's (1981a) discrimination methodology. In this procedure, two types of stimuli are constructed. In a *replaced* stimulus, a section of a word is digitally replaced by white noise; the section corresponds to one phoneme plus its transitions to neighbouring phonemes. In an *added* stimulus, the white noise is digitally added to the speech segment; the noise is superimposed on the phoneme, leaving the word intact. On each trial, the subject hears a single stimulus and must judge whether or not the noise replaced a phoneme. To the extent that replaced phonemes are perceptually restored, listeners should perceive them as intact (with noise superimposed), which should make it very difficult to discriminate between *added* and *replaced* stimuli. The strength of the illusion is thus indexed by the signal detection measure of discriminability, d', with low d's signifying strong restoration effects.

Experiments 1 and 2 include extensive training procedures (with feedback) on the discrimination task. Such training could potentially allow listeners to modify their normal tendency to attend primarily to lexical-level representations, and thus improve performance. In Experiment 3, several attentional cue conditions are compared. Each cue is presented visually immediately before a test stimulus and can potentially affect the level of representation that is attended to. Across the set of experiments, the goal is to determine whether listeners can control the level of analysis that is used to make the required intactness judgement. The results will be used to develop the model of speech processing outlined by Samuel and Ressler, a model in which control processes are included in a partially interactive theory.

EXPERIMENT 1

In the initial experiments using the discrimination methodology, *added* and *replaced* versions of approximately 100 English words were presented to each listener (Samuel, 1981a, 1981b), for a total of about 200 trials without feedback (subjects received ten practice trials with feedback). Samuel and Ressler (1986) suggested that this did not provide listeners with an opportunity to develop optimal processing procedures. To provide such an opportunity, Samuel and Ressler ran their subjects through three sessions of the task, for a total of 972 trials with feedback. Despite such extensive practice, subjects showed few signs of improvement, suggesting that the tendency to rely on a lexical code is difficult to overcome. However, the results are problematic because we cannot distinguish between two possibilities: (1) listeners cannot learn to direct attention to sublexical representations, or (2) listeners did not have sufficient opportunity to develop the necessary control.

In Experiment 1, the training was increased by an order of magnitude—each subject received almost 10,000 word training trials with feedback. Training on this scale has the virtue that even a null result should be informative—with this much practice, a failure to improve would indicate that attentional control over the illusion is not realistically possible. Schneider (personal communication) has suggested that in attentional training experiments, if a stimulus fails to produce improvement within 200 presentations, the discrimination is not going to improve with additional practice. In the present experiment, each word was presented 180 times through the course of training, a level of practice that should reveal any improvement that is likely to occur.

Experiment 1 included an additional manipulation that was intended to examine the role that pre-existing lexical representations might play in focusing attention. Subjects received training on *added* and *replaced* versions of both real English words and pseudowords. The latter, while phonologically legitimate, had no pre-existing lexical representations. Over the course of scores of presentations, a pseudoword might be expected to develop some sort of lexical-like code (without any semantic or syntactic information). The pseudoword condition thus might be expected to produce different results initially, and over training, to converge with the word condition as the pseudowords became more word-like.

Method

Stimuli. One hundred and eight English words were initially recorded on audiotape by the author. The 108 included four sets of 27 words, with each set representing the factorial crossing of three word lengths (two, three, or four syllables) with three critical phoneme classes (fricative, nasal, or liquid) and three critical phoneme positions (word-initial, word final, or word-medial). The words were lowpass filtered (4.8 kHz), digitized at 10 kHz (12-bit A/D), and stored in a PDP-11 disc file. *Added* and *replaced* stimuli were constructed using the procedures described in Samuel (1987) and Samuel and Ressler (1986): Critical segments were located with a waveform editor and either replaced by signal-correlated noise (*replaced*) or superimposed with the noise (*added*). The signal-correlated noise was constructed by randomly flipping the sign (+ or −) of half of the samples. This creates a waveform with a flat spectrum (noise) but preserves the magnitude and shape of the amplitude envelope. The manipulated segments were chosen to include the critical phoneme, and its transitions into the adjacent phonemes. Some of the important properties of the stimuli are summarized in DeWitt and Samuel (1990).

The word stimuli were used to construct 108 pseudowords. The pseudowords were made by selecting pairs of words, digitally splitting each word into two pieces, and swapping the halves (see Samuel, 1987, for details of the procedure). For example, "familiar" and "domestic" were split and swapped to produce "famestic" and "domiliar". Note that this procedure produces pseudowords that include exactly the same critical phonemes as the words because they are literally copies. The original 108 words were chosen in pairs that either shared a medial phoneme, or that had a medial stop closure; this minimized any acoustic-phonetic discontinuities due to the splicing procedure.

Apparatus and Procedure. Each subject participated in 30 sessions, with sessions generally run once a day, Monday through Friday. The 108 words and 108 pseudowords were each split into sets of 54 stimuli, and one set of 54 words and 54 pseudowords was designated as the training set for each subject; the other half of each stimulus type was reserved for a baseline and transfer test (see below). The assignment of stimuli to training and transfer sets was counterbalanced across subjects.

Each session consisted of 648 trials. This total represents three passes through 108 stimuli (54 words and 54 pseudowords), with each stimulus occurring in two forms (*added* and *replaced*). Thus, each subject received 19,440 trials (30 × 648). Half of these trials involved words and half involved pseudowords. Word and pseudoword trials were randomly mixed. Each session lasted approximately 45 minutes.

The first session for each subject was used as a baseline measure. The "other" 108 stimuli—that is, the words and pseudowords that were *not* going to be used in training for that subject—were presented in this session. In Sessions 2–29, the training stimuli were used. Finally, in Session 30, the baseline stimuli were presented again. The last session served as a transfer test, to see whether any gains observed on the training set would transfer to other stimuli. This test assesses whether any learning that occurs is item-specific.

Each subject was tested individually in a sound-attenuating chamber. Stimuli were converted to analog form (12-bit D/A), lowpass filtered (4.8 kHz), amplified, and presented over high-quality headphones. Subjects responded by pushing buttons labelled "added" or "replaced". After the subject responded, the correct answer was displayed for 1 sec on a computer terminal in front of the subject. Approximately 1 sec later the next test stimulus was presented.

At the beginning of the experiment, the nature of the stimulus types was fully explained to the subjects. They were informed that the discrimination was often difficult, and that we were interested in how well people could learn to make the distinction.

Subjects. Four individuals living in the New Haven area participated in Experiment 1. All were native English speakers with no known hearing problems. They were paid for their participation.

Results and Discussion

Two types of errors were considered. A *false alarm* was defined as the report of an objectively intact stimulus (*added*) as not intact (*replaced*); a *miss* was the reverse (a *replaced* stimulus being identified as *added*). Percentages of misses and false alarms were computed for each session for each subject, broken down by word versus pseudoword stimuli. These two error types were then used to calculate d' scores. As noted previously, strong perceptual restoration should cause *replaced* stimuli to sound intact, making discrimination difficult and therefore producing low d' values.

For purposes of analysis, the 28 training sessions were treated separately from the baseline and transfer sessions. The 28 sessions were grouped into seven blocks of four consecutive sessions (Days 2–5, 6–9, . . . , 26–29); each block included 2592 trials per subject. The discriminability scores were submitted to a two-way analysis of variance. The two factors in the analysis were block (1–7) and stimulus type (word verusus pseudoword). Figure 1 presents the mean d' scores for each subject individually, and for the subjects collectively. Note that in the figure, the baseline session and transfer session are called Blocks 1 and 9, and the training sessions are numbered 2 through 8.

The central question in Experiment 1 is, can listeners learn to attend to low levels of analysis through practice on the discrimination task? The flat functions shown in Figure 1 suggest that any such learning is minimal at best. The analysis of variance confirms this impression: the main effect of training block did not approach significance [$F(6, 18) < 1$], nor did its interaction with Stimulus type [$F(6, 18) < 1$]. Given the null training effects, any comparison of the baseline session (Day 1) to the transfer one (Day 30) is moot.

The results for words and pseudowords were quite similar overall, and across training. The analysis of variance did not reveal any differences in processing the two stimulus types ($F(1, 3) = 1.03$, n.s.]. However, this is clearly a weak test, and a subject-by-subject analysis indicates that there was some differentiation. For each subject, a matched-pairs t-test was conducted, using the word and pseudoword d' scores for each of the seven training blocks. For two of the subjects (S1 and S3) no difference was found. However, for the other two (S2 and S4), discriminability was significantly better for words, $t(6) = 3.91$, $p < 0.01$ [S2] and $t(6) = 8.82$, $p < 0.001$ [S4]. Note that these two subjects had higher d' scores overall. It appears that the other

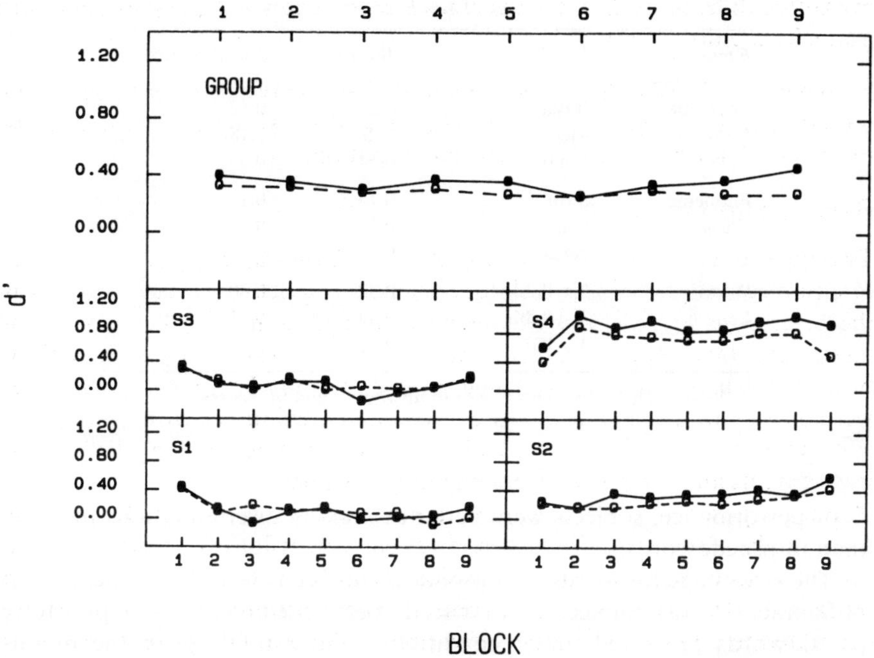

FIG. 1. Discrimination scores (d') for the four subjects in Experiment 1 individually (bottom four panels) and as a group (top panel). Block 1 was a baseline session, Blocks 2–8 were training sessions, and Block 9 was a transfer test. Performance on word stimuli is indicated by solid lines, and data for the pseudowords are connected by dashed lines.

two subjects were largely unable to make the discrimination, regardless of stimulus type.

Table 1 presents discrimination performance, broken down by the three stimulus factors: position of the critical phoneme, class of the critical phoneme, and length of the test word. For each of these factors, a three-way analysis of variance was conducted, pairing the factor with block (1–7) and lexicality (word versus pseudoword). The results of these analyses were straightforward: In no analysis did the training factor (block) produce a reliable main effect or interaction with any other factor [the largest such effect was the interaction of block and phoneme class, with $F(12, 36) = 1.62$, n.s.]. Thus, the general pattern of results described above is not qualified by any interactions with the stimulus factors. There were two reliable effects that did not involve the training factor: Performance was best for final-position stimuli, $F(2, 6) = 8.80$, $p < 0.02$, and lexicality interacted with phoneme class, $F(2, 6) = 5.26$, $p < 0.05$. The latter effect reflects the better performance on nasals in words than in pseudowords, coupled with no difference on the more difficult stops and fricatives. When stimulus factors did not produce near-

TABLE 1

Factor	*Level*	*Words*	*Pseudowords*
Phoneme	Initial	0.24	0.17
Position	Medial	0.26	0.18
	Final	0.54	0.55
Phoneme	Stop	0.14	0.15
Class	Fricative	0.25	0.22
	Nasal	0.65	0.51
Word	2-syllable	0.32	0.30
Length	3-syllable	0.34	0.21
	4-syllable	0.35	0.35

Note: The values shown are in absolute units (d' scores).

floor performance, subjects were better at making discriminations in words than in pseudowords.

The advantage for words over pseudowords is consistent with the findings of Samuel (1981a). Subjects in that study performed comparably poorly on pseudowords presented under conditions similar to those in the present study. The difficulty of the task with pseudowords stems in part from listeners' well-established inability to localize extraneous noise relative to the speech stream. This problem would lead to the noise being heard before or after the pseudoword, which puts subjects in the position of having to make an impossible judgement. For example, if "famestic" is presented, and subjects hear "famestic" with a following noise, they must decide whether "famestic" was the whole stimulus, or whether some other pseudoword (e.g. "famestics") had been presented with a phoneme deleted. In Samuel's (1981a) study this problem was overcome by including an additional condition in which the intact pseudoword was presented before the *added* or *replaced* version, to provide the listener with a target stimulus. The present study did not use this procedure because it seemed likely that after pseudowords had been repeated dozens of times subjects would know their identities. The data suggest that this was only partially true.

Part of the difficulty the subjects had may have been due to the mixed design: From trial to trial, subjects could not predict whether a test item would be a word or a pseudoword. The analysis just presented suggests that different strategies are needed for word and pseudoword trials, because words can be judged relatively ("was what I heard an intact word?"), whereas pseudowords must be judged absolutely ("did the noise coincide with a phoneme?"). The random presentation order precluded the optimization of these strategies. This, in turn, might have precluded the optimization of attentional allocation. If so, the null result found in Experiment 1 would not reflect people's true abilities to control attention in perceiving speech.

EXPERIMENT 2

Experiment 2 was essentially identical to Experiment 1, with one critical exception: No pseudowords were used. As in the first experiment, the subjects received approximately 10,000 word trials with feedback. Eliminating the pseudowords should allow subjects to develop a single optimal strategy for doing the task. The fundamental question remains the same: Can listeners learn to attend to low-level phonemic representations well enough to reduce the strength of the phonemic restoration effect?

Method

Stimuli. The same word stimuli used in Experiment 1 were used in Experiment 2. The pseudowords were not used.

Apparatus and Procedure. Each subject participated in 15 sessions, with sessions generally run once a day, Monday through Friday. The 108 words were split into two sets of 54, and one set was used for training; the second set was used on the first and last days (baseline and transfer). The assignment of word sets to training versus baseline/transfer was counterbalanced across subjects.

As in Experiment 1, each session included 648 trials. In this case, the 648 derived from six passes through the two versions (*added* and *replaced*) of the 54 words in a set. Across 15 sessions, each subject received 9720 trials. The structure of a trial was as in Experiment 1, including feedback on the correct answer; the same audio equipment was used.

Subjects. Four new subjects were recruited to participate in Experiment 2. All were native English speakers with no known hearing problems. They were paid for their participation.

Results and Discussion

The data were analysed as in Experiment 1. The resulting d' scores for each subject were again grouped into seven training blocks. Six blocks were formed by collapsing together scores from Days 2–3, 4–5, 6–7, 8–9, 10–11, and 12–13; the seventh was based on Day 14. The baseline (Day 1) and transfer (Day 15) data were not included in the analysis of training effects. Figure 2 presents the results.

The seven d' scores for each subject were submitted to a one-way analysis of variance. As is clear in Figure 2, training did not produce any reliable

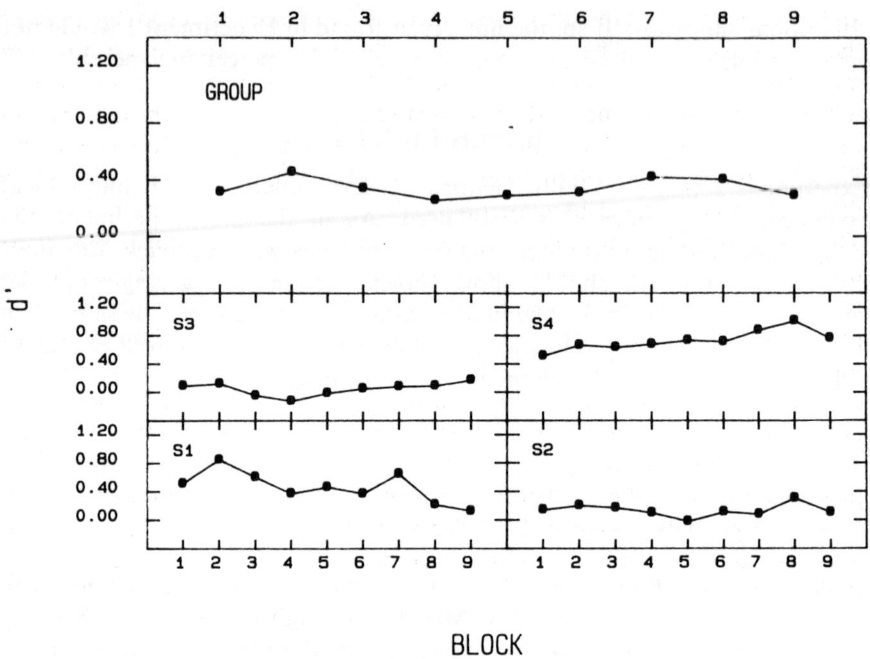

FIG. 2. Discrimination scores (d') for the four subjects in Experiment 2 individually (bottom four panels), and as a group (top panel). Block 1 was a baseline session, Blocks 2–8 were training sessions, and Block 9 was a transfer test.

increase in discrimination performance; the effect of training block did not approach significance [$F(6, 18) < 1$]. Thus even without the complications introduced by the inclusion of pseudoword trials, subjects were generally unable to direct attention well enough to judge whether a word was intact. As in Experiment 1, this failure to improve makes further consideration of the baseline and transfer sessions unnecessary.

The results of Experiments 1 and 2 are extremely clear-cut. In both experiments, subjects received extensive training with feedback on the discrimination task. In both experiments, subjects failed to improve despite this extensive practice. This failure to improve can be interpreted in at least three ways: (1) the training may have been insufficient in scale; (2) the restoration effect might not reflect a failure to attend appropriately for the task; and (3) the training might not be of a type that can affect control processes in speech perception.

It is not logically possible to reject the first alternative, but it seems very implausible. As noted previously, other work on attentional learning suggests that effects should be seen in the first 200 training trials per stimulus, and none were found in either experiment. Thus, it seems reasonable to reject the first possibility. The second case is theoretically more interesting and more difficult to reject on the basis of the data. If the basic illusion does not reflect attentional failures, then no amount of attentional training should reduce the strength of the effect. The strongest critique of this view is that Samuel and Ressler (1986) have already shown that the strength of the illusion can be affected by experimentally manipulating attentional factors. This leads us to the third interpretation, that long-term training is simply not usable by the attentional processes that may be responsible for aspects of the restoration illusion. Samuel and Ressler were able to attenuate the illusion by providing subjects with *trial-by-trial* attentional cues, rather than by providing long-term *general* training. Interestingly, in the visual domain Posner (1980) has also reported that long-term (block-by-block) attentional set did not produce reliable shifts in performance, whereas trial-by-trial cues did. Thus it may be a general property of control processes mediating perceptual processing that moment-to-moment information is much more useful than long-term perceptual learning. Experiment 3 examines such local cues and addresses the issue of how attention can be distributed to detailed aspects of the signal.

EXPERIMENT 3

As Samuel and Ressler (1986) noted, many illusions can be considered as cases in which the global percept interferes with accurate perception of more local information. For example, in the Mueller–Lyer illusion (<——> vs. >——<), observers cannot accurately judge the relative length of the horizontal lines; the global percept, based on the figure formed by the combination of horizontal lines with arrowheads, dominates. If observers can focus attention on the lower-level aspects of the stimulus, the illusion is diminished. For example, the horizontal lines can differ from the arrowheads in colour or brightness, or they can be spatially separated, and length judgement accuracy improves (Coren & Girgus, 1972; Dewar, 1967).

Samuel and Ressler argued that the phonemic restoration illusion could be similarly construed as a failure to attend to low-level aspects of the stimulus because of global dominance. In particular, they suggested that listeners primarily have access to lexical representations, and that it is difficult to gain access to components of such representations. To test this hypothesis, they provided listeners with pre-cues designed to enhance access to the lower-level codes needed to make the intactness judgement (*added* versus *replaced*). Each cue was presented visually shortly before a test stimulus.

There were four conditions: (1) Baseline performance was measured by providing an uninformative pre-cue (a set of dashes) before the *added* or *replaced* stimulus. (2) A phonemic/positional cue provided information about the critical phoneme in the test stimulus. For example, if the /v/ in "overdue" was replaced with noise, the subject would see "–v———" before the test stimulus. This would inform the subject that /v/ was the critical phoneme, and that the critical phoneme was near the beginning of the word (but was not word-initial). This information might allow listeners to focus attention on the critical phonemic information and thereby reduce the illusion's strength. (3) A lexical cue informed the subject of what word was coming but gave no local information (e.g. "overdue" would be shown on the screen). This cue should not help if the illusion results from a failure to access low-level information. (4) The final condition provided both lexical and phonemic/positional information. Thus, the subject would see "o*verdue" before hearing "overdue" with the /v/ replaced by noise.

The results supported an attentional interpretation of phonemic restoration. As expected by this view, the lexical cue did not improve performance relative to the baseline. Interestingly, neither did the phonemic/positional case. However, providing subjects with *both* types of information led to significantly improved discrimination. Either type alone was useless, but together they allowed subjects to control processing more effectively. Samuel and Ressler argued that this pattern of results may be best interpreted as reflecting a significant constraint on attentional control processes: Listeners appear to be unable to attend to a phoneme in the abstract (e.g. "–v———"). Instead, they appear to require a lexical address, and to focus attention on a particular phoneme within the lexical representation. Thus, on this account, the lexicon plays a critical role as the conduit of attention.

Samuel and Ressler's claim was a very strong one, stronger in fact than their data definitively support. Experiment 3 was designed to test the strongest part of their claim: Is a lexical code really necessary to direct attention when making a difficult discrimination? The test consists of considering the sufficiency of the most plausible alternative level of representation. On linguistic and psycholinguistic grounds, the syllable seems to be an excellent alternative. Syllables are pronounceable and easily encoded; they bear the same superset/subset relationship to phonemes as do lexical representations. In Experiment 3 the central question is thus, can a syllabic attentional cue serve as a conduit for attention in a way that is analogous to the role demonstrated for lexical codes?

Method

Stimuli. The 108 words used by Samuel and Ressler (1986) were used in Experiment 3. The words were all three or four syllables long and were balanced for location of primary stress. Critical phonemes varied factorially in phone class (fricative, nasal, or vowel) and position (first, second, or third syllable). *Added* or *replaced* versions of each word were constructed using the technique described previously. The 108 words were assigned to two balanced sets of 54 words.

Apparatus and Procedure. The same apparatus was used as in Experiments 1 and 2. Testing was done in groups of up to four subjects at a time. Each trial began with the presentation of an attentional cue on a computer terminal in front of each subject. The cue remained visible for 750 msec and was followed by a 250-msec preparation period in which the screen was blank. A test stimulus in *added* or *replaced* form was then presented, and the subjects responded by pushing one of two labelled buttons. Feedback was provided on the screen after all subjects had responded. Approximately one second after the feedback was terminated, the next trial was initiated.

Subjects were assigned to one of four conditions. The *baseline* condition was the same as Samuel and Ressler's: a set of dashes was displayed as the pre-cue. The number of dashes corresponded to the number of letters in the word, a cue that should not provide any attentional advantage. The second condition was a replication of the *lexical plus phonemic/position* case that proved successful in Samuel and Ressler's study. This condition provides an upper bound on what we might expect to find for syllabic cueing. Two syllabic cue conditions were included. The *syllabic* case provided subjects with the identity and location of the syllable containing the added/replaced phoneme. For example, with a replaced /v/ in "overdue", the precue would be "–/ver/——". Subjects were told that slashes denoted syllable boundaries, so this cue would inform them that the critical phoneme would occur in the syllable "ver", and that this syllable would be the second of a three-syllable word. This condition thus provides definitive, encodable syllabic information, and some positional information. The final condition, *syllabic plus phonemic/position*, provided additional positional information. In the "overdue" example, the cue would be "–/$\overset{*}{\text{v}}$er/—". Note that this provides subjects with the syllabic code and the critical phoneme. This condition is modelled directly on the lexical plus phonemic/position case, with the substitution of the syllabic code for the lexical one.

Subjects participated in one session lasting approximately 45 min. The session was divided into three blocks of 108 trials each. Each block included the *added* and *replaced* versions of one set of 54 words. The stimuli in the first block were, of course, new to the subjects: half the subjects started with one set of 54 words, and the other half started with the other. In the second block, half the subjects received the same set of 54 words (108 stimuli); these subjects received the other set of 54 in their final block. For the other subjects, the new set of 54 words was introduced in Block 2, followed by the original set in Block 3). This design ensured that stimuli were unknown in

Block 1 for all subjects, and unknown for half the subjects in Blocks 2 and 3. This was controlled because of concern that subjects might learn, for example, that "–/ver/—" would be followed by "overdue". This would allow implicit lexical effects to appear in what was intended to be a syllabic condition. To foreshadow, this problem did not arise.

Subjects. Sixty-four students enrolled in Introductory Psychology participated in Experiment 3. All were native English speakers, with no known hearing problems. All subjects had normal or corrected-to-normal vision. They received course credit for their participation. Sixteen subjects were assigned to each cue condition; within each condition, four subjects were assigned to each of the four stimulus set counterbalancing orders.

Results and Discussion

The responses of each subject were analysed as in the first two experiments to yield d' scores. These discrimination scores were submitted to a three-factor analysis of variance. Test block (1–3) was a within-subject factor; attentional cue condition (baseline, syllabic, syllabic plus phonemic/position, and lexical plus phonemic/position) and order (stimulus set order 1, 1, 2; 1, 2, 1; 2, 2, 1; or or 2, 1, 2) were between-subjects factors. Neither block nor order had a significant effect on discrimination [larger $F(2, 96) = 1.58$, n.s.]; neither did any interaction involving these factors [largest $F(9, 48) = 1.06$, n.s.].

The unimportance of these procedural factors allows us to focus on the theoretically important factor of attentional cue condition without the need to qualify its interpretation. This factor produced a reliable effect, $F(3, 48) = 3.69, p < 0.02$. Table 2 displays the d' scores for the four conditions. To assess which cues provided a significant advantage over baseline performance, the three cue conditions were each compared to the baseline d' of 0.47. Neither the syllabic cue alone nor the syllabic plus phonemic/position condition approached significance [for both, $F(1, 30) < 1$]. In contrast, discrimination with the lexical plus phonemic/position cue differed reliably from the baseline, $F(1, 30) = 6.68$, $p < 0.02$.

TABLE 2

Cue Condition			
Baseline	*Syllable*	*Syllable and Position*	*Lexical and Position*
0.47	0.43	0.53	0.69

Note: The values shown are in absolute units (d' scores).

The results thus replicate Samuel and Ressler's finding that the phonemic restoration illusion can be attenuated by providing both lexical and phonemic/positional information. The efficacy of this type of attentional cue stands in contrast to the failure of both syllabic cue types. Even when the subjects knew what syllable to expect and which phoneme would be critical within it, they could not improve their discrimination performance. This failure is particularly striking in light of the easy encodability of syllables: Subjects should have no more trouble forming an auditory representation or image of "ver" than of "overdue", yet such representations were apparently not useful on the task.

Why should syllabic codes prove useless, while lexical ones enhance performance? If the restoration effect does stem in part from an attentional failure, then the difference in efficacy could be attributed to differences in the utility of attentional allocation. Samuel and Ressler suggested that lexical representations play a fundamental role in speech processing, and that attentional control is mediated via the lexicon. The results of Experiment 3 are in accord with this view. On this account, simply having an encodable cue is not sufficient. Rather, because the lexicon is central to speech perception, control processes have developed that use lexical representations to allocate processing resources. From this perspective, the syllabic cues with positional information did not help because the system did not have an effective means to focus attention on the phonemic representations. With a lexical route, such a focus appears to be more attainable.

GENERAL DISCUSSION

The results of Experiments 1–3 help to specify listeners' limits of control over their speech processing. In the first two experiments, subjects were given very extensive training on the discrimination task. Despite such extended practice, performance remained very poor; the phonemic restoration illusion is very powerful and apparently not amenable to a *general* shift in attentional control. That is, people are fundamentally suited to deriving lexical representations, and even 10,000 trials cannot shift this predilection.

However, Experiment 3's results, along with those of Samuel and Ressler (1986), indicate that *some* attentional control is possible; under some conditions, listeners can in fact pay more attention to phonemic representations and less to lexical ones. For the difficult discrimination task used in these studies, both lexical and phonemic/position information must be provided for such an attentional shift. The strongest alternative candidate—a syllabic code—proved to be inadequate for supporting the refocusing of attention. These results bolster Samuel and Ressler's contention that lexical representations are normally the focus of attention, and that a finer focus can be achieved by narrowing attention to a particular subset of the phonological code in the lexical representation. On this account, in order for attention to enhance performance, the listener must know *where* in the word the critical phoneme will occur; with words that vary in length and stress pattern, "where" can only be well-defined by also knowing *what* the word will be.

This analysis converges well with two related research efforts. Nusbaum, Walley, Carrell, and Ressler (1982) used the restoration discrimination task with a small stimulus set (10 three-syllable words) in which the critical phoneme always occurred word-finally. They found that with relatively modest training (scores of trials, rather than thousands), subjects improved on the task. This result indicates that listeners are capable of learning to focus attention on a particular location, if that location is consistently maintained through training (cf, Schneider & Shiffrin, 1977; Shiffrin & Schneider, 1977). Because all words were of a consistent structure and critical phonemes were always word-final, listeners could focus attention on the critical phoneme and reduce lexically-mediated restoration.

Watson and his colleagues (Watson, Wroton, Kelly, & Bebasset, 1975; Watson, Kelly, & Wroton, 1976; Espinoza-Varas & Watson, 1986) have conducted a series of studies that share some important features with the present study. Subjects in these studies were required to make a difficult auditory discrimination, under varying levels of stimulus uncertainty, and with varying amounts of practice (over ten thousand training trials). The stimuli in these experiments were ten-note sequences approximately 500 msec long, a duration roughly comparable to the words used in the present study. Subjects made a same–different judgement on pairs of sequences that could differ in frequency of one tone (Watson et al., 1975, 1976) or in duration of a tone (Espinoza-Varas & Watson, 1986). The critical role of stimulus uncertainty is highlighted by Watson et al.'s (1976, p. 1182) summary of a large set of experiments in which discrimination performance under highly uncertain conditions is two orders of magnitude worse than discrimination when the target note's location and identity are known. Tens of thousands of training trials, coupled with a stimulus set size restriction to a handful of tone locations/identities, improves performance by one order of magnitude. The results of Watson's research program make it clear that perceptual processing of complex auditory stimuli is highly dependent on having access to a pre-stored representation of the complex pattern, and to having knowledge of the probable location of the critical portion of the pattern. Clearly, this conclusion is entirely consistent with the results of Experiment 3. The relevance of Watson's research with musical stimuli is supported by DeWitt and Samuel's (1990) recent report that perceptual restoration of musical notes occurs (see also Sasaki, 1980) and appears to follow many of the same principles as phonemic restoration.

For both speech and music, there is now evidence to suggest that some higher-level sources of information are used by the perceptual process, whereas others are not. In the speech domain, it appears that lexical-level knowledge does become incorporated perceptually, but that sentential-level information does not (Connine & Clifton, 1987; Fodor, 1983; Samuel, 1981a, 1986; Tanenhaus & Lucas, 1987). In music, a similar architecture is suggested by the significant perceptual restoration effects found for similarly "precompiled" representations (scales and chords), coupled with an absence of such effects for less entrenched structures, such as melodies (DeWitt & Samuel, 1990). In both stimulus domains, the architecture is best captured by a partially interactive model (Samuel, 1981a, 1986, 1990). This model class includes the top-down information flow characteristic of fully interactive models (e.g. McClelland & Elman, 1986; Marslen-Wilson & Welsh, 1978). However, the top-down flow is restricted; no supra-lexical information is postulated to be used by the perceptual process. In this respect, the partially interactive model shares features with more bottom-up or autonomous models (e.g. Cutler & Norris, 1979; Cutler, Mehler, Norris, & Segui, 1987; Massaro, 1989). As noted in the Introduction, recent attempts to support autonomous models have relied on the relatively straightforward way that these models can invoke differential access to lexical or sublexical representations (e.g. Cutler et al., 1987). The results of Experiment 3 indicate that in order to model human performance accurately, some sort of attentional control mechanisms must be included. Given that the restoration literature has been most consistent with a partially interactive model, it seems appropriate to suggest that such a control mechanism should be incorporated into the model, as Samuel and Ressler (1986) argued. This control mechanism could take the form adopted in autonomous theories, in which an executive process is hypothesized to link output processes to one level of representation rather than another (e.g. lexical rather than phonemic) as a function of task parameters. Alternatively, the attentional control could be thought of in terms that are more consistent with interactive models by postulating a modulation of the overall gain or activation associated with one level versus another. In this conception, "attending" to a phonemic code would involve the assignment of a higher weighting to the output of phonemic representations. The data in hand do not currently provide any strong basis for choosing between the two conceptions; either could be accommodated in a partially interactive model.

The most promising route for providing a basis to flesh out the details of attention's role and mechanisms will probably come from developing converging methodologies. Currently, there are at least two methodologies (apart from the restoration discrimination paradigm) that are being widely used to examine information flow and control during speech perception. Ganong's (1980) identification paradigm has emerged as a fertile testing ground for contrasting autonomous, partially interactive, and fully interactive model classes. Fox (1984) and Connine (1987; Connine and Clifton 1987) have developed reaction-time variations of the task; Connine's analyses converge very well with the restoration results in supporting a partially interactive architecture. Burton, Baum, and Blumstein (1989) have examined the role that stimulus quality plays in the appearance of lexical effects in Ganong's paradigm and have suggested that lexical influences only appear under difficult listening conditions. They argued that this pattern is most consistent with autonomous models. However, both fully and partially interactive models can easily accommodate this finding by assuming that top-down effects will only be evident when the bottom-up path is poor; when the signal is very clear, bottom-up analyses can complete before top-down influences can affect responses. Note that the sort of control processes examined in the present study are well suited to the task of affecting which path will dominate in a given testing situation. A final recent use of Ganong's paradigm is Elman and McClelland's (1988) examination of perceptual compensation for coarticulation effects. This study demonstrated that lexical context can alter the perception of an ambiguous phoneme, and that the lexically-driven percept is "real" enough to in turn drive low-level adjustments for coarticulation effects. This result is another demonstration that lexical information can constrain lower-level (phonemic) perception, as predicted by both fully and partially interactive models.

In addition to Ganong's paradigm, the phoneme-monitoring technique continues to be widely used. This paradigm has provided much of the evidence for autonomous theories (e.g. Cutler et al., 1987; Frauenfelder, Segui, & Dijkstra, 1990). The method has also been adopted to explore attentional allocation. For example, target detection times are faster for phonemes in syllables that are expected to be stressed (Shields, McHugh, & Martin, 1974), even when local acoustic cues for stress have been eliminated (Cutler, 1976; Pitt & Samuel, 1990a). With the elimination of an acoustic basis to the advantage, the most parsimonious account of the effect is that listeners differentially allocate processing resources to aspects of the signal that are expected to provide the most stable analysis; stressed syllables also tend to coincide with high-information content words. Most recently, Pitt and Samuel (1990b) have incorporated cost–benefit analyses (Posner, 1980) into the phoneme-monitoring technique in order to develop an "attentional profile" during speech perception. In this version of the task, probability manipulations are used to induce subjects to expect targets at certain points in an utterance. Detection times for targets occurring at either an expected location or at an unexpected location were compared to detection times in a control condition in which no localized expectations were induced. The data revealed substantial benefits in reaction time to targets in expected locations and substantial costs for targets in unexpected locations. Moreover, the technique provides a phoneme-by-phoneme profile of attentional allocation, a profile that indicated very fine tuning of expectations, particularly for word-initial and word-final phonemes. This procedure seems very promising as a converging operation with the techniques used in the present study. Along with the other methodologies noted above, these procedures show promise of helping to delineate both the flow of information during speech perception, and the processes that control this flow.

REFERENCES

Burton, M.W., Baum, S.R., & Blumstein, S.E. (1989). Lexical effects on the phonetic categorization of speech: The role of acoustic structure. *Journal of Experimental Psychology: Human Perception and Performance, 15*, 567–575.

Connine, C.M. (1987). Constraints on interactive processes in auditory word recognition: The role of sentence context. *Journal of Memory and Language, 26*, 527–538.

Connine, C.M. & Clifton, C., Jr. (1987). Interactive use of lexical information in speech perception. *Journal of Experimental Psychology: Human Perception and Performance, 13*, 291–299.

Coren, S. & Girgus, J.S. (1972). Differentiation and decrement in the Mueller-Lyer illusion. *Perception and Psychophysics, 12*, 466–470.

Cutler, A. (1976). Phoneme-monitoring reaction time as a function of preceding intonation contour. *Perception & Psychophysics, 20*, 55–60.

Cutler, A., Mehler, J., Norris, D., & Segui, J. (1987). Phoneme identification and the lexicon. *Cognitive Psychology, 19*, 141–177.

Cutler, A. & Norris, D. (1979). Monitoring sentence comprehension. In W.E. Cooper & E.C.T. Walker (Eds.), *Sentence processing: Psycholinguistic studies presented to Merrill Garrett* (pp. 113–134). Hillsdale, NJ: Lawrence Erlbaum Associates, Inc.

Dewar, R.E. (1967). Stimulus determinants of the magnitude of the Mueller-Lyer illusion. *Perceptual and Motor Skills, 24*, 708–710.

DeWitt, L. & Samuel, A.G. (1990). The role of knowledge-based expectations in music perception: Evidence from musical restoration. *Journal of Experimental Psychology: General, 119*, 337–374.

Elman, J.L. & McClelland, J.L. (1984). Speech as a cognitive process: The interactive activation model. In N. Lass (Ed.), *Speech and Language* (Vol. 10). New York: Academic Press.

Elman, J.L. & McClelland, J.L. (1988). Cognitive penetration of the mechanisms of perception: Compensation for coarticulation of lexically restored phonemes. *Journal of Memory and Language, 27*, 143–165.

Espinoza-Varas, B. & Watson, C.S. (1986). Temporal discrimination for single components of nonspeech auditory patterns. *Journal of the Acoustical Society of America, 80*, 1685–1694.

Fodor, J.A. (1983). *The Modularity of Mind.* Cambridge, MA: MIT Press.

Fox, R.A. (1984). Effect of lexical status on phonetic categorization. *Journal of Experimental Psycholoy: Human Perception and Performance, 10*, 526–540.

Frauenfelder, U.H., Segui, J., & Dijkstra, T. (1990). Lexical effects in phonemic processing: Facilitatory or inhibitory? *Journal of Experimental Psychology: Human Perception and Performance, 16*, 77–91.

Fujimura, O. (1976). Syllables as concatenated demisyllables and affixes. *Journal of the Acoustical Society of America*, S55.

Ganong, W.F. (1980). Phonetic categorization in auditory word perception. *Journal of Experimental Psychology: Human Perception and Performance, 6*, 110–125.

Judd, C.H. (1902). Practice and its effects on the perception of illusions. *Psychological Review, 8*, 27–39.

Lewis, E.O. (1908). The effect of practice on the perception of the Mueller-Lyer illusion. *British Journal of Psychology*, *2*, 294–306.

Marslen-Wilson, W.D. & Welsh, A. (1978). Processing interactions and lexical access during word recognition in continuous speech. *Cognitive Psychology*, *10*, 29–63.

Massaro, D.W. (1975). Preperceptual images, processing time, and perceptual units in speech perception. In D.W. Massaro (Ed.), *Understanding language: An information-processing analysis of speech perception, reading, and psycholinguistics*. New York: Academic Press.

Massaro, D.W. (1989). Testing between the TRACE model and the fuzzy logical model of speech perception. *Cognitive Psychology*, *21*, 398–421.

McClelland, J.L. & Elman, J.L. (1986). The TRACE model of speech perception. *Cognitive Psychology*, *18*, 1–86.

Norris, D. & Cutler, A. (1988). The relative accessibility of phonemes and syllables. *Perception & Psychophysics*, *43*, 541–550.

Nusbaum, H.C. & Schwab, E.C. (1986). The role of attention and active processing in speech perception. In E.C. Schwab & H.C. Nusbaum (Eds.), *Pattern recognition by humans and machines: Speech perception* (Vol. 1, pp. 113–157). New York: Academic Press.

Nusbaum, H.C., Walley, A.C., Carrell, T.D., & Ressler, W.H. (1982). *Controlled perceptual strategies in phonemic restoration* (Research on Speech Perception Progress Report 8, pp. 83–103). Bloomington, IN: Department of Psychology, Indiana University.

Pitt, M.A. & Samuel, A.G. (1990a). The use of rhythm in attending to speech. *Journal of Experimental Psychology: Human Perception and Performance*, *16*, 564–573.

Pitt, M.A. & Samuel, A.G. (1990b). Attentional allocation during speech perception: How fine is the focus? *Journal of Memory and Language*, *29*, 611–632.

Posner, M.I. (1980). Orienting of attention. *Quarterly Journal of Experimental Psychology*, *32*, 3–25.

Samuel, A.G. (1981a). Phonemic restoration: Insights from a new methodology. *Journal of Experimental Psychology: General*, *110*, 474–494.

Samuel, A.G. (1981b). The role of bottom-up confirmation in the phonemic restoration illusion. *Journal of Experimental Psychology: Human Perception and Performance*, *7*, 1124–1131.

Samuel, A.G. (1986). The role of the lexicon in speech perception. In E.C. Schwab & H.C. Nusbaum (Eds.), *Pattern recognition by humans and machines: Speech perception* (Vol. 1, pp. 89–112). New York: Academic Press.

Samuel, A.G. (1987). The effect of lexical uniqueness on phonemic restoration. *Journal of Memory and Language*, *26*, 36–56.

Samuel, A.G. (1990). Using perceptual restoration effects to explore the architecture of perception. In G. Altman (Ed.), *Cognitive Models of Speech Processing: Psycholinguistic and Computational Perspectives* (pp. 295–314). Cambridge, MA: MIT Press/Bradford Books.

Samuel, A.G. & Ressler, W.H. (1986). Attention within auditory word perception: Insights from the phonemic restoration illusion. *Journal of Experimental Psychology: Human Perception and Performance*, *12*, 70–79.

Sasaki, T. (1980). Sound restoration and temporal localization of noise in speech and music sounds. *Tohoku Psychologica Folia*, *39*, 79–88.

Sawusch, J. (1977). Peripheral and central processes in selective adaptation of place of articulation in stop consonants. *Journal of the Acoustical Society of America*, *62*, 738–750.

Schneider, W. & Shiffrin, R.M. (1977). Controlled and automatic human information processing: I. Detection, search, and attention. *Psychological Review*, *84*, 1–66.

Shields, J.L., McHugh, A., & Martin, J.G. (1974). Reaction time to phoneme targets as a function of rhythmic cues in continuous speech. *Journal of Experimental Psychology*, *102*, 250–255.

Shiffrin, R.M. & Schneider, W. (1977). Controlled and automatic human information processing: II. Perceptual learning, automatic attending, and a general theory. *Psychological Review*, *84*, 127–190.

Tanenhaus, M.K. & Lucas, M.M. (1987). Context effects in lexical processing. *Cognition*, *25*, 213–234.

Warren, R.M. (1970). Perceptual restoration of missing speech sounds. *Science*, *167*, 392–393.

Watson, C.S., Wroton, H.W., Kelly, W.J., & Benbasset, C.A. (1975). Factors in the discrimination of tonal patterns. I. Component frequency, temporal position, and silent intervals. *Journal of the Acoustical Society of America*, *57*, 1175–1185.

Watson, C.S., Kelly, W.J., & Wroton, H.W. (1976). Factors in the discrimination of tonal patterns. II. Selective attention and learning under various levels of stimulus uncertainty. *Journal of the Acoustical Society of America*, *60*, 1176–1186.

Revised manuscript received 7 October 1990

THE QUARTERLY JOURNAL OF EXPERIMENTAL PSYCHOLOGY, 1991, *43A* (3) 701–731

The Interlingual Identification of Spanish and English Vowels: Orthographic Evidence

James Emil Flege
University of Alabama at Birmingham, Alabama, U.S.A.

When someone who is learning a second language (L2) produces a sound in the L2 using a familiar, native-language (L1) category, the L2 sound is said to have been "identified with" an L1 sound. Although interlingual identification exerts a powerful influence on L2 pronunciation, it is still poorly understood. Orthographic classification was used here to assess the interlingual identification of Spanish and English vowels. Sixty native speakers of Spanish in three experiments judged the vowels /i/, /ɪ/, /ɛ/, and /æ/ in multiple tokens of English words ("beat", "bit", "bet", "bat") spoken by ten native speakers of American English. The subjects labelled each English vowel by circling one of the five letters used to spell the vowel phonemes of Spanish (viz. <i>, <e>, <a>, <o>, <u>) or by circling "none" if they thought they had heard a vowel not found in Spanish. Subjects who spoke English as an L2 used the "none" label more often than did Spanish monolinguals, suggesting that L2 learning heightens bilinguals' awareness of cross-language phonetic differences. Experienced Spanish speakers of English did use the "none" label more often than did inexperienced subjects (42% vs. 18%). A few subjects used the "none" label consistently for /æ/ and /ɪ/, suggesting that they may have regarded these vowels as "new" (i.e., non-Spanish). However, the group data provided little support for the hypothesis that the adult Spanish learners of English treated either /æ/ or /ɪ/ as new. The great majority of subjects, even those highly experienced in English, identified English /æ/ with their Spanish /a/.

It is widely believed that adults will inevitably speak a language learned after childhood with a foreign accent (Lenneberg 1967). Scovel (1969, 1988) claimed that foreign accents occur because of lost "plasticity" in "neuropsy-

Requests for reprints should be sent to James Emil Flege, Department of Biocommunication, University of Alabama at Birmingham, Box 503 University Station, Birmingham, Alabama 35294–0019 USA.

This study was supported by NIH grant DC00257. The author thanks O.-S. Bohn, L. Cueva, C. Mena, and L. Skelton for their contributions to the study. Thanks are also extended to S. Fletcher and M. Munro for comments on an earlier version of this article.

chological mechanisms" deriving from the completion of cerebral lateralization at around the age of 12 (see also Patkowski, 1990; but cf. Flege, 1987a, Flege & Fletcher, submitted). Precisely *which* aspect(s) of speech learning changes with age has not been identified by advocates of the critical period hypothesis, but it is often implied that processes that underlie sensorimotor learning may become less effective as the result of neural maturation (Sapon 1952; Scovel, 1988, p. 62). Some L2 production errors do, in fact, seem to have a motoric basis (Flege, 1988c; Flege, McCutcheon, & Smith, 1987),[1] but many others may arise from the inaccurate *perception* of L2 sounds.[2] The results of certain speech perception experiments suggest that adult learners of an L2 do not have representations for some sounds in an L2, at least not at first (e.g. Miyawaki et al., 1975. Mochizuki, 1981; Sheldon & Strange 1982). For other L2 sounds, adult learners have been observed to perform consistently, albeit not precisely like native speakers of English. In these instances, the adult learners appear to make use of native language (L1) representations that differ from those of native speakers (e.g. Flege & Hillenbrand, 1985, 1987; Flege & Eefting, 1986; Flege, 1989b; Flege & Wang, 1990).

It is generally agreed that speech perception is an obligatory process. L2 learners attempt to make perceptual sense of the sounds making up L2 words, regardless of whether or not they have an accurate (i.e. native-like) perceptual representation for the L2 sounds. Unless they have managed to establish phonetic categories for L2 sounds (see Flege, 1990; in press, a, b), adult learners will tend to identify unfamiliar L2 sounds in terms of an L1 category (Weinreich, 1953; Wode, 1977, 1978; see also Butcher, 1976). This process, called "interlingual identification", often amounts to fitting square pegs into round holes. Adult learners' perceptual "errors" may not be evident, however, because they often comprehend the L2 in the absence of accurate phonetic perception by exploiting semantic context and their knowledge of the world.

The occurrence of perceptual errors or mismatches in the processing of L2 words may be inferred, however, from how adult learners *pronounce* the L2. When an unfamiliar L2 sound has been identified with an acoustically

---

[1] Flege (1988c) and Flege et al. (1987) examined the production of the word-final English /p/–/b/ contrast by native speakers of Chinese. A significant difference in peak oral air pressure between English /p/ and /b/ suggested that the Chinese subjects produced these sounds with different laryngeal articulations. However, they failed to sustain closure voicing in /b/ for as long as native speakers, apparently because they had not learned to enlarge the supraglottal cavity actively during labial closure for /b/.

---

[2] The term "sound", as used here, refers to a class of phones that can be used to contrast meaning. It is a terminological convenience that obviates the need to draw a distinction constantly between the phonetic and phonemic levels. For an exposition of this theoretically important distinction, see Flege (in press, a).

different sound in the L1, the L1 sound may be used in place of the L2 sound (Valdman, 1976). Table 1 summarizes six studies that have reported on vowel substitution errors in Spanish-accented English. The target vowels in this table are those examined in the present study (viz. /i/, /ɪ/, /ɛ/, and /æ/). The six studies differed in many ways, including the L2 experience of the Spanish subjects examined, speech materials, and elicitation techniques. It is unclear in many instances whether the "substitutes" reported were English vowels, Spanish vowels, or a phonetic approximation of the intended English target vowel. Several conclusions can nevertheless be drawn from Table 1: (1) Spanish speakers usually produce English /i/ as an [i]-quality vowel; (2) if they mispronounce /ɪ/, it is usually as an [i]-quality vowel; and (3) if they mispronounce /ɛ/, it is as an [e]-quality vowel.

One might also conclude from the data in Table 1 that Spanish learners of English are more variable in their mispronunciation of /æ/ than that of other front, monophthongal English vowels. In producing /æ/, they manifest both mid-vowel ([e], [eᶦ], [ɛ]) and back-vowel ([a]) substitutes. The use of multiple L1 substitutes for an unfamiliar L2 sound, especially in early stages of learning (Hammarberg, in press), may mean that an unfamiliar L2 sound has been judged to be perceptually equidistant from two or more L1 sounds. It might also be taken to mean that a particular L2 vowel does not have a readily identifiable counterpart in the L1.

None of the five Spanish vowels (/i, e, a, o, u/) seems to match any of the 15 vowels of English. Flege (1989a) found that the tongue is lower for English /i/ and /u/ than for the corresponding vowels of Spanish, and the tongue is lower for English /ɑ/ than for Spanish /a/ (suggesting a narrower pharyngeal cavity for the English vowel). English /oᵁ/ and especially /eᶦ/ are more diphthongized than Spanish /e/ and /o/ (Stockwell & Bowen, 1965;

TABLE 1
Vowel Substitution Errors in Spanish-Accented English

Target English Vowel	*Most Frequent Substitute Reported*	*Other Reported Substitutes*
/i/	[i][2]	
/ɪ/	[i][1,2,3,4,5,6]	[e][2]
/ɛ/	[e][2,4,5,6]	
/æ/	[a][1,3,4,5] [ɛ][6]	[ɛ][4] [e][2] [eᶦ][6]

[1] Brennan & Brennan (1981);
[2] Hammond (1986);
[3] Flege (1990)
[4] Amastae (1978);
[5] Ornstein (1974);
[6] MacDonald (1989).

Dalbor, 1980; Quiles, 1981; Flege, 1989a). Also, English vowels are generally longer than Spanish vowels because they are lengthened more under stress and in pre-pausal position (Delattre, 1966).

Wode (1977, 1978) suggested that there is a threshold beyond which an L2 sound will be recognized as distinct from any sound in the L1. A distinction between "new" L2 sounds and those that are merely "similar" to sounds in the L1 has been drawn by researchers for several decades (Delattre, 1964, 1969; Brière, 1968), but no satisfactory metric now exists for determining whether an L2 vowel will be treated as new or similar (see below).[3] Unlike consonantal sounds, vowel sounds are discriminated readily even if they are not classified differently.[4] One obstacle to classifying L2 vowels as new vs. similar has been uncertainty as to whether the distance between vowels in two languages is judged in terms of an auditory,[5] phonetic, or phonemic metric (see below). The question raised in this study was whether Spanish speakers would come to recognize that any of the front, monophthongal vowels of American English are new (i.e. non-Spanish).

Orthographic Classification

The present study examined patterns of interlingual identification that might be responsible for vowel production errors like those in Table 1. Native Spanish subjects were asked to label English vowels with one of the letters used to write the five vowel phonemes of Spanish (<i>, <e>, <o>, <a>, <u>). The vowels they were asked to label (viz. /i/, /ɪ/, /ɛ/, /æ/) occurred in CVC words spoken by native speakers of American English.

---

[3] Flege (in press, a) discussed methods that might be used to operationalize the distinction between new and similar L2 sounds. A similar L2 sound may be defined as a sound that is represented by the same IPA symbol as a sound in the L1, provided it can be shown to differ auditorily from the corresponding L1 sound. New sounds, on the other hand, may be defined as L2 sounds that are represented by an IPA symbol not used for any sound in the L1 (and, of course, which differ auditorily from the nearest L1 sound). Problems with this approach do exist, however, especially with the "symbol" test (see, e.g., Footnote 4).

[4] Phoneticians have long debated whether transcriptions of vowels should be detailed enough to represent any *auditorily detectable* difference between vowels or just differences that underlie word contrasts in a particular language. It is uncertain how many different distinct vowel "types" there are. Ladefoged (1989) estimated that an expert phonetician might be capable of identifying as many as 200 vowels in absolute terms.

[5] The use of an auditory-based metric to evaluate the relationship between vowels in two languages cannot be discounted. Spanish and English listeners in the Flege et al. (in preparation) study gave much the same responses to pairs of vowels that were labelled differentially. For example, both groups rated Spanish /i/–/a/ pairs to be more dissimilar than /i/–/e/ pairs; and both groups rated the /i/–/e/ pairs as more dissimilar than /e/–/a/ pairs. Such agreement between groups implies the existence of a universal auditory-based distance metric. Interlingual comparisons based on auditory representations would be expected to differ at times from those based on representations of phonetic quality (see, e.g., Klatt, 1987, Figure 34).

Orthographic classification was a plausible technique for investigating interlingual identification because Spanish vowels (unlike those in English) stand in a one-to-one relationship with letters. It has been used successfully by Wiik (1965, cited by Flege, 1988b) to examine the classification of English vowels by native speakers of another language with "phonemic" spelling (i.e. Finnish).

Subjects in the present study were also permitted to use the label "none". This label provided a means for determining whether any of the English vowels were judged to fall outside the bounds of the Spanish vowel system. Results obtained by Butcher (1976) suggested that adult subjects can use "none" appropriately. In that study, French and English subjects were asked to label a set of cardinal vowels that differed to varying degrees from L1 vowels. The English but not the French subjects used "none" frequently to label front rounded (/y/, /o/, /œ/) and nasalized vowels (/ɛ̃/, /ɑ̃/, /ɔ̃/). These vowels differed substantially from any English vowel but were similar to vowels in French.

Level of Analysis

Perception research suggests that speech sounds are processed at three successive levels: auditory, phonetic, and phonemic (see Elman, Diehl, & Buchwald, 1977; Repp, 1981; Pisoni, Aslin, Perey, & Hennessey, 1982; Werker & Logan, 1985; Werker, Klein, & Logan, 1986; Mann, 1986). It is uncertain at which level(s) interlingual identification occurs. Bilinguals judge interlingual distances by comparing incoming L2 phones to perceptual prototypes in long-term memory (Best, McRoberts, & Sithole, 1988; Flege, 1984, 1988a, 1988b).[6] The orthographic classification technique employed in the present study probably favoured the use of phonemic representations (Mann, 1986), but it was also possible that the subjects would be influenced by representations at other processing levels.

Catford (1968) stated that the basis for interlingual identification is "substantial rather than formal" (p. 164). This implies that the L1 prototype against which L2 phones are gauged may be phonetic in nature (Brière, 1966), not phonemic, as usually supposed (e.g. Trubetzkoy 1939; Scholes, 1968a, 1968b; Best et al., 1988). The distinction between phonetic and phonemic levels can be illustrated with reference to Spanish /e/, a vowel phoneme with two allophones.[7] Spanish /e/ is realized as an [ɛ]-quality vowel

---

[6] Bilinguals might assess the distance between L1 and L2 sounds by implicitly comparing the *gestures* needed to produce them (see Scholes, 1968b), but there is as yet no evidence for this.

[7] The allophones of Spanish /e/ are in complementary distribution—that is, they occur in mutually exclusive phonetic contexts. Because of this, [e] and [ɛ] cannot be used to contrast meaning in Spanish.

in most closed syllables. These variants are said to "match" the vowel in English "bet" (Dalbor, 1980), a claim supported by a recent L2 vowel intelligibility study (Flege, 1990).[8] As suggested by the symbol used to represent it, Spanish /e/ may be implemented as [e] in other contexts (most open syllables except those preceding /r/, and in closed syllables ending in /s/ or /z/). American English /eᶦ/, on the other hand, is implemented with a single allophone (viz. [eᶦ]).[9]

Spanish /e/ shows some formant movement, but not nearly as much as the diphthongal English /eᶦ/ (Flege, Munro, & Fox, in preparation). In a study using glossometry, Flege (1989a) found that the average tongue position used for the [e] allophone of Spanish /e/ was intermediate between the tongue positions observed in the "onglide" and "offglide" of English /eᶦ/. It is uncertain whether bilinguals will identify a diphthongal L2 vowel with a monophthongal L1 vowel. It is also uncertain how they will deal with differing *distributions* of allophones for phonemes in their two languages. If interlingual identification occurs at a *phonemic* level, then Spanish speakers of English should consistently identify the realizations of English /ɛ/ in terms of the Spanish /e/ phoneme. The error data in Table 1 indirectly supports this view.

There is reason to suppose, however, that interlingual identification does not occur *exclusively* at an abstract, phonemic level. If Spanish speakers compare English vowels to the Spanish /e/ phoneme, then their judgements should be influenced by the properties of both the [e] and [ɛ] allophones of that phoneme. A recent study by Flege et al. (in preparation) suggests that this does not happen, at least not in certain tasks. Spanish and English subjects used a 9-point scale to rate pairs of CV syllables for degree of dissimilarity. Some pairs contained realizations of English /æ/ and /ɛ/. Had the Spanish subjects based their judgements on a phonemic representation, they should have judged the [æ]–[ɛ] pairs to be more dissimilar than the English subjects because, for them, [ɛ] phones would be associated via phonemic representations with [e] phones. However, the Spanish subjects judged the [æ]–[ɛ] pairs to be *less* dissimilar than did the native English subjects (3.1 vs. 4.2, $p=0.003$).[10]

---

[8] In that study, Spanish speakers produced English "beat", "bit", "bet", and "bat". Their [ɛ] attempts were identified correctly by native English listeners in most instances, but not their attempts at English /i/, /ɪ/, and /æ/. It remains to be seen whether Spanish learners of English will be successful in producing /ɛ/ in phonetic contexts in which the [e] allophone of Spanish /e/ would be expected, for example in words like "Bess", "mess", "says".

[9] The quality of this vowel varies, of course—for example, the offglide of /eᶦ/ may not be reached at a fast speaking rate.

[10] This same kind of reasoning can be applied to CV pairs containing realizations of English /ɛ/ and Spanish /e/. If subjects used phonemic-level representations exclusively for such pairs, one would expect *less* perceived dissimilarity for Spanish than English subjects because the [ɛ]

Changes in Interlingual Identification

In addition to unresolved questions pertaining to the processing level(s) at which interlingual identification occurs, it is uncertain whether patterns of interlingual identification will change as L2 learners grow familiar with the L2 sound system. A change in interlingual identification may be more likely for certain L2 sounds than others.

Some L2 sounds are virtually identical to those in the L1 (Bohn & Flege, submitted), but most differ from any L1 sound, if only in the details of timing, amplitude, or placement of articulatory constrictions. It was once believed that cross-language differences were the primary source of speech learning difficulty (e.g. Stockwell & Bowen, 1965; Brière, 1968). This leads one to expect that L2 sounds that match an L1 sound closely will be produced authentically whereas those that do not match an L1 sound closely will be produced poorly. It may be, however, that a "U"-shaped rather than a linear function best describes the effect of varying differences between L1 and L2 sounds. That is L2 sounds that match an L1 sound closely, or else differ *considerably* from any sound in the L1 may be produced authentically, whereas L2 sounds that *partially* resemble an L1 sound may be pronounced poorly.

I have hypothesized that "new" L2 sounds will stop being identified with L1 sounds at some point in L2 learning, whereas "similar" L2 sounds will continue being identified with an L1 sound (Flege, 1988b; 1990; in press, a, b; see also Oller & Ziahosseiny, 1970; Wode, 1977, 1978). As a result, adult learners may be able to establish phonetic categories for new L2 sounds and eventually produce them authentically. Similar L2 sounds may prove to be the most difficult kind of sound for adult learners because, by hypothesis, they continue to be identified with L1 sounds (which blocks the phonetic category formation needed for authentic production). In support of this, several studies have shown that vowels not found in the L1 inventory are produced more authentically than are L2 vowels that differ acoustically from a counterpart in the L1 (Mueller & Niedzielski 1963; Flege, 1987b; Major,

---

allophone of Spanish /e/ is said to match English /ɛ/ realizations. Instead, the Spanish listeners rated [ɛ]–[e] pairs as more dissimilar than English listeners (4.8 vs. 3.9, $p=0.011$). One other recent study points to the operation of phonetic-level processes. In a study by Flege (submitted), Spanish and English subjects estimated degree of rhyme in English words. Both groups rated pairs of English words with /eⁱ/ and /ɛ/ (e.g. "mate"–"met") to rhyme equally, but they gave different ratings for other word pairs. It was assumed that the Spanish subjects would identify English /eⁱ/ with their Spanish /e/, and that vowels classified as being the same "will rhyme more than those classified as different". Had the rhyming judgements been made at a phonemic level, therefore, the Spanish subjects should have perceived a greater degree of rhyme than did the English subjects.

1987; Bohn & Flege, 1990; but cf. Flege, 1990). There is also some preliminary evidence that L2 consonants that are unlike any in the L1 may be produced more authentically than L2 consonants that differ acoustically from an L1 counterpart.[11]

Figure 1 shows the distribution of formant values for six English vowels (/i,ɪ,ɛ,æ,ɑ,u/) spoken by 30 male native speakers of American English (Peterson & Barney, 1952) and the five Spanish vowels spoken by 16 native Spanish males (Godinez, 1978). In agreement with articulatory data (Flege, 1989a), English /i/ and /u/ are lower in the F_1–F_2 space than Spanish /i/ and /u/, and English /ɑ/ is posterior to Spanish /a/. The data in Figure 1 largely agree with a study of Argentine Spanish (Guirao & de Manrique, 1972, 1975), which showed that the distribution for Spanish /i/ fell within the ellipse for American English /i/ (Peterson & Barney, 1952). Data reported by Skelton (1969; see also Quiles, 1981; Navarro Tomas, 1950) suggest that this would not be true if the relatively open allophone of /i/ in closed syllables had been included. The data in Figure 1 agree with the Argentine Spanish data in showing that realizations of /e/ fell entirely within the space occupied by American English /ɪ/ (see also Papçun, 1976; Ladefoged, 1975). The Argentine data for /e/ and that shown in Figure 1 may be misleading, however, because only the [e] allophone of /e/ was examined. Had [ɛ] allophone tokens been included, the Spanish /e/ ellipse in Figure 1 would probably have encompassed much of the F_1–F_2 space occupied by English /ɛ/ (see Skelton, 1969).

If interlingual identification were based on proximity in a psychological space resembling the F_1–F_2 space in Figure 1, we might expect the following:

1. English /i/ will be identified with Spanish /i/;
2. English /ɪ/ will be identified with Spanish /e/, /i/;
3. English /ɛ/ will be identified with Spanish /e/;
4. English /æ/ will not be identified consistently with a Spanish vowel.

---

[11] Best et al. (1988) provided perceptual evidence that Bantu clicks may be sufficiently distinct from any English consonant that they are not identified in terms of an English category. No L2 production study, to my knowledge, has examined click production. Such a study would be problematical, however, because clicks are likely to occur seldom in human langauges because they are complex articulatorily. (This would work against the hypothesis that new L2 sounds will be mastered.) Several studies examined the production of English /r/ and /l/ by Japanese speakers. These sounds might be regarded as new, for there is no /l/ in Japanese and the Japanese /r/ is realized as a voiced tip-alveolar flap (see Flege, 1988*b*, for a review). Speech production and perception research has suggested that at least some native speakers of Japanese can master the /r/–/l/ contrast of English (MacKain et al., 1981; Mochizuki, 1981; Sheldon & Strange, 1982; see also Flege, 1988b). Research examining similar L2 stops, on the other hand, indicate that they will seldom if ever be mastered by adult learners (Flege, 1991).

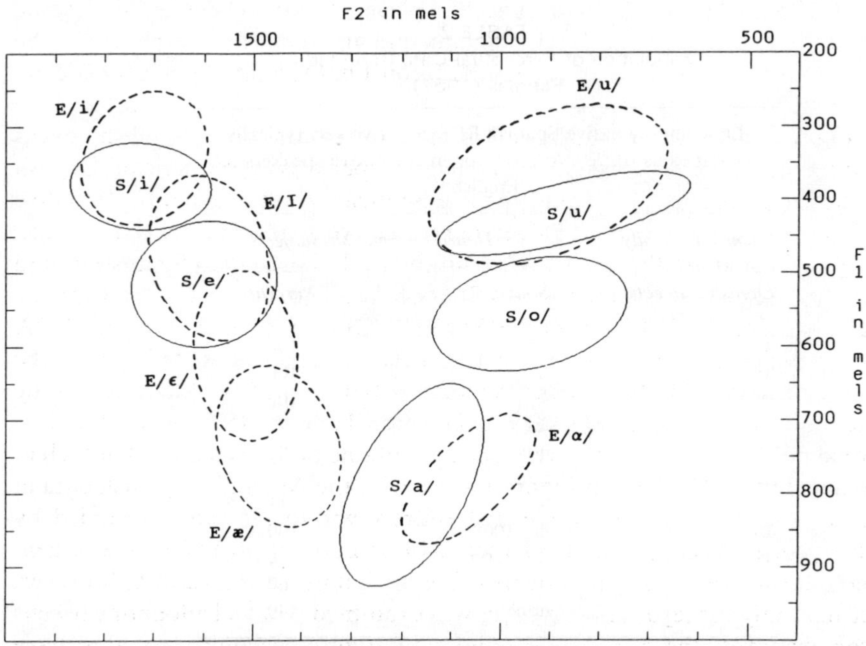

FIG. 1. Formant frequency values for six English vowels (/i/, /ɪ/, /ɛ/, /æ/, /ɑ/, /u/) spoken by 30 male native speakers of American and English (Peterson & Barney, 1952) and five Spanish vowels (/i/, /e/, /a/, /o/, /u/) spoken by 16 male native speakers of Spanish (Godinez, 1978), in mels. The ellipses define 95% confidence limits; they are based on the two principle components of variation in F_1 and F_2 values.

Prediction (1) agrees with results obtained in a cross-language perceptual study by Scholes (1967), summarized in Table 2. In that study, English and Spanish subjects used keywords from their L1, or the label "none", to identify a matrix of 69 isolated synthetic vowels in which F_1 and F_2 frequencies were varied. The vowels typically heard as /i/ by native English subjects were also heard as /i/ by the Spanish subjects. In agreement with the error analyses in Table 1, but in apparent disagreement with Prediction (2) above, [ɪ]-quality vowels were always heard as /i/ by Scholes' Spanish subjects, never as /e/.[12] Prediction (3), as stated, would be true only if interlingual judgements are made exclusively at a phonemic level. The finding that [ɛ]-quality vowels were sometimes identified as "none" by

[12] One reason for caution in regards to Scholes' (1967) /ɪ/ data is that just one of the 69 synthetic vowel stimuli was heard consistently by English subjects as /ɪ/, probably because the stimuli were 400 msec long.

TABLE 2
Tabulation of Perceptual Data Reported by Scholes (1967).

Labelling by native Spanish listeners of vowels typically classified as /i/, /eⁱ/, /ɑ/, /oᵁ/, or /u/ by native speakers of English

Sounds Typically Classified by English Subjects	*Heard by Spanish Subjects*	
	Sound	*Percent*
/i/	/i/	100
/ɪ/	/i/	100
/eⁱ/	/e/	100
/ɛ/	/e/	72
	none	28
/æ/	none	89
	/e/	11
/ɑ/	/a/–100%	100
/oᵁ/	/o/–100%	100
/u/	/u/	60
	none	40

Labelling by native English listeners of vowels typically classified as /i/, /e/, /a/, /o/, or /u/ by native Spanish speakers

Sounds Typically Classified by Spanish Subjects	*Heard by English Subjects*	
	Sound	*Percent*
/i/	/i/	70
	/ɪ/	20
	/ɛ/	10
/e/	/eⁱ/	41
	/ɛ/	29
	/æ/	18
	none	12
/a/	/ɑ/	88
	/ʌ/	12
/o/	/o/	50
	none	33
	/ɑ/	17
/u/	/u/	50
	/U/	50

Scholes' Spanish subjects suggested that their judgements were based, at least in part, on phonetic-level representations.[13]

Perhaps the most interesting observation to be drawn from Scholes' (1967) data is that the Spanish subjects seemed to use the "none" response predominantly to label [æ]-quality vowels. This agrees with the acoustic data in Figure 1 and is consistent with the observation that Spanish speakers of English mispronounce English /æ/ in a variety of ways (Table 1). This may mean that /æ/ emerges as a new vowel for native Spanish learners of English. Such a conclusion is be no means certain, however, because Scholes made use of isolated synthetic vowels. The subjects might have used the "none" response because some incidental property of the stimuli (e.g. duration) diverged from values specified in their central representation of the closest Spanish vowel.

Decisions as to whether a vowel is "different" from any L1 vowel may be influenced by response biases and perhaps subtle aspects of experimental design, such as the wording of instructions. The criterion used here to determine whether an English vowel emerges as "new" was the pattern of behaviour observed for groups of native Spanish subjects differing in English-language experience. Experiment 1 examined Spanish subjects who had little or no prior exposure to English (i.e. Spanish monolinguals). Experiments 2 and 3 examined Spanish speakers of English who differed in L2 experience. Experiment 3 differed from the first two experiments in using instructions that encouraged subjects to use the "none" label. If English /æ/ emerges as a new vowel, we would expect Spanish speakers of English to use the "none" label for /æ/ more often than Spanish monolinguals but not to differ from the monolinguals in the frequency with which "none" is applied to other English vowels. If L2 learners recognize only gradually that certain L2 vowels are new, we might see no difference between inexperienced Spanish speakers of English and Spanish monolinguals, but observe the kind of difference just described between relatively experienced and inexperienced Spanish speakers of English.

EXPERIMENT 1

Method

Ten native speakers of English (5 males, 5 females) living in Birmingham, Alabama, read a randomized list containing multiple repetitions of English "beat", "bit", "bet", and "bat". The first three repetitions of each word were

---

[13] This is especially true given that the Spanish subjects were offered two Spanish keywords with which to label the synthetic vowels—one that contained the [ɛ] allophone (viz. *ser*) and one with the [e] allophone (viz. *de*).

lowpass-filtered at 4.8 kHz and digitized at 10 kHz with 12-bit amplitude resolution. The formant frequencies of all 120 words (10 talkers × 4 vowels × 3 repetitions) were estimated using LPC analysis (14 coefficients for males, 12 for females) by placing a 25.6-msec Hamming window at the acoustic midpoint. Fundamental frequency (F0) measurements were based on the duration of three successive glottal periods at the vowel midpoint. "Vowel" duration was measured (in msec) from the onset to the offset of periodicity in each waveform.

Table 3 presents the mean acoustic values for the five female talkers who produced the English /bVt/ words used as stimuli in Experiments 1–3. Table 4 presents the mean values for the five male talkers. As expected, /i/ was longer than /ɪ/, and /æ/ was longer than /ɛ/. Also as expected, F0 was slightly higher for the two high vowels (/i/, /ɪ/) than for the two non-high vowels (/ɛ/, /æ/). For the most part, the formant frequency values reported in Tables 3 and 4 correspond to values published for American English by Peterson and Barney (1952).

In Figure 2 the 15 tokens of each vowel obtained from the male talkers are plotted in an F_1–F_2 space along with ellipses defining native Spanish males' productions of the Spanish vowels /i/, /e/, /a/, /o/, and /u/ (Godinez, 1978). All but one English /i/ token fell within the ellipse for Spanish /i/. Most of the English /ɪ/ tokens fell within the Spanish /e/ ellipse. One English /ɛ/ token fell within the /e/ ellipse, but most fell outside any Spanish ellipse (usually closer to Spanish /e/ than /a/). None of the English /æ/ tokens fell within a Spanish vowel ellipse, but most were slightly closer to Spanish /a/ than /e/.

The 120 English /bVt/ words were normalized for peak intensity, then recorded on audio tape (Marantz PMD 420) for later playback to subjects. Two randomizations of the 12 words spoken by each talker (4 words × 3 repetitions) were recorded. The five male talkers were recorded on Side A of the tape, the five females on Side B. The interval between each word was fixed at 2.5 sec. The interval between talkers was 10 sec. Sides A and B were presented binaurally over headphones in a sound-booth to 20 monolingual speakers of Spanish. The paid subjects (11 males, 9 females) had a mean age of 27 years (*S.D.* = 9). Each reported having normal hearing. Most subjects had been in the United States for only several weeks at the time of testing. Fourteen were from Mexico, five were from El Salvador, and one was from Argentina. It is not known what influence, if any, the variations in native dialect of Spanish may have had on the results.

A native Spanish research assistant read instructions in Spanish to the subjects. They were told to identify the vowel in each word by circling <i>, <e>, <a>, <o>, or <u> on a specially prepared answer sheet, or by circling "ninguno" (none) if they heard a vowel "not found in Spanish". The subjects were told to guess if they were uncertain. The words spoken by one talker (24 stimuli) were presented for practice before the experiment began.

TABLE 3
Duration[a] and Frequency[b] in the Vowels Found in "Beat", "Bit", "Bet", and "Bat" as Spoken by Five Adult Female Native Speakers of American English

Vowel	*Talker*	*Dur.*	*F0*	*F1*	*F2*	*F3*
/i/	1	125	143	329	2698	3228
	2	153	179	358	3107	3620
	3	197	213	352	2982	3681
	4	136	193	376	2728	3471
	5	246	192	384	2502	3058
	M	171	184	360	2803	3412
/ɪ/	1	96	144	415	2096	2861
	2	122	187	571	2340	3184
	3	143	204	469	2237	3065
	4	118	205	417	2152	2850
	5	214	198	416	2089	2790
	M	139	188	458	2182	2949
/ε/	1	145	137	530	2043	2856
	2	182	175	731	2033	3070
	3	206	186	684	1928	2988
	4	147	184	506	2100	2925
	5	266	194	559	2082	2763
	M	189	175	602	2037	2921
/æ/	1	195	135	656	2062	2866
	2	216	159	792	1900	2863
	3	289	192	822	1823	3043
	4	209	161	817	1915	2787
	5	285	168	742	2047	2673
	M	239	163	766	1949	2846

[a] Duration in msec.
[b] Frequency in Hz. *Note*: Each talker mean is based on three tokens.

Half of the subjects heard a male talker on Side A for practise, the other half a female talker on Side B. This may have been insufficient in a few instances. A total 5.5% of the data, all from three subjects, had to be discarded because of missing responses.[14]

[14] Each listener marked 24 answers in response to the vowels of the 10 talkers, as required, but the three listeners just mentioned probably did not respond to every word *as it was presented*

(continued overleaf)

TABLE 4
Duration[a] and Frequency[b] in the Vowels Found in "Beat", "Bit", "Bet", and "Bat" as Spoken by Five Adult Male Native Speakers of American English

Vowel	*Talker*	*Dur.*	*F0*	*F1*	*F2*	*F3*
/i/	1	131	111	263	2523	3171
	2	164	115	322	2486	2989
	3	202	104	312	2044	2764
	4	195	84	319	2512	2876
	5	234	129	279	2260	3007
	M	185	109	299	2365	2962
/ɪ/	1	108	102	436	1929	2739
	2	120	111	458	1993	2746
	3	158	117	461	1555	2451
	4	146	80	471	1768	2695
	5	225	125	389	1933	2648
	M	151	107	443	1835	2656
/ɛ/	1	116	93	621	1821	2643
	2	161	110	590	1837	2709
	3	214	105	549	1430	2288
	4	160	80	536	1758	2694
	5	247	119	475	1825	2579
	M	180	101	554	1734	2582
/æ/	1	182	98	711	1926	2604
	2	175	98	766	1683	2615
	3	273	103	697	1530	2219
	4	223	81	701	1739	2549
	5	300	110	661	1840	2738
	M	231	98	707	1744	2545

[a] Duration in msec.
[b] Frequency in Hz.
Note: Each talker mean is based on three tokens.

---

in the few blocks. It appears that these listeners missed a response but attempted to conceal this fact by marking an answer(s) at the end of the answer sheet after the last word had been presented, resulting in responses that were out of sequence with the stimuli. All data obtained in response to a particular talker were discarded if two or more obviously inappropriate responses were obtained for that talker. "Inappropriate" was defined here as an <a> response for either "beat" (/bit/) or "bit" (/bɪt/). It seems highly unlikely that such a response could be anything other than a mistake.

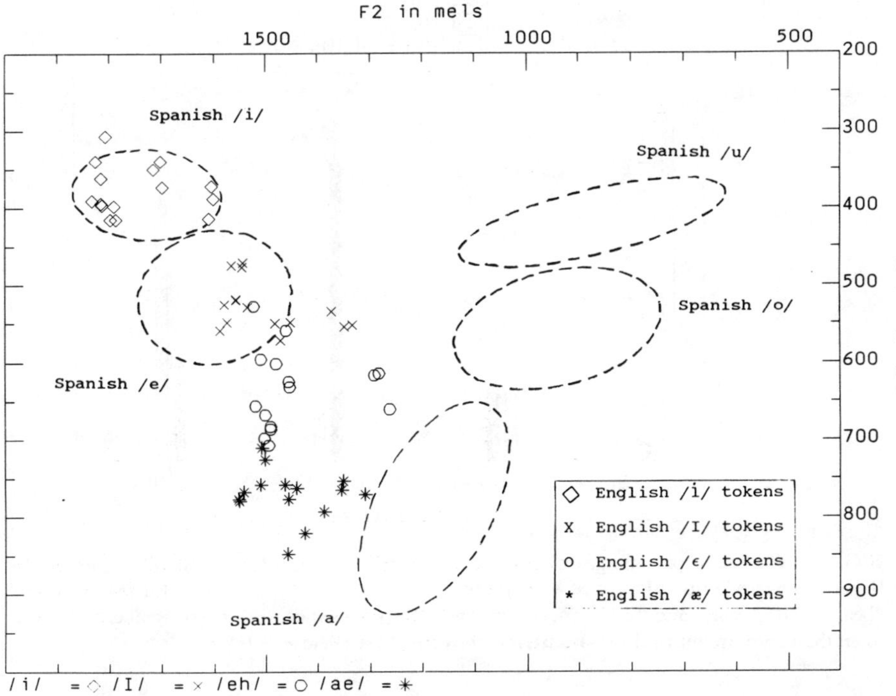

FIG. 2. The F_1–F_2 values (in mels) in vowel tokens spoken by 5 male native speakers of American English that were used as stimuli in Experiments 1–3. The ellipses define the Spanish vowels /i/, /e/, /a/, /o/, /u/) as spoken by 16 male native speakers of Spanish (Godinez, 1978).

The frequency with which <i>, <e>, <a>, <o>, <u>, and "none" were used by each subject to label the four English vowels was computed. For all but the three subjects just mentioned, the frequencies for each vowel were based on 60 responses (10 native English talkers × 3 replicate tokens × 2 randomizations). T-tests were performed to determine whether a particular response was used to label each vowel at a rate significantly exceeding zero. Since 24 *t*-tests were performed (4 vowels × 6 possible response labels), an alpha level of 0.004 was used to give an experiment-wise error rate of 0.10 (Snedecor & Cochran, 1980).

Results and Discussion

Figure 3 shows the mean frequency with which <i>, <e>, <a>, <o>, <u>, or "none" was used to label the English vowels. An asterisk in this figure and those to follow indicates that a response label was used at a significantly above-chance rate ($p < 0.10$). The Spanish subjects' most frequent response for both English /i/ and /ɪ/ vowels was <i> (94%, 68%),

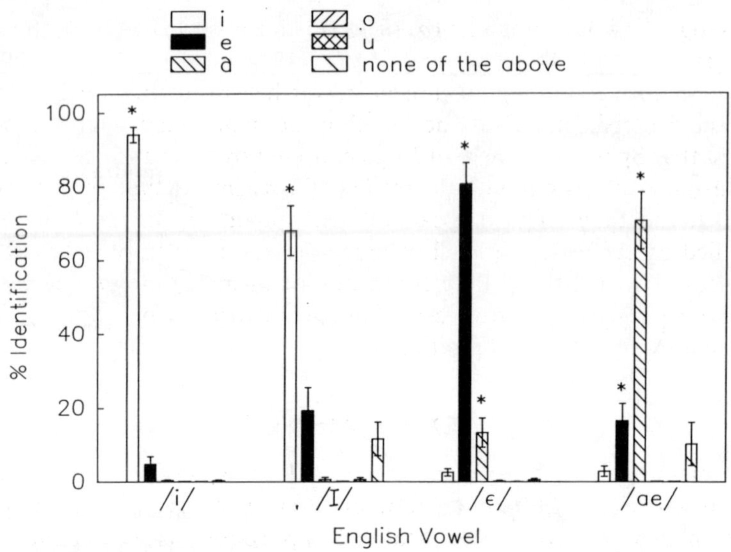

FIG. 3. The mean percentage of instances in which the monolingual Spanish subjects in Experiment 1 used the <i>, <e>, <a>, <o>, <u>, and "none" labels for the vowels in "beat", "bit", "bet", and "bat" (/i/, /ɪ/, /ɛ/, /æ/). Responses that were given significantly more often than zero are marked by an asterisk; the error bars enclose ± 1 *S.E.*

suggesting that they identified both English vowels in terms of the Spanish /i/ phoneme. The subjects also gave a few <e> and "none" responses for /ɪ/ (19%, 12%), but not at above-chance rates. The most frequent response for English /ɛ/ was <e> (81%). The subjects also used <a> to label English /ɛ/ in a small (13%) but significant number of instances. The most frequent response for /æ/ was <a> (71%), but <e> was also used at an above-chance rate (17%).

The results for /i/ and /ɛ/ agree with the acoustic and perceptual results presented in the Introduction. The results for /ɪ/ agree better with Scholes' (1967) perceptual data than an inference drawn from acoustic data, viz. that /ɪ/ would be identified frequently with Spanish /e/. Perhaps the relatively short duration of the English /ɪ/, or its centring offglide (Flege et al., in preparation), distinguished it from Spanish /e/. The most surprising result was the one obtained for /æ/. Previously published acoustic data showed that this English vowel is about midway between Spanish /e/ and /a/ in an F_1–F_2 space (Figure 1)—that is, /æ/ does not seem to occupy a portion of the acoustic vowel space exploited by a Spanish vowel. The particular /æ/ tokens used here (at least the males') fell outside any Spanish vowel ellipse. They were only slightly closer, perhaps, to the Spanish /a/ than /e/. This, taken together with the finding that the Spanish subjects in Scholes' (1967) study often applied the "none" label to [æ]-quality vowels, suggests that Spanish monolinguals would not identify English /æ/ in terms of a Spanish vowel category.

The Spanish monolingual subjects nevertheless identified /æ/ consistently with the Spanish /a/. Thus the labelling data obtained in this experiment suggest that Spanish learners of English do *not* treat English /æ/ as new. This conclusion is consistent with the results of a recent intelligibility study. Flege (1990) found that Spanish speakers' attempts at /æ/ in the word *bat* were identified by American English listeners as /^/ or /ɑ/ in over one-fourth of instances. This relatively high frequency of misperceptions does not prove that Spanish learners fail to establish a category for /æ/, but it is at least consistent with that interpretation.

EXPERIMENT 2

Experiment 2 further explored the extent to which Spanish speakers of English will note a difference between English /i/, /ɪ/, /ɛ/, /æ/ and vowels found in their L1. More specifically, the purpose of Experiment 2 was to determine whether native Spanish speakers of English would use the "none" label significantly more often than the monolingual subjects in Experiment 1, and significantly more often for /æ/ than for the other three English vowels examined.

Method

The stimuli from Experiment 1 were presented to 20 native Spanish speakers of English living in Birmingham, Alabama. The mean age of the subjects (10 male, 10 female) was 29 years ($S.D.=6$). They had arrived in the United States at an average age of 25 years ($S.D.=6$) and estimated using English about 65% of the time on a daily basis ($S.D.=19$). The subjects differed considerably in terms of L2 experience. Length of residence in the United States ranged from 4 months to 10 years ($M=5$ years, $S.D.=5$). Ten "inexperienced" subjects had lived in the United States for only 0.8 years, on the average, and 10 "experienced" subjects had lived in the United States for 6.8 years. A total of 4% of the data was declared missing (see Footnote 14). The frequency with which the six response categories (<i>, <e>, <a>, <o>, <u>, "none") were used to label the four English vowels was calculated as before.

Results and Discussion

A series of Mann–Whitney tests were carried out on the frequency data to determine whether the 10 experienced and the 10 inexperienced subjects responded differently. In many instances a response label was not used at all, or only marginally. Tests were carried out only if a label was used in at least 5% of instances overall. This criterion was met in 12 instances. A 0.004 alpha level was used for the 12 tests to give an experiment-wise error rate of 0.05 (Snedecor & Cochran, 1980).

No difference between the experienced and inexperienced speakers of English was significant. Only two between-group differences approached significance. The experienced subjects gave more <e> responses to /ɛ/ than did the inexperienced subjects (57% vs. 31%); conversely, they gave fewer <a> responses to /ɛ/ than did the inexperienced subjects (26% vs. 53%) [$U=21.5, p=0.028$; $U=18.0, p=0.015$]. These tendencies suggest that Spanish subjects who are relatively inexperienced in English may have difficulty in relating English /ɛ/ to the [ɛ] allophone of Spanish /e/ if it occurs in an unfamiliar phonetic context (i.e. preceding a word-final stop).

The responses obtained for the experienced and inexperienced speakers of English have been combined in Figure 4 because none of the between-group differences was statistically significant. English /i/ was labelled as <i> in 84% of instances. English /ɪ/ received the following responses at above-chance rates: <e> (39%), <i> (36%), and "none" (21%). An inference drawn from acoustic analyses of Spanish and English vowels in the Introduction was that English /ɪ/ might be identified more closely with Spanish /e/ than with Spanish /i/. The response pattern obtained here in Experiment 2 is more consistent with this inference than is the response pattern obtained in

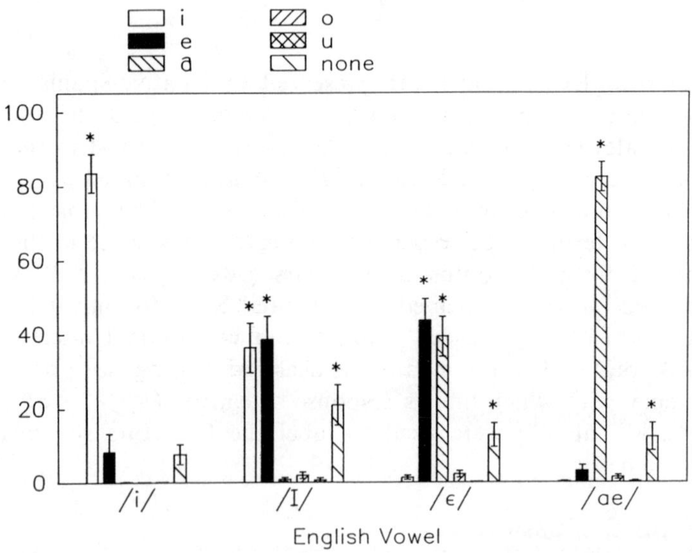

FIG. 4. The mean percentage of instances in which the Spanish speakers of English in Experiment 2 used <i>, <e>, <a>, <o>, <u>, and "none" as labels for the vowels in "beat", "bit", "bet", and "bat" (/i/, /ɪ/, /ɛ/, /æ/). Data for experienced and inexperienced native Spanish speakers of English have been pooled because these subgroups did not differ significantly. Frequencies that significantly exceeded zero are marked by an asterisk; the error bars enclose ± 1 *S.E.*

Experiment 1. Thus, the Experiment 2 data for /ɪ/ suggest indirectly that Spanish speakers of English may be better able to appraise the *phonetic* characteristics of English vowels than subjects without such familiarity. Three responses were obtained at above-chance rates for English /ɛ/: <e> (44%), <a> (39%), and "none" (13%). One might expect English /ɛ/ to be identified with Spanish /e/ because this phoneme has an [ɛ] allophone. "None" responses might be expected because the /ɛ/ realizations in "bet" occurred in an unaccustomed phonetic context (i.e., preceding a word-final stop). The only explanation that comes to mind for why English /ɛ/ was sometimes labelled <a> is the acoustic similarity of some of the English /ɛ/ realizations to Spanish /a/ (see Figure 2). Two responses at above-chance rates were obtained for English /æ/: <a> (82%) and "none" (12%). This finding does not support a conclusion that might be drawn from Scholes' (1967) perceptual study, viz. that Spanish speakers judge English /æ/ to be a new vowel.

"None" responses were obtained more often from bilinguals in the present experiment than from the monolingual subjects in Experiment 1. The frequencies of none responses obtained in Experiments 1 and 2 were: /i/ (0% vs. 8%), /ɪ/ (12% vs. 21%), /ɛ/ (1% vs. 13%), /æ/ (10% vs. 12%). The differences between experiments were all significant at the 0.05 level [$U=107.0$, 119.0, 65.0, 118.0]. The same procedures were used for the bilinguals and monolinguals, so these results suggest that the Spanish speakers of English had begun to note some of the acoustic differences between English and Spanish vowels. However, although the Spanish/English bilinguals used the "none" label more often than did the Spanish monolinguals, few bilinguals used it as their predominant response for the English vowels. The rate of "none" never exceeded an average 20% for any vowel in Experiment 2; and only 12 of the 20 individual subjects used "none" in more than 10% of instances in responding to the four vowels. If we consider all 40 subjects who participated in Experiments 1 and 2, the rate of "none" responses exceeded 50% in only 10 of the 160 possible instances (40 subjects × 4 vowels). Six subjects used "none" as their predominant label for /ɪ/, and four used it predominantly for /æ/ (see Figure 7 below).

Of the four American English vowels examined, /ɪ/ and /æ/ are probably the least like a Spanish vowel phoneme in acoustic phonetic terms. We reexamined the data obtained for those subjects from Experiments 1 and 2 who were not reluctant to use the "none" response. The "non-reluctant" subjects were defined as all those who responded "none" in more than 10% of instances overall. The frequencies with which the "none" response was used in labelling /ɪ/ and /æ/ by these 18 subjects were compared to the frequencies for /i/ and /ɛ/. The combined frequency of "none" response for the non-reluctant subjects was significantly greater for /ɪ/–/æ/ than /i/–/ɛ/ (28% vs. 13%) [$H=12.1$, $df=3$, $p=0.007$]. Still, had the Spanish subjects established phonetic categories for English /ɪ/ and /æ/, we would have expected "none" responses to be used more consistently. Thus the results obtained in the first two experiments do not strongly support the hypothesis that any of the English vowels examined here will be treated as "new" by adult Spanish learners of English.

EXPERIMENT 3

The inter-subject variation in the use of "none" suggests that it may be difficult to determine, in an absolute sense, whether bilinguals judge an English vowel to be phonetically or phonemically distinct from vowels in the L1 inventory. The orthographic classification of L2 vowels in Experiments 1 and 2 resembles an experiment described recently by Johnson (1990), where subjects were asked to determine whether words synthesized with different F0 values had been spoken by the same talker or by different talkers. One listener identified only those words produced with an *identical* F0 values as having been produced by the same talker. Other listeners had a more liberal standard. Some, in fact, seemed willing to attribute *any* detectable F0 difference to a difference in speaker identity.

It is possible that some subjects in the Experiments 1 and 2 were more willing to use the "none" label than other subjects as the result of a general response bias. If so, it should be possible to manipulate the frequency of "none" responses. We attempted to do so in Experiment 3 by using instructions that were quite different from those used in the two earlier experiments. The new instructions encouraged subjects to use the "none" label. Under the new instructions, "none" might be used often enough to warrant concluding that an English vowel emerges as "new" for Spanish speakers of English.

Method

The stimuli used in Experiments 1 and 2 were again used here. The only important change in procedures was in the instructions read in Spanish to the subjects. The subjects in Experiments 1 and 2 were told that the purpose of those experiments was to "compare" Spanish and English vowels. Here, they were told that the purpose of the experiment was to identify *differences* between Spanish and English vowels. The Experiment 1 and 2 subjects were told to circle one of five vowel letters, but to use "none" if they did not hear a vowel from Spanish. Included in the instructions for Experiment 3 was the observation that "many English vowels are unlike any vowel in Spanish". The subjects were told to use "none" if they heard one of these "different" English vowels, but to use one of the five letters if they thought they had heard a Spanish vowel.

Twenty additional native Spanish speakers of English were drawn from the same population as in Experiment 2. The average age of the subjects (10 male, 10 females) was 28 years (*S.D.* = 6). These subjects had arrived in the United States at an average age of 25 years (*S.D.* = 7), had studied English for an average of 5 years (*S.D.* = 5), and estimated that they used English about 56% of the time on a daily basis (*S.D.* = 31). A subgroup of ten inexperienced subjects had lived in the United States for only 0.4 years on the average at the time of the study; 10 relatively experienced subjects had lived in the United States for an average of 6.4 years.

Results and Discussion

A series of Mann–Whitney tests was carried out to test for between-group differences. Tests were not carried out when a label was used in less than 5% of instances. The alpha level was set at 0.0045 for the 11 tests that were performed to ensure an experiment-wise error rate of 0.05. No between-group difference reached significance. The largest difference observed was for the "none" response as applied to /ɪ/. The experienced subjects used "none" more often than did the inexperienced subjects (51% vs. 25%) (U=23.0, p=0.043]. A non-significant trend in the opposite direction was observed for "none" responses to /æ/ (13% vs. 23%) [U=49.0, p=0.971].

The data for the experienced and inexperienced subjects have been combined in Figure 5 because the differences between the two subgroups were non-significant. The "none" response was used more often here than in

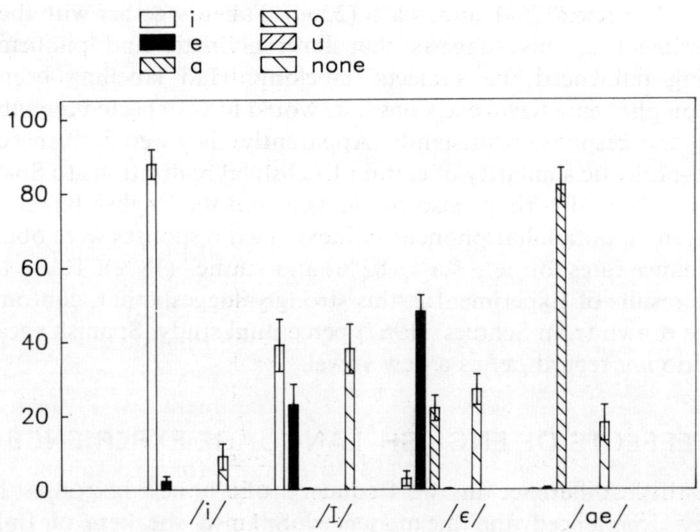

FIG. 5. The mean percentage of instances in which the Spanish speakers of English in Experiment 3, where instructions encouraged "none" reponses, used <i>, <e>, <a>, <o>, <u>, and "none" to label the vowels in "beat", "bit", "bet", and "bat". Data for experienced and inexperienced speakers of English have been pooled because these subgroups did not differ significantly. An asterisk indicates above-chance frequencies; the error bars enclose ± 1 *S.E.*

Experiment 2 (23% vs. 14%), but the difference was smaller than expected, given the major change in instructions (see above). Mann–Whitney tests were used to test for differences in the frequency of "none" responses in Experiments 2 and 3. The difference between Experiment 2 and Experiment 3 was non-significant for /i/ (8% vs. 9%) and for /æ/ (12% vs. 18%) [$U=190.0$, 180.0]. The difference for /ɪ/ (21% vs. 38%) was marginally significant, $U=133.5, p=0.072$; the difference for /ɛ/ (13% vs. 27%) reached significance at the 0.05 level, $U=111.5$, $p=0.016$. Recall that the Spanish speakers of English in Experiment 2 used "none" more often than did the Spanish monolinguals in Experiment 1 (14% vs. 6% overall). It thus appears that manipulating instructions had about as much influence on subjects' likelihood to use "none" for an English vowel as did learning to speak English.

The subjects in Experiment 3 used <i> to label the English /i/ realizations in most instances (88%). For /ɪ/, three responses were used at above-chance rates: <i> (39%), none (38%), and <e> (23%). Taken together with the results of Experiment 2, this suggests that Scholes' (1967) 400-msec synthetic stimuli probably did not permit an accurate assessment of how Spanish speakers identify English /ɪ/. Apparently, the acoustic overlap between English /ɪ/ and Spanish /e/ realizations is sufficient to cause at least some Spanish/English bilinguals to identify the two vowels with one another perceptually.

Three responses were obtained at above-chance rates for English /ɛ/: <e> (48%), none (27%), and <a> (22%). Taken together with the results of Experiment 2, this suggests that both phonetic and phonemic-level processing influenced the subjects' labelling. Had labelling been based entirely on phonemic-level decisions, one would have expected the subjects to use the <e> response consistently. Apparently, they were influenced by the acoustic–phonetic similarity of certain English [ɛ] realizations to Spanish /a/ (see Figure 2), and perhaps also by the fact that the English [ɛ] realizations occurred in an unfamiliar phonetic context. Two responses were obtained at above-chance rates for /æ/: <a> (82%) and "none" (18%). Taken together with the results of Experiment 2, this strongly suggests that, contrary to an inference drawn from Scholes' (1967) perceptual study, Spanish speakers of English do *not* regard /æ/ as a new vowel.

EFFECTS OF ENGLISH-LANGUAGE EXPERIENCE

We saw little difference in the frequency of "none" responses between relatively experienced and inexperienced Spanish speakers of English in Experiments 2 and 3. The possibility existed that significant effects of L2 experience might be evident if the data from these two experiments were combined. That was the purpose of this section. Characteristics of the 20 experienced and 20 inexperienced subjects from Experiments 2 and 3 are

TABLE 5
Characteristics of the Native Spanish Subjects in Experiments 1–3

	Monolingual Spanish	*Inexperienced in English*	*Experienced in English*
N:	20 (11 M/9 F)	20 (10 M/10 F)	20 (10 M/10 F)
Age	26.8 (8.8)	28.9 (6.2)	28.8 (6.5)
AOA[1]	—	28.1 (6.2)	22.5 (5.9)
LOR[2]	—	0.6 (0.4)	6.6 (2.5)
YRS[3]	—	5.6 (4.1)	6.4 (4.6)
PER[4]	—	59% (28)	62% (24)

[1] Age of arrival in the United States, in years.
[2] Length of residence in the United States, in years.
[3] Years of classroom instruction in English, in years.
[4] Self-estimated percentage daily use of English.
Note: "M" indicates male, "F" indicates female.

summarized in Table 5. The experienced subjects had arrived in the United States at an earlier average age than the inexperienced subjects (22.5 vs. 28.1 years) and had lived there longer (6.6 vs. 0.6 years). The two groups were matched fairly closely, however, in terms of chronological age, amount of formal education in English, and self-estimated daily usage of English.

One-half of the experienced Spanish speakers of English received the "neutral" Experiment 2 instructions, whereas the other half received the instructions from Experiment 3, which encouraged the use of "none". The same proportion of inexperienced and experienced Spanish subjects received the two types of instruction, so it is possible to draw valid comparisons between the two groups. It would *not* be valid, on the other hand, to compare either group of bilinguals to the 20 Spanish monolinguals, whose characteristics are also summarized in Table 3. This is because all of the monolinguals received the "neutral" instructions. The monolinguals' results are nevertheless juxtaposed to those of the bilinguals in Figure 6 for the sake of completeness.

Inspection of Figure 6 reveals that the subjects in all three groups used <i> predominantly to label English /i/, and <a> predominantly to label /æ/. There was not a systematic increase in "none" responses for /æ/, suggesting that /æ/ does *not* emerge as a new vowel. The greatest effects of L2 experience seemed to be for /ɪ/ and /ɛ/. Use of the <i> label for English /ɪ/ decreased, and use of "none" responses for English /ɪ/ increased, as function of L2 experience. This suggests that /ɪ/ may be treated as a new vowel by at least some experienced Spanish speakers of English.

Compared to the monolinguals, the Spanish speakers of English were more likely to judge the English vowel /ɛ/ in "bet" as non-Spanish. For some

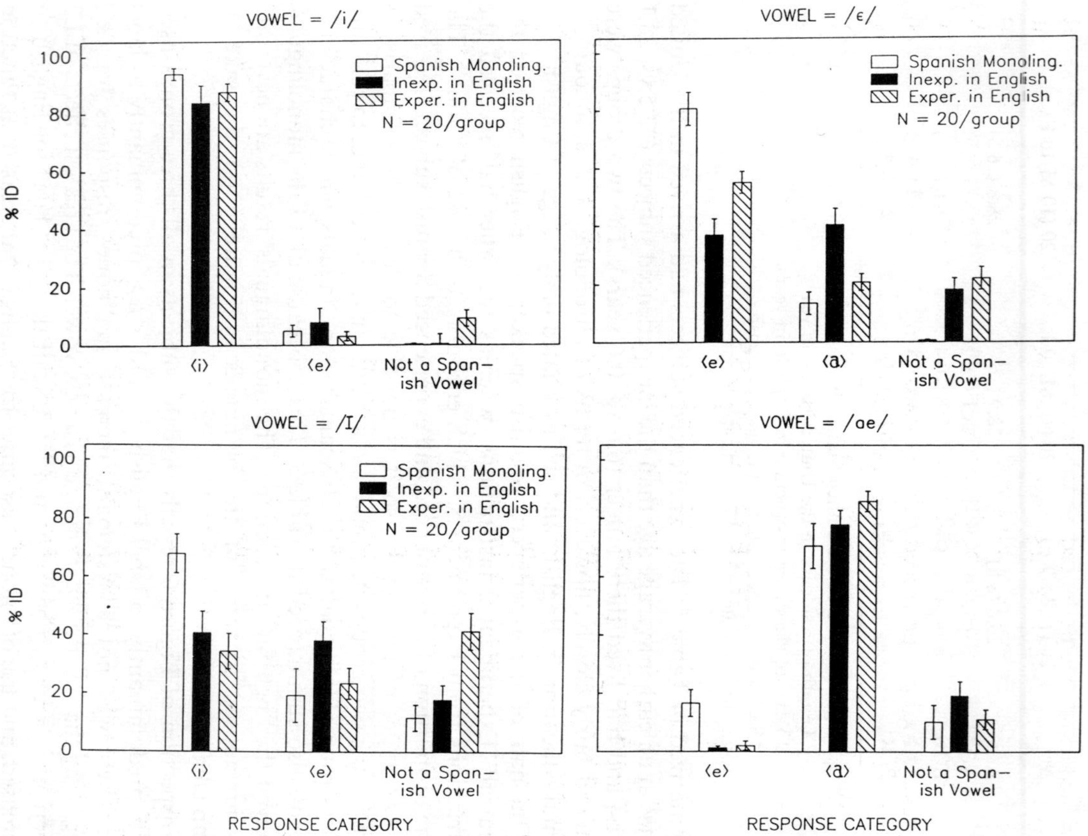

FIG. 6. Comparison of the results obtained in Experiments 1–3.

reason, the inexperienced subjects who had just begun learning English seemed to identify English /ɛ/ with Spanish /a/ at a relatively high rate. The experienced speakers of Spanish did so at a lower rate, thereby resembling the Spanish monolinguals.

Mann–Whitney tests were carried out to test for differences between the experienced and inexperienced Spanish subjects. The alpha level was set at 0.0045 because a total of 11 tests was performed. (Tests were not carried out in the 13 instances where a label was used in fewer than 5% of instances.) None of the between-group difference reached significance. It is worth noting, however, that the difference in the frequency with which the experienced and inexperienced subjects used "none" in labelling /ɪ/ (42% vs. 18%) came very close to reaching significance [$U=99.5$, $p=0.0056$], as did the between-group difference in <a> responses for /ɛ/ (21% vs. 40%; $U=105.0$, $p=0.0095$].

GENERAL DISCUSSION

Spanish monolinguals and Spanish speakers of English who differed in English-language experience used one of the five vowel letters of "none" to classify the American English vowels in "beat", "bit", "bet", "bat" (i.e., /i/, /ɪ/, /ɛ/, and /æ/) Their response patterns were, for the most part, predictable on the basis of the acoustic relationship between Spanish and English vowels as described in the Introduction.

The study yielded several important findings. Changing instructions so as to encourage the use of "none" resulted in a 9% increase in the frequency of "none" responses. The size of the increase was of about the same magnitude as the difference between Spanish monolinguals and Spanish speakers of English who received the same instructions (6% vs. 14%). Apparently, learning English heightens native Spanish speakers' awareness of acoustic–phonetic differences between Spanish and English vowels. Directing subjects' attention to cross-language vowel differences via experimental instructions may result in a similar heightened awareness. This will need to be explored further, however, as the observed effect may simply have been due to a change in response bias (i.e. an overall greater propensity to respond "none").

There was little evidence that Spanish learners of English will judge /æ/ in the context of word-final /t/ to be a "new" (non-Spanish) vowel. Even experienced Spanish speakers of English seem to continue identifying English /æ/ realizations in terms of their Spanish /a/ category. In this sense they differ from native speakers of German, another language that has no /æ/ phoneme. Germans seem to identify English /æ/ with German /ɛ/ or /ɛː/ (Bohn & Flege, 1990). Native speakers of Mandarin Chinese and Korean also seem to identify English /æ/ with an /ɛ/ (or /ɛ/-like) category in their L1 (Flege, 1990).

Some Spanish subjects in the present study seemed to be aware of the difference between English /ɪ/ and vowels in the Spanish inventory. Inexperienced Spanish speakers of English applied the "none" (i.e., non-Spanish) label to English /ɪ/ more often than did Spanish monolinguals. Also experienced Spanish speakers of English used "none" for /ɪ/ more often than did inexperienced Spanish speakers of English. The difference between the experienced and inexperienced subjects (42% vs. 18%) just missed reaching significance, however ($p = 0.0056$).

The results obtained here for /ɪ/ and /æ/ provide insight into results obtained in a forced-choice identification experiment by Flege and Bohn (1989). The members of synthetic continua ranging from "beat" to "bit" (/i/–/ɪ/) and "bet" to "bat" (/ɛ/–/æ/) were presented to native speakers of English and to experienced and inexperienced Spanish speakers of English. Only a few Spanish subjects resembled the native English subjects in showing a clear crossover from /i/ to /ɪ/ responses as a function of spectral changes. (Those who did not use spectral changes divided the continuum on the basis of duration differences.) However, nearly all of the Spanish subjects resembled the native English subjects in showing a clear crossover from /ɛ/ to /æ/ responses as a function of spectral changes in the stimuli. The results obtained here suggest that the Spanish subjects tested by Flege and Bohn (1989) probably did not succeed on the /ɛ/–/æ/ continuum as a result of having formed an /æ/ category. They may simply have appeared to resemble native English subjects as a result of identifying the /æ/ endpoint of the synthetic continuum in terms of their Spanish /a/ category. The few Spanish subjects who resembled the native English subjects for the /i/–/ɪ/ continuum, on the other hand, may have succeeded as the result of having formed an /ɪ/ category (unless, of course, they identified the /ɪ/ endpoint with Spanish /e/).

An examination of responses to English /ɛ/ suggested that the orthographic responses may not have been based entirely on phonemic level classifications. Had this been so, we would have expected the <e> label to have been applied consistently to realizations of English /ɛ/. This is because Spanish /e/ has an [ɛ] allophone said to match the English /ɛ/ in "bet" (Dalbor, 1980). However, the subjects often used <a> and "none" responses for English /ɛ/. Of the 20 bilingual subjects in Experiment 2 (where use of the "none" response was not specifically encouraged), four used <e> in more than 75% of instances to identify English /ɛ/, three used <a> in more than 75% of instances, and the remaining 13 used both <e> and <a>. The <a> responses might be attributed to the acoustic phonetic similarity of certain realizations of English /ɛ/ and Spanish /a/ (see Figures 1 and 2). The "none" responses to English /ɛ/ might be attributed to the fact that the English /ɛ/ realizations occurred in a phonetic context in which such vowels are not found in Spanish (i.e. preceding a word-final /t/).

The study did not provide strong support for the hypothesis that certain

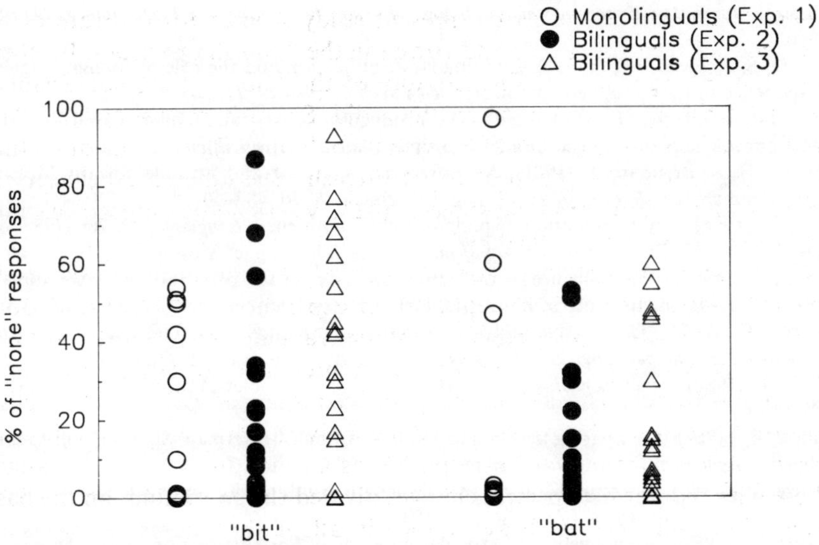

FIG. 7. The percentage of times the subjects in Experiments 1–3 used the "none" (i.e. not Spanish) to label the English vowels /ɪ/ and /æ/ (in *bit*, *bat*). The mean values for most subjects is based on 60 responses (10 native English talkers × 3 tokens × 2 randomizations) in most instances.

English vowels will be treated as "new" by adult native speakers of Spanish. There was, however, a high degree of inter-subject variability in the use of the "none" response, especially for /ɪ/ and /æ/. Figure 7 shows the frequency with which the "none" label was applied to these vowels by the 60 subjects who participated in Experiments 1–3. It appears that English /æ/ and especially English /ɪ/ fell outside the bounds of the Spanish vowel system for at least some subjects. It has been hypothesized that the authentic production of L2 sounds that are not identical to sounds in the L1 requires the formation of additional phonetic categories, and that L2 phonetic category formation is blocked when interlingual identification persists (Flege, 1988b; 1990; in press, a, b). The possibility therefore exists that the subjects who frequently judged English /æ/ and /ɪ/ to be non-Spanish were better at producing these vowels than were the subjects who seldom used the "none" label. Production was not tested in this study, however. It would be useful to examine production and orthographic classification together in a future experiment.

REFERENCES

Amastae, J. (1978). The acquisition of English vowels. *Papers in linguistics*, *11*, 423–457.

Best, C., McRoberts, G., & Sithole, N. (1988). Examination of perceptual reorganization for nonnative speech contrasts: Zulu click discrimination by English-speaking adults and infants. *Journal of Experimental Psychology: Human Perception and Performance, 14*, 345–360.

Bohn, O.-S. & Flege, J. E. (1990). Interlingual identification and the role of foreign language experience in L2 vowel perception. *Applied Psycholinguistics, 11*, 303–328.

Bohn, O.-S. & Flege, J.E. (submitted). The production of new and similar vowels by adult German learners of English. *Studies in Second Language Acquisition.*

Brennan, E. & Brennan, J. (1981). Measurement of accent and attitude toward Mexican American speech. *Journal of Psycholinguistic Research, 10*, 487–501.

Brière, E. (1966). An investigation of phonological interference. *Language, 42*, 769–796.

Brière, E. (1968). *A phonological study of interference.* The Hague: Mouton.

Butcher, A. (1976). The influence of the native language on the perception of vowel quality. *Arbeitsberichte, 6* (Institute of Phonetics, University of Kiel).

Catford, J.C. (1968). Contrastive analysis and language teaching. In J. Alatis (Ed.), *Contrastive linguistics and its pedagogical implications.* Washington: Georgetown University Press.

Dalbor, J. (1980). *Spanish pronunciation, theory and practice.* New York: Holt, Rinehart, & Winston.

Delattre, P. (1964). Comparing the vocalic features of English, German, Spanish, and French. *International Review of Applied Linguistics, 2*, 71–97.

Delattre, P. (1966). A comparison of syllable length conditioning among languages. *International Review of Applied Linguistics, 4*, 183–198.

Delattre, P. (1969). An acoustic and articulatory study of vowel reduction in four languages. *International Review of Applied Linguistics, 7*, 295–323.

Elman, J., Diehl, R., & Buchwald, S. (1977). Perceptual switching in bilinguals. *Journal of the Acoustical Society of America, 62*, 871–974.

Flege, J.E. (1981). The phonological basis of foreign accent. *TESOL Quarterly, 15*, 443–455.

Flege, J.E. (1984). The detection of French accent by American listeners. *Journal of the Acoustical Society of America, 76*, 692–707.

Flege, J.E. (1987a). A critical period for learning to pronounce foreign languages? *Applied Linguistics, 8*, 162–177.

Flege, J.E. (1987b). The production of "new" and "similar" phones in a foreign language: evidence for the effect of equivalence classification. *Journal of Phonetics, 15*, 47–65.

Flege, J.E. (1988a). Factors affecting degree of perceived foreign accent in English sentences. *Journal of the Acoustical Society of America, 84*, 70–79.

Flege, J.E. (1988b). The production and perception of speech sounds in foreign languages. In H. Winitz (Ed.), *Human communication and its disorders. A review 1988* (pp. 224–401). Norwood, NJ: Ablex.

Flege, J.E. (1988c). The development of skill in producing word-final /p/ and /b/: Kinematic parameters. *Journal of the Acoustical Society of America, 84*, 1639–1652.

Flege, J.E. (1989a). Differences in inventory size affect the location but not the precision of tongue positioning in vowel production. *Language and Speech, 32*, 123–147.

Flege, J.E. (1989b). Chinese subjects' perception of the word-final English /t/–/d/ contrast: Performance before and after training. *Journal of the Acoustical Society of America, 86*, 1684–1697.

Flege, J.E. (1990). Speech learning in a second language. In C. Ferguson, L. Menn & C. Stoel-Gammon (Eds.), *Phonological development: models, research, and application.* Parkton, MD: York Press.

Flege, J.E. (1991). Age of learning affects the authenticity of voice onset time (VOT) in stop consonants produced in a second language. *Journal of the Acoustical Society of America, 89*, 395–411.

Flege, J.E. (in press a). The intelligibility of English vowels spoken by British and Dutch talkers. In R. Kent (Ed.), *Intelligibility in speech disorders: theory, measurement, and management.* Philadelphia: John Benjamins.

Flege, J.E. (in press b). Perception and production: The relevance of phonetic input to L2 phonological learning. In C. Ferguson & T. Huebner (Eds.), *Crosscurrents in second language acquisition and linguistic theory*. Philadelphia: John Benjamins.

Flege, J.E. (submitted). The use of rhyming judgments to evaluate interlingual identification of Spanish and English vowels. *Journal of Phonetics*.

Flege, J.E. & Bohn, O.-S. (1989). The perception of English vowels by native Spanish speakers. *Journal of the Acoustical Society of America, 85*, S85 (Abstract).

Flege, J.E. & Eefting, W. (1986). Linguistic and developmental effects on the production and perception of stop consonants. *Phonetica, 43*, 155–171.

Flege, J.E. & Eefting, W. (1988). Imitation of a VOT continuum by native speakers of English and Spanish: Evidence for phonetic category formation. *Journal of the Acoustical Society of America, 83*, 729–740.

Flege, J.E. & Fletcher, K. (submitted). At what age of learning (AOL) does a foreign accent first become perceptible? *Journal of the Acoustical Society of America*.

Flege, J.E. & Hillenbrand, J. (1985). Differential use of temporal cues to the [s–z] contrast by native and non-native speakers of English. *Journal of the Acoustical Society of America, 79*, 508–517.

Flege, J.E. & Hillenbrand, J. (1987). Differential use of closure voicing and release burst cues to stop voicing by native speakers of French and English. *Journal of Phonetics, 15*, 203–208.

Flege, J.E., McCutcheon, M., & Smith, S. (1987). The development of skill in producing word-final English stops. *Journal of the Acoustical Society of America, 82*, 433–447.

Flege, J.E., Munro, M., & Fox, R. (in prep.). *The interlingual identification of Spanish and English vowels: Dissimilarity ratings*. Department of Biocommunication, University of Alabama at Birmingham.

Flege, J.E. & Wang, C. (1990). Native-language phonotactic constraints affect how well Chinese subjects perceive the word-final English /t/–/d/ contrast. *Journal of Phonetics, 17*, 299–315.

Godinez, Jr. M. (1978). A comparative study of some Romance vowels. *UCLA Working Papers in Phonetics, 41*, 3–19 (Department of Linguistics, University of California at Los Angeles).

Guirao, M. & de Manrique, B. (1972). Identification of Argentine Spanish vowel. In A. Rigault & R. Charbonneau (Eds.), *Proceedings of the 7th international congress of phonetic sciences*. The Hague: Mouton.

Guirao, M. & de Manrique, B. (1975). Identification of Argentine Spanish vowels. *Journal of Psycholinguistic Research, 4*, 17–25.

Hammarberg, B. (in press). Conditions on transfer in phonology. In J. Leather & A. James (Eds.), *New sounds 90, proceedings of the Amsterdam symposium on second-language speech*. Dordrecht: Foris.

Hammond, R. (1986). Error analysis and the natural approach to teaching foreign languages. *Lenguas Modernas, 13*, 129–139.

Johnson, K. (1990). The role of perceived speaker identity in F0 normalization of vowels. *Journal of the Acoustical Society of America, 88*, 642–654.

Klatt, D. (1987). Review of text-to-speech conversion for English. *Journal of the Acoustical Society of America, 82*, 737–793.

Ladefoged, P. (1975). *A course in phonetics*. New York: Harcourt, Brace Jovanovich.

Ladefoged, P. (1989). Representing Phonetic Structure. *UCLA Working Papers in Phonetics, 73* (Department of Linguistics, University of California at Los Angeles).

Lenneberg, E. (1967). *The biological foundations of language*. New York: Wiley.

MacDonald, M. (1989). The influence of Spanish phonology on the English spoken by United States Hispanics. In P. Bjarkman & R. Hammond (Eds.), *American Spanish pronunciation*. Washington, DC: George Washington University Press.

MacKain, K., Best, C., & Strange, W. (1981). Categorical perception of English /r/ and /l/ by

Japanese bilinguals. *Applied Linguistics*, *2*, 369–390.

Major, R.C. (1987). Phonological similarity, markedness, and rate of L1 acquisition. *Studies in Second Language Acquisition*, *9*, 63–82.

Mann, V. (1986). Distinguishing universal and language-dependent levels of speech perception: Evidence from Japanese listeners' perception of English "l" and "r". *Cognition*, *24*, 169–196.

Miyawaki, K., Strange, W., Verbrugge, R., Liberman, A., Jenkins, J., & Fujimura, O. (1975). An effect of linguistic experience: The discrimination of /r/ and /l/ by native speakers of Japanese and English. *Perception & Psychophysics*, *18*, 331–340.

Mochizuki, M. (1981). The identification of /r/ and /l/ in natural and synthetic speech. *Journal of Phonetics*, *9*, 283–303.

Mueller, T. & Niedzielski, H. (1963). The influence of discrimination training on pronunciation. *Modern Language Journal*, *52*, 410–416.

Navarro Tomas, T. (1950). *Manual de pronunciation española* (6th ed.). Madrid: C.S.I.C.

Oller, J. & Ziahosseiny, S. (1970). The contrastive analysis hypothesis and spelling errors. *Language Learning*, *20*, 183–189.

Ornstein, J. (1974). Mexican–American sociolinguistics. In B. Hoffer & J. Ornstein (Eds.), *Sociolinguistics in the southwest*. San Antonio, TX: Trinity University Press.

Papçun, G. (1976). How may vowel systems differ? *UCLA Working Papers in Phonetics*, *31*, 38–45 (Department of Linguistics, University of California at Los Angeles).

Patkowski, M. (1990). Age and accent in a second language: A reply to James Emil Flege. *Applied Linguistics*, *11*, 73–89.

Peterson, G. & Barney, H. (1952). Control methods used in a study of the vowels. *Journal of the Acoustical Society of America*, *24*, 175–184.

Pisoni, D., Aslin, R., Perey, A., & Hennessey, B. (1982). Some effects of laboratory training on identification and discrimination of voicing contrasts. *Journal of Experimental Psychology: Human Perception and Performance*, *8*, 297–314.

Quiles, A. (1981). *Fonetica Acustica de la Lengua Española*. Madrid: Biblioteca Romanica Hispanica.

Repp, B. (1981). Two strategies in fricative discrimination. *Perception and Psychophysics*, *30*, 217–227.

Repp, B., Healy, A., & Crowder, R. (1979). Categories and context in the perception of isolated steady-state vowels. *Journal of Experimental Psychology: Human Perception and Performance*, *5*, 129–145.

Sapon, S. (1952). An application of psychological theory to pronunciation problems in second language learning. *Modern Language Journal*, *36*, 111–114.

Scholes, R. (1967). Phoneme categorization of synthetic vocalic stimuli by speakers of Japanese, Spanish, Persian, and American English. *Language and Speech*. *10*, 46–68.

Scholes, R. (1968a). Phonemic interference as a perceptual phenomena. *Language and Speech*, *11*, 86–103.

Scholes, R. (1968b). Perceptual categorization of synthetic vowels as a tool in dialectology and typology. *Language and Speech*, *11*, 194–207.

Scovel, T. (1969). Foreign accents, language acquisition, and cerebral dominance. *Language Learning*, *28*, 129–142.

Scovel, T. (1988). *A time to speak. A psycholinguistic inquiry into the critical period for human speech*. New York: Newbury House.

Sheldon, A. & Strange, W. (1982). The acquisition of /r/ and /i/ by Japanese learners of English: Evidence that speech production can precede speech perception. *Applied Psycholingistics*, *3*, 243–261.

Skelton, R. (1969). The pattern of Spanish vowel sounds. *International Review of Applied Linguistics*, *7*, 231–237.

Snedecor, G.W. & Cochrane, W.G. (1980). *Statistical methods*. Ames, IA.: Iowa State University Press.

Stockwell, R. & Bowen, J. (1965). *The sounds of Spanish and English*. Chicago: University of Chicago Press.

Trubetzkoy, N. (1939). *Grundzuge der phonologie*. Berkeley: University of California Press (English translation by C. Baltaxe, 1969).

Valdman, A. (1976). *Introduction to French phonology and morphology*. Rowley, MA: Newbury House.

Weinreich, U. (1953). *Languages in contact, findings and problems*. The Hague: Mouton.

Werker, J. & Logan, J. (1985). Cross-language evidence for three factors in speech perception. *Perception & Psychophysics*, *37*, 35–44.

Werker, J., Klein, R., & Logan, J. (1986). *Auditory, phonetic, and phonemic processing of non-native speech: Optional or obligatory?* Manuscript, Dalhousie University.

Werker, J. & Tees, R. (1983). Developmental changes across childhood in the perception of non-native sounds. *Canadian Journal of Psychology*, *37*, 35–44.

Werker, J. & Tees, R. (1984). Phonemic and phonetic factors in adult cross-language speech perception. *Journal of the Acoustical Society of America*, *75*, 1866–1878.

Wiik, K. (1965). Finnish and English Vowels. *Annals of the University of Turku*, *94* (Turku, Finland).

Wode, H. (1977). The L2 acquisition of /r/. *Phonetica*, *34*, 200–217.

Wode, H. (1978). The beginning of non-school room L2 phonological acquisition. *International Review of Applied Linguistics*, *16*, 109–125.

Revised manuscript received 1 January 1991

THE QUARTERLY JOURNAL OF EXPERIMENTAL PSYCHOLOGY, 1991, *43A* (3) 733–758

The Use of Prosody in Highlighting Alterations in Repairs from Unrestricted Speech

Peter Howell and Keith Young

University College London, University of London, London, U.K.

A speaker has several ways in which he or she may highlight the fact that an error or imprecision of speech has been made and subsequently altered. The three principal ones are by signalling through the structure of the speech that surrounds the error (the repair-syntax), by the use of prosody, and through the semantic content. The role of prosody in the correction process is investigated in the current studies. Analysis of the prosody of a number of errors and their alterations drawn from unrestricted speech are reported. The analysis shows that pauses occur at the moment of interruption and that an increase in stress occurs at the start of the alteration. Pauses could indicate the moment of interruption, and stress could highlight what has been altered. Two sets of perceptual experiments were carried out to assess whether these cues are salient for listeners who hear constructions containing an error and its alteration. Two paradigms were employed in each set of experiments: (1) direct judgement about the comprehensibility of sentences containing errors and alterations, and (2) repeating a message that had an error and alteration without the error. The effects of stress and pauses on (Experiments 1A and 1B) or pauses around (Experiment 2A and 2B) the alterations were assessed. In the first set of experiments it was shown that pauses and stress help listeners process repairs. When a word is spoken in error, the speaker may repeat a section of speech immediately preceding the alteration and/or a section immediately following that word. Inclusion of these repeated sections allows assessment of whether pauses signal where the interruption occurred. The second experiment shows that the placing of the pause before the retrace, rather than at other locations, indicates to listeners where the repair starts.

Requests for reprints should be sent to Peter Howell, Department of Psychology, University College London, Gower Street, London WC1E 6BT, U.K.

This research was supported by grants from the procurement executive of the Ministry of Defence and the Science and Engineering Research Council (SERC) GR/F 92923. The C version of the JSRU synthesizer was written by Mike Johnson, who was supported by a grant from the Wellcome Trust to the first author. Thanks to Helen Jefferson-Brown and Karima Kadi-Hanifi, who helped at many stages, and to Anne Cutler and two anonymous reviewers for helpful comments. Finally, thanks to Quentin Summerfield for his influence on the speedy editorial processing of this manuscript.

When speakers make errors in their speech, they often correct them spontaneously. The entire grammatical structure containing an error can be considered to consist of an original utterance and a repair (Levelt, 1983). Thus, a speaker wanting to say, "Then you turn left at the end of the street", might make an error and produce: "Then you turn right at the, no, turn left at the end of the street". The original utterance in this example starts at the first "turn" and is interrupted after the first "at the". The speaker then gives an explicit indication that a repair is going to be made by use of the word "no". Terms like this are referred to generically as "editing terms".

The repair starts at the second "turn" and continues as far as the second "at the". The type of repair in this example is a lexical error repair (the word "right" is used instead of "left"). In lexical error repairs, the word that is changed is referred to as the reparandum ("right"), and the substituted word as the alteration ("left") (Levelt, 1983). Note that parts of the sentence have been repeated. Thus, in the original utterance, the speaker has continued past the word that is in error (the overshoot, here the first "at the", which is termed the "repeat" on its second saying). In the repair, the speaker has repeated the part of the sentence that preceded the reparandum in the original utterance (in the example the word "turn", referred to when it is placed before the alteration as the retrace). In lexical error repairs, all the components except the reparandum and alteration are optional. However, repeated sections of speech are important as they define the extent and syntax of the repairs. Thus, the overshoot plus repair starts at the first word in the section that will be retraced and the end of the repeat indicates the point at which the repair has been completed.

The question addressed in the present study is what source (or sources) of information a listener uses in such constructions in order to follow the message the speaker intended. There are at least three possible types of information that could be used: semantic, structural (repair-syntactic), and prosodic.[1]

The first type of information, semantic, was investigated by Levelt and Cutler (1983). There are several types of repair besides lexical error repairs, and pertinent for understanding the Levelt and Cutler (1983) study are "appropriateness" repairs. In this type of repair, the speaker does not correct an error but breaks off to replace an utterance with something more precise, as when replacing "brown box" by "big brown box".

Levelt and Cutler (1983) point out that lexical error and appropriateness repairs differ on the semantic dimension and that it is more important to draw attention to information that is incorrect (as in a lexical error repair)

[1] The structural aspects of a repair are to do with its syntax, but the term "structure" is used in preference so as to avoid confusion with wider usage of the term "syntax".

than to something that has been merely elaborated upon (as in an appropriateness repair). Thus, they use the difference in type of repair as a way of deducing how the repairs are arrayed at different points on the semantic dimension. There are other ways in which repairs can differ in their semantic content. For example, an indication of the semantic dimension can occur in speech when a speaker gives an explicit verbal gesture that signals that something has been changed (that is, by use of an editing term such as the "no" used in the example given earlier). These editing terms can often provide a sign that an error is being repaired rather than something more appropriate being said, and, therefore, editing terms play a semantic role. Editing terms might be used when the speaker has to be precise. Therefore, error repairs with editing terms would be higher on the semantic dimension than those without editing terms.

The second source of information that a repair is being made is structural. Levelt (1983, 1989) has given a "well-formedness" rule to characterize the structure of repairs. The rule states that

> An original utterance plus repair ⟨OR⟩ is well formed if and only if there is a string C such that the string ⟨OC or R⟩ is well formed, where C is a completion of the constituent directly dominating the last element of O (or is to be deleted if that last element is itself a connective such as "or" or "and"). [Levelt, 1989, p. 486]

In "There you can park at the left-hand side of the, the right-hand side of the road," the original utterance is "park at the left-hand side of the". The VP "park at the left-hand side of the" can be completed with "road" (=C). The repair (R) is "park at the right-hand side of the road". The coordination thus becomes:

There you can park at the left-hand side of the road or
park at the right-hand side of the road

Depending what original utterance is taken, other well-formed repairs that can be produced are:

There you can park at the left-hand side of the road or
at the right-hand side of the road

There you can park at the left-hand side of the road or
the right-hand side of the road

Retracing to other points is not acceptable by this rule, as the coordinations that result are ill-formed. An example from the sentence being considered is: "There you can park at the left-hand side of the road or can park at the right-hand side of the road". Thus, the rule specifies the relationship between the original utterance and the repair, showing, in particular, what points are possible locations where a speaker could restart after an interruption. If listeners have some knowledge about the association of these structures with the form of repairs, it could be used to predict whether a repair is being made in a stretch of speech.

The third and most apparent indication that a repair is being made is in the prosody of the speech. Prosody is a suprasegmental phenomenon, and schemes for transcribing it allow the patterning of stresses, pauses, and pitch movement, as well as rate variation, nasalization of stretches of speech, and the like to be represented in groups of words. Pauses and pitch movement are self-explanatory; stress refers to an increase in prominence usually due to an increase in loudness of a particular syllable (Crystal, 1985).

Levelt and Cutler (1983) investigated prosodic alterations in lexical error repairs to see how they might indicate to a listener that a repair was being made. The authors looked at the frequency with which the corrections were marked; by "marked" they meant when the alteration differed prosodically from the reparandum (Levelt & Cutler, 1983, p. 212). They found a high incidence of marking on lexical error repairs compared with appropriateness repairs. For Levelt and Cutler (1983), this finding is important, as the two types of repairs differ on the semantic dimension. Thus, for them, prosodic markedness in repairs is related to the semantic dimension. They went on to show that marking is not related to the point at which the interruption occurs, and concluded that speakers do not use intonational marking to indicate to the listener where the item occurred relative to the interruption. Thus, this result appears to show that the marking of a repair is not governed by the structure of a repair.

Speakers need to do two things when they make a repair: (1) indicate that the forward flow of speech has stopped, and (2) make the alteration in such a way that it is intelligible to a listener. Prosody could be used in both of these processes. (1) Often there is a pause when speakers interrupt the flow of speech, which could indicate where the repair starts. The position of such pauses relative to the alteration would depend upon whether or not a retrace occurs. Thus, when a retrace occurs, a pause should occur prior to it, whereas when there is no retrace, the pause should occur prior to the first word of the alteration. (2) Speakers may mark the start of the alteration, as the work of Levelt and Cutler (1983) shows for the case of lexical error repairs. Here we examine the more specific question of whether stress is used to indicate the start of an alteration in an unrestricted set of repairs. It is predicted that in all cases there will be a tendency for the first word of the alteration to be stressed. In the cases where there is no retrace, the alteration will occur immediately after the pause, but the pause will be separated from the alteration by the retrace when such a section occurs. The two sets of perceptual experiments that follow investigate whether the prosody on these constructions aids listeners' perception of what the speaker intended.

REPAIRS IN UNRESTRICTED SPEECH

Levelt's (1983) task involved speakers describing coloured dot patterns arranged rectilinearly, so that a person listening could reproduce the pattern. Here, analysis of a corpus of repairs drawn from unrestricted speech is reported. Pauses that occur at the beginning of a retraced section when none occurred at the corresponding part of speech in the original utterance are compared with the incidence of pauses dropped before the retrace, again in relation to the corresponding position in the original utterance. The first words of the alteration for repairs with and without a retrace are compared to see whether there is a tendency to stress syllables in this word in comparison with the first word of the reparandum. Finally, comparison of pauses and stresses in repairs without a retrace and in those with a retrace allows an assessment of whether pauses indicate where the repair starts, and addition of stress where the alteration begins. In the former case pause and stress should coincide, whereas in the latter pauses should occur at the beginning of the retrace and stress on the (later-occurring) first word of the alteration.

Method

Material Selection. The current corpus of repairs is drawn from the Survey of English Usage (Svartvik & Quirk, 1980). These data comprise conversations between groups of two or more speakers who were not aware that they were being recorded at the time the recordings were being made.[2] The first 391 repairs were selected by one judge and then examined independently by a second judge. Note that no selection was made contingent on the type of repair. Care was taken to ensure that what appeared to be a repair was not a reply to an interruption by another speaker.

In 19 cases (4.9%)[3] it appeared that rather than "repairing" and completing an utterance, the speaker simply abandoned the idea he/she was expressing and began again with a new sentence. This corresponds roughly

[2] The transcriptions are performed by one transcriber and checked by a second, with particular attention being given to prosodic factors (Svartvik & Quirk, 1980, p. 19). No statistical analysis of reliability is available. It is unlikely that any transcriptional biases would influence the current results, as the transcribers could not have been aware that this material would be extracted for specific analysis in this manner.

[3] Percentages are expressed relative to the initial total repairs (391) throughout this article.

with Levelt's D-repairs (where the current message replaces a different one), which account for 1% of his data. The much higher incidence in our corpus is probably accounted for by the fact that Levelt's subjects had a much clearer idea of what it was they intended to say. In unrestricted speech, this is not always the case. Though D repairs could legitimately be considered as part of the repair corpus assembled for other purposes, they are excluded here, as it is likely that the prosody on an abandonment differs from the prosody on other types of repair. In addition, sequences involving overlapping (2, 0.5%) and multiple repairs where a repair was repaired (33, 8.4%) were excluded, again on the basis that there are good reasons to suppose that their prosody would differ from isolated single repairs. The multiple and overlapping repairs were counted as single repairs in the total of 391.

The "disagreements" between judges were invariably about alternative readings of a repair, and each judge admitted these alternative readings: These can be classified into those where it is possible to argue that the utterance was not a repair at all (37 cases—9.5%—including 8 cases where the speaker produced a sequence of the words "yes" and "no") and instances where it was difficult to tell what was intended (13 cases—3.3%). In total, 104 (26.6%) of the original repairs were excluded, 50 because they are open to alternative interpretations (12.8%) and 54 (13.8%) because our taxonomic categories differ from Levelt's.

Finally, the data were partitioned into those with and those without editing terms. In three cases, the editing term occurred after the alteration (1%). These were excluded, as they may be atypical. After these exclusions, a total of 284 repairs remained.[4]

Prosody. The data from the Survey of English Usage are in orthographic form, with prosody marked following Crystal's (1969) scheme. The repairs were phonemically transcribed into a machine-readable form using a convention based upon that used by the Joint Speech Research Unit (JSRU). The JSRU convention allows for primary and secondary stress and pauses of specified duration. The prosodic transcriptions were mapped from those given in the Survey of English Usage to the JSRU convention directly. Kinetic pitch movements, which are marked in the Survey of English Usage, include an obligatory increase in intensity that is equivalent to an increase in stress (Crystal, 1969, p. 143). Therefore all pitch glides that occurred in the

[4] Levelt includes filled pauses (i.e. pauses filled with "erm"s, etc.) as editing terms. However, as their name suggests, they can also be categorized as a type of pause. In the present study it was decided not to count filled pauses as editing terms and to total them separately from unfilled pauses. Any unfilled pause before a filled pause was also ignored, as the convention was to count pauses immediately prior to the designated word.

data were converted to primary stresses. An example of the prepared transcription of the repair "about six months later three months later" is:

/a-bout :siks :munths :"lai-ta ~ = :"three :munths :"lai-ta ~ =

The double quote denotes primary stress (a secondary stress would have been indicated by a single quote). Syllabification within words is shown explicitly by the hyphen unless a primary or secondary stress occurs. An oblique (/) before a word indicates that it is a function word, and a colon (:) that it is a content word. Tone unit boundaries are indicated either by punctuation (none in the above example) or by the symbols ~ =.

Results and Discussion

Table 1 shows the distribution of repairs with and without editing terms. These are classified to show whether the repair contains a retrace, an overshoot, neither, or both (i.e. the structure of the repair). Table 1 shows that there is a marked imbalance in the proportion of repairs with and without editing terms, with only 12 (4.2%) having editing terms. As repairs with editing terms may differ from those without (see the introduction), these were omitted from the following analyses.

The repairs were parsed by computer using a set of symbols designed to distinguish repairs with retraces from those without.[5] The parsing decomposed each repair into the retraced section and the first occurrence of this section of speech, the overshoot and its repeat, and the reparandum and alteration.

Analysis of Retraces. In the introduction it was predicted that pauses would be added at the beginning of the retrace section relative to the occurrence of pauses at this position in the original utterance. No systematic changes in stress pattern (measured by comparison of the first word of the retrace with the corresponding word in the original utterance) would be expected, as no alterations have been made in the retrace section.

TABLE 1
Classification of Repairs with Respect to Whether They Contained a Retrace, an Overshoot, Both, or Neither.

	No Overshoot or Retrace	*Overshoot*	*Retrace*	*Overshoot and Retrace*	*Total*
With editing term	3	4	4	1	12
No editing term	119	43	93	17	272

[5] The parser deals with concatenated and, more importantly, embedded repairs.

The first and second occurrences of the retraced section were aligned syllable by syllable. All prosodic alterations were measured relative to the original utterance (containing the reparandum)—e.g. when no pause (or stress) occurred at a corresponding position in the repaired speech, the pause (or stress) was said to be dropped; if a pause (or stress) only occurred in the repaired speech, it was said to be added.[6] Comparisons were made of corresponding syllables with respect to whether stress was added or dropped or a pause inserted or removed.

The results for pauses and stresses added before the first word of the retrace and on the first word of the retrace (for pauses and stresses, respectively) are shown in Table 2. The three rows at the left of the table give the results for pauses, and these are (in order) the number of repairs where pauses were added or dropped before the first word of the retrace and the total number of repairs (*N*). The data show clearly that, as predicted, there was a marked tendency to add pauses before the first word of the retraced portion. A one-tail sign test shows that there are significantly more added pauses than dropped pauses ($p < 0.001$). The corresponding data on stresses are shown in the three rows on the right. These show that there is no systematic tendency to add stresses ($p > 0.05$). Thus it appears that pauses are used by speakers to indicate the point where the repair starts; stress is not used for this purpose.

TABLE 2
Analysis of Pauses and Stresses on Retraced Sections

	Pauses	*Stresses*
Added	27	1
Dropped	2	2
N	110	110

Note: Comparison was made of the retraced section with its first occurrence. In the left column of the table, the rows present the number of pauses added or dropped before the first word of the retrace relative to the first occurrence of the retraced section. N = total number of repairs with a retraced section. The data for stresses are arranged in similar fashion in the right-hand column.

[6] Increases in stress from no stress to secondary, from secondary to primary, and from no stress to primary stress were counted separately. Similarly decreases in stress from secondary to no stress, from primary to secondary, and from primary to no stress were also counted separately. However, in the analyses reported, only the direction of the change is reported (increase or decrease of stress).

Analysis of First Words of Reparandum/Alteration. It was not possible to classify the type of repair because much depends on a prediction of what the speaker would have continued to say, especially where the moment of interruption occurs within a word. In a constrained task such as Levelt (1983) used, prediction may be possible. In our data, however, it would have involved far too many guesses. Because of this difficulty in assessing the exact relationship of the alterations to the reparanda, and because syntactic structures and number of words often differed in the two, we decided to examine only changes in prosody between the first word following a retrace (or, where no retrace was present, the first word of the repair) and the first word of the reparandum.

To carry out this analysis, it was necessary to exclude more data. Where the "repair" consisted of the insertion of a word or a short phrase ($N=17$, 4.3%), alteration/reparandum comparisons were not made (although the retrace comparisons, reported above, were where applicable). The reason that these data were excluded is that it could be argued that the inserted word does not replace anything.

Because the words to be compared frequently had a differing number of syllables, syllable alignment, as done with retraced sections, was not possible. The pause comparison was therefore made on the pauses before the first syllable of each word, and the stress comparison on the highest stress on any syllable of each word.

The data for the first word of the alteration are presented in Table 3 in a similar way to the retrace data (Table 2). Here, though, the data are also displayed depending on whether there had been a retrace prior to the alteration or not.

For the cases that had no retrace (and had no editing term), there was a significant tendency to add rather than drop pauses before the alteration

TABLE 3
Analysis of Pauses and Stresses on the First Word of the Reparandum and Alteration

	Pauses		*Stresses*	
	No Retrace	*Retrace*	*No Retrace*	*Retrace*
Added	38	5	41	19
Dropped	5	4	7	4
N	149	106	149	106

Note: Comparison was made of the first word of the alteration with the first word of the reparandum. In the left-hand columns of the table, the rows present the number of pauses added or dropped before the first word of the retrace relative to the first occurrence of the retraced section. N = total number of repairs with a retraced section. The data for stresses are arranged in similar fashion in the right-hand columns.

($p < 0.01$ by sign test), but there was no such tendency when there had been a retrace ($p > 0.05$). In the former case the pause is occurring at the point where the repair is starting, but this point is not the start of the repair in the latter. Thus, taken in conjunction with the data on retraces, it appears that a pause serves the function of indicating that a repair is being made.

It can be seen in Table 3 that stresses were added on the alteration, whether or not a retrace had occurred. In both cases significantly more stresses were added than dropped on the first word ($p < 0.001$ by sign test in each case). Moreover, the tendency to add stresses is particularly marked when a retrace occurs. The addition of stress on the first word of the alteration shows that this factor is used by speakers to indicate that the speech being altered has started.

In summary, the data show that a pause is produced by a speaker to indicate that the forward flow of speech has been interrupted; the first word of the alteration carries higher stress than does the first word of the reparandum.

PERCEPTUAL ASSESSMENT OF PROSODY IN REPAIRS

The cues that speakers use to indicate where a repair starts and what has been altered may also be used by listeners to ascertain whether and at what point information is being changed in a repair. The following experiments examined the role of prosodic factors in aiding listeners in their perception of repaired speech. In Experiments 1A and 1B, the original utterance contained a one-word reparandum, and the repair was also one word. Thus the contribution that an increase in stress or the addition of a pause around an alteration makes to the ease with which a message is perceived was addressed. In Experiments 2A and 2B, a retrace was included in the repair, and the influence of pauses at the beginning of the retrace was examined. In these experiments, prosodic alterations were systematically introduced onto repairs by editing the transcriptions of actual spoken sentences. These transcriptions were then used to drive a synthesis-by-rule system to produce stimuli for perceptual assessments. Assessments could than be made about what prosodic factors influence listeners with repairs of different structures.

Improvements in comprehension due to the prosodic alterations are assessed in two ways: (1) A group of speakers was asked for a direct judgement about which of two versions of the same sentence would be the easier to comprehend (direct assessment of comprehensibility). The two versions of the sentence presented to the listener were the baseform and one of the versions with prosody altered. The pattern of preferences for the prosodically altered versions of the sentences indicates which prosodic factor or factors influence judged comprehensibility of repaired sentences. This procedure was adopted in Experiments 1A and 2A. (2) In the second test procedure (speech repair task) the listeners first heard a synthesized sentence. The sentence might contain either an altered or repeated word, and, in each case, the speaker had to respond by repeating the message the speaker intended without the erroneous or duplicated material. The measure taken was the time to initiate speech (Sternberg, Monsell, Knoll, & Wright, 1978). In this task, subjects have to monitor the speech until they hear a tone indicating that the sentence is complete. They then make their response. The time from indication that the complete speech has been delivered to the speaker's initiation of the response reflects the amount of time taken up in processing the sentence and organizing the response. Earlier speech initiations indicate, therefore, that the speaker is able to disambiguate the speech more rapidly. Shorter initiation time with the sentences that have prosody altered would indicate that the speaker is able to process that type of speech more rapidly and, therefore, would show what prosodic factors aid processing of repairs. This procedure was adopted in Experiments 1B and 2B.

It is hypothesized that pauses indicate the start of the repair and stress the start of the alteration. In Experiments 1A and 1B the positions of pauses and stresses were correlated: There the intention is to assess whether either or both cues influence these judgements. In Experiments 2A and 2B the influence of pauses on processing, when they are placed at locations other than immediately before the alteration, is assessed.

GENERAL PROCEDURE FOR STIMULUS PREPARATION: EXPERIMENTS 1A AND 1B

The types of repairs used in Experiments 1A and 1B contain neither an overshoot nor a retrace. An example is: "She moved to a different school class in Barnet." The baseline version of such a sentence would have no pause after the reparandum (school), nor any stress on the alteration (class). Prosody can then be systematically added on and around the alteration, to create three further versions of each sentence, one with an added stress on the alteration, one with a pause preceding the alteration, and one with both of these additions. In this section the material used in Experiments 1A and 1B is described.

Materials

The original sentences from which the test materials were derived were extracted from recorded dictation. These sentences were available on dictaphone tapes that were being made as part of the speaker's normal work. Dictaphone material was used because it is spontaneous speech, with the added advantage that the speaker is motivated to speak grammatically. Recordings from four male speakers who were experienced dictaphone users were available. None of these speakers dictated from notes nor, in the recordings used, switched off the dictaphone machine during the parts of the message that were selected. The content of the tapes was routine letters/memoranda about academic and associated administrative matters.[7]

Conditions imposed for selection of sentence material for the experiment were that there should be equal numbers of sentences from each of the four speakers. No names were allowed in the sentences in order to maintain the anonymity of the speaker. To ensure that the sentences sounded natural, recordings that contained instructions concerning number of copies, punctuation, etc. were excluded. The original sentences did not include any errors, so the repair and prosody in the immediate vicinity of a repair were all introduced.

Seventy-two sentences were used in the current experiment. The same selection criteria (detailed below) applied to all sentences. These sentences were split into one group of 36 in which an altered word was introduced, and a second group of 36 in which a word was repeated.

The sentences were transcribed according to the conventions described in connection with the analysis of the Survey of English Usage data. The transcription of the example "She moved to a different school class in Barnet" is:

/shee :"muuvd /tuu /a :'dif-rant :skuul /in :"bar-nit.

The word selected as reparandum had to be a single-syllable noun, verb, or adverb (a noun in the example). These were at the end of a constituent (here, at the end of the NP "to a different school"). The constituents were not at tone-unit boundaries, and the nucleus occurred in the remainder of the sentence. These constraints guaranteed that when the alteration was inserted and the prosodic manipulations introduced, the prosody sounded natural. All repairs were "well-formed" according to Levelt's rule. The latter constraint was included so that when the repairs were constructed, the structure was appropriate.

---

[7] The tapes were collected but not used for preparation of experimental material, nor listened to until permission to use them had been given. Thus, at the time of making the recordings, the speaker did not know that the tapes would be used for anything other than the purpose intended. The speakers were then offered the opportunity of checking that the tapes contained no confidential material before anyone was allowed to listen to them. All speakers gave permission for their tapes to be used.

The alteration had to be a single-syllable word. The types of reparandum-to-alteration changes were opposites (as in the right/left example used in the introduction), exchange of common nouns (school/class), and change in numerals. Changes in verbs included tense changes (e.g. "was"/"is") and inter-substitution of full verbs (e.g. "have"/"spend", "see"/"find"). In the example, "She moved to a different school in Barnet", "class" was inserted as the alteration to produce the repair:

/shee :"muuvd /tuu /a :'dif-rant :skuul :klars /in :"bar-nit.

To produce the repetition material, the alteration was not included, and the word used as the reparandum was repeated. The constraints imposed on selection of position of the alteration always led to a sentence with a repeated word such as a speaker would produce. This type of material is appropriate as a control as it is similar in all respects to the alteration with regard to its influence on the temporal, prosodic, lexical, and syntactical properties.

Preparation of Prosodic Variants

So far the baseform sentences (including the altered or repeated word) have been described. Three additional versions of each baseform sentence were produced by editing symbols on to the transcription which indicated (Version a) a pause of 200-msec duration between alteration and reparandum, (Version b) a loudness increase and durational change corresponding to a primary stress on the alteration, (Version c) adding both a pause and stress at these positions. (The rules for durational change are given in Edward, 1982. The increase in loudness was an introduced modification.)

ORIGINAL

/shee :"muuvd /tuu /a :'dif-rant :skuul :klars /in :"bar-nit.

VERSION WITH ADDED PAUSE

/shee :"muuvd /tuu /a :'dif-rant :skuul QQQQ :klars /in :"bar-nit
where the Qs are used here to indicate a pause (multiples of 50 msec).

VERSION WITH ADDED STRESS

/shee :"muuvd /tuu /a :'dif-rant :skuul :"klars /in :"bar-nit.

VERSION WITH ADDED PAUSE AND STRESS

/shee :"muuvd /tuu /a :'dif-rant :skuul QQQQ :"klars /in :"bar-nit.

Synthesis

The transcriptions of the sentences were used to drive a synthesis-by-rule programme based on the Joint Speech Research Unit synthesis-by-rule scheme (Edward, 1982; Holmes, 1988; Holmes, Mattingly, & Shearme, 1964). Phonemes are specified in the programme as target formant frequency values. In the case of vowels, these targets specify the ideal frequency that would be aimed for in long isolated utterances. Consonants are specified as locus formant frequencies (Delattre, Liberman, & Cooper, 1955) and transition rules for changing between targets. A rank is specified which governs the influence of a particular phoneme when it is part of a group of phonemes that would result in the sounds having overlapping transitions.

The output of the synthesis-by-rule programme produces a frame of control parameters at 10-msec intervals, which represent the time-varying values for a parallel formant synthesizer. The parallel formant synthesizer is based on that described in Holmes (1983) and can be either a hardware (Loughborough Sound Images) or software version. The hardware version was used for the recordings where a direct judgement task was made and the software version when speakers had to repeat the sentence. Both versions of the synthesizer are controlled by ten parameters—amplitude and formant frequency of three vocal tract and one nasal formant; the amplitude of a higher pole correction factor and a voicing switch. The fundamental frequency of excitation is calculated in a similar fashion, with a declination over a tone unit and local variations superimposed on the nuclear syllables as specified by the punctuation (e.g. rising for a question). The altered or repeated words were not close to these pitch movements and, so, were not influenced by them.

EXPERIMENT 1A

In Experiment 1A subjects were presented with the baseline version of each sentence and one of the versions with prosody altered. They were asked to indicate which of the two sentences would be the easier to comprehend. The pattern of preferences for the sentences would indicate whether pauses, stresses, or both are judged to aid comprehension of the repair.

Method

Subjects. Twelve undergraduate volunteers, seven female and five male, were paid for participating.

Procedure. The control parameter output was used to control the hardware synthesizer directly. Listeners were told that they would hear synthesized copies of real speech that sometimes had a word that had been altered and sometimes had a repeated word. They were told that they would hear two versions of each sentence, after which they would have to indicate which of the sentence forms they would judge to be the easier to comprehend if it were spoken in real speech.

Each listener made judgements on all 36 sentences including an alteration and all 36 including a repetition (all received 12 pairs per prosodic-alteration version). Each sentence was presented to the listener in two forms, one with no prosodic change introduced on the alteration, the other being one of the other three versions of the sentence in which the prosody was altered. The type of the non-baseform version of each sentence was counterbalanced across listeners, so each sentence was heard with the different prosodic types an equal number of times across the group of listeners. The order of occurrence of baseform/non-baseform type was counterbalanced across sentences and listeners. The order of sentences with altered or repeated words was randomized across listeners. There was a 2-sec pause between each sentence in a pair and a 5-sec pause between sentence pairs.

Results and Discussion

The number of occasions on which a preference was indicated by a listener for each of the altered versions over the baseform of the sentence was ascertained. The scores so obtained are out of a maximum of 12 for each prosodic alteration/baseline pair. Thus, for each listener, scores for sentences that include an altered or repeated word separately for the three types of prosodic alteration were obtained. The data, averaged across listeners, are presented in Table 4 (the mean number of preferences for the baseline condition in a pair is 12 minus the tabulated value). The data were analysed by a repeated measures analysis of variance (ANOVA), with factors alteration condition (alteration versus repetition) and prosodic alteration (stress, pause preceding, or both stress and a preceding pause on the alteration or repetition).

Sentences with altered prosody were preferred on a greater number of occasions when an altered word was included compared with when the sentence had a repeated word (the mean number of preferences for prosodically altered versions in the alteration condition was 9 and 6.3 in the

TABLE 4
Mean Preferences Across Twelve Listeners for the Conditions in Experiment 1A

	Pause Added	*Stress Added*	*Pause and Stress Added*
Alteration	9.33	8.00	9.67
Repetition	6.25	6.17	6.50

Note: All values are out of a maximum of 12.

repetition condition, with both scores out of a maximum of 12), $F(1, 11) = 23.8$, $p < 0.01$. Note that in the repetition condition sentences with no prosodic alteration were preferred about as often as prosodically altered sentences (5.7 out of 12 occasions, compared with 6.3 out of 12, respectively).

There was a significant main effect of type of prosodic alteration, $F(2, 22) = 5.8$, $p < 0.05$, and this factor interacted with alteration/repetition condition, $F(2, 22) = 7.5$, $p < 0.01$. The interaction was decomposed using a Newman–Keuls test. This showed that there were no significant differences between the types of prosodic alteration in the repetition conditions (all $ps > 0.05$), but that all had significantly lower scores than those for each of the prosodic alterations made on the alteration material ($p < 0.05$ or better in all cases). Material where there was addition of a pause, or a pause and stress, was significantly different from that which only had a stress on the alteration ($p < 0.05$). The material with alteration to stress alone was judged as less comprehensible than the other types.

In summary, the evidence from this experiment indicates that judgements about the comprehensibility of repaired speech are affected by two prosodic factors: stress and pauses. In Experiment 1B this finding is examined further using a different experimental task.

EXPERIMENT 1B

An indication about which form of prosody on two otherwise identical sentences containing a repair makes the sentence most comprehensible offers little indication about speakers' ability to process the repair on-line. In Experiment 1B, to verify the conclusions from Experiment 1A, subjects were required to repeat sentences that contained altered or repeated words with the form of that sentence which excludes these materials.

As in experiment 1A, pauses and stresses were added around the altered and repeated words. Utterance initiation time was measured; if pauses and stress aid the processing of repairs, shorter initiation times would be expected when sentences included these prosodic cues than when no such cues occurred in the sentences. As the concern is whether prosody helps listeners process repairs, initiation times to sentences with reparanda/alterations but no introduced pauses or stresses were compared with responses to prosodically altered forms of the sentences.

It could be argued that the addition of pauses increases the presentation time of sentences and that this allows more time for processing the sentences. Similarly, arguments could be made about the durational changes associated with syllables that carry stress (Edward, 1982). In each case, the longer processing time allowed might result in faster initiation times. Material that contained a repeated word controls for this possibility: If the initiation times are associated with processing of prosody irrespective of the type of construction, differences should occur in material that contains either an altered or a repeated word. If differences in initiation times contingent on prosody are due to extra processing time associated with the alteration, then these should occur only for sentences containing an altered word

Method

Subjects. Eight undergraduate volunteers, four speakers of each sex, were paid for participating.

Materials. The sentences used were as for Experiment 1A.

Procedure. Control parameter outputs were used as input to the software synthesizer to produce a digital version of the speech, which was stored as a computer file for further processing.

In preliminary work, it was found that the task was too easy if speech was played straight from the synthesizer, giving no differences in reaction time. Speech-correlated noise (Schroeder, 1968) was synthesized and added to the speech before the recording was made. The speech-correlated noise was produced by randomly reversing the polarity of speech samples so that positive values became negative and vice versa. The reversing was determined by the value of a random varying binary variable (Schroeder, 1968). This produces noise whose intensity varies directly with that of speech. The latter is important here to ensure that the speech:noise ratio is constant when, for example, comparing responses to stressed and unstressed syllables that vary in their intensity. A speech:noise ratio of +6 dB was used.

The type of alteration to be made to each sentence (inclusion of an altered or repeated word), and the type of prosodic change for each subject was established. Once this had been decided, the order in which sentences would occur was randomized, and a test tape was prepared for each subject.

The sentences were recorded on tape, and a 200-msec duration, 1-kHz tone indicated that the trial had started; 200 msec later, the synthetic version of the sentence with added signal-correlated noise was played, and 200 msec after the end of the sentence the 200-msec tone was played again, to indicate that the subject could start his/her response. After the tone, there was a 20-sec gap before the next sentence was played. A practice tape was prepared in the same way, consisting of eight sentences (one of each type of alteration and prosodic change). This tape was the same for all subjects. The practice and test tapes were played to the subjects from a Revox B77 over headphones.

Subjects were informed that they would hear a synthetic version of a sentence, after which they would hear a tone burst. This tone burst indicated that the sentence was complete, and that they should begin their response.

The experimenter drew attention to the fact that each sentence would include either an altered or a repeated word, although subjects would not know which would occur before they heard the sentence. Each subject was instructed that his/her task was to repeat the sentence, but with the repeated word or reparandum excluded. The subjects were told that they had to perform this task as quickly as possible, but they should not make any mistakes such as missing material out. No mention was made of prosodic variation between sentences, nor was any mimicking of prosody noted in the subjects' responses.

Each listener made responses to all 72 sentences. A particular sentence could be spoken in one of eight ways—with a repetition or alteration and with one of the four forms of prosodic change—no change, added stress, pause, or both. Each subject heard and responded to only one of these forms of each sentence. For each subject, repetitions and alterations were presented an equal number of times across sentences, as were versions with each of the four prosodic alterations (each of the eight conditions was presented nine times). In addition, type of alteration (repeated/altered word) and type of prosodic change were balanced across subjects, so that all of the eight versions of a sentence were presented once to each of the eight subjects.

The sentence the subject heard and response (from a microphone) were recorded on two tracks of a Revox B77. The experimenter monitored the subject's accuracy at the time of the recordings. This monitoring showed that subjects could perform this task without error.

Results and Discussion

Each sentence was digitised at 10 kHz for timing measurements. For each of the sentences, the time from the start of the tone to the start of speech was measured from displayed digital oscillograms.

The data from each alteration condition (repetition or alteration) and prosodic change type within these (no alteration to prosody, added stress, added pause, stress and pause added) were extracted. The mean initiation time for each of these eight conditions was calculated for the individual subjects. Averages of these values over the eight subjects are shown in Table

TABLE 5
Mean Initiation Times for Repetition of Repaired Speech for Sentences Containing an Alteration or Repetition in Experiment 1B

	No Prosodic Change	*Pause Added*	*Stress Added*	*Pause and Stress Added*
Alteration	3.45	2.75	3.06	2.68
Repetition	2.33	2.11	2.09	2.15

Note: Mean initiation times in seconds.

5. The data were analysed by a repeated-measures ANOVA with factors alteration condition (two levels), prosodic change type (four levels), and subjects.

The main effect of alteration condition was significant, $F(1, 7) = 13.9$, $p < 0.01$. This was due to the initiation times being shorter for repetition than for alteration. The difference between the prosodic change types was significant, $F(3, 21) = 4.7$, $p < 0.05$. The main differences between these occurred when the sentence contained an alteration as shown by the interaction between alteration condition and prosodic change type, $F(3, 21) = 6.8$, $p < 0.01$.

The latter interaction was examined by a Newman–Keuls test. This showed that there were no significant differences between prosodic alterations when the material contained a repeated word (all ps > 0.05), although the initiation times in the repetition conditions were significantly shorter than all the initiation times when an alteration had occurred in the material. Comparisons showed that sentences containing alterations that had introduced prosody had significantly different initiation from those where there was no prosodic alteration. Similarly, initiation times to sentences with change made to stress alone were significantly longer than when either of the other prosodic alterations was made. There was no difference between the initiation times when alteration had been made to pause or pause and stress.

Thus the results substantially confirm those obtained from direct judgements about comprehensibility (Experiment 1A); those conditions with an altered word that had received the higher ratings concerning comprehensibility were responded to faster than those with lower ratings. One additional finding here is that the prosodic change condition with addition of stress alone was repeated significantly faster than when no prosodic change was made. Thus, stress appears to aid repetition of repaired speech. Finally, the faster responses to the material with a repeated word indicate that the process of understanding speech with an altered word is more difficult than repeating material with a repeated word.

Summary

In sum, the results of Experiments 1A and 1B show that processing of repairs is influenced by the presence of a pause prior to the alteration. Though it is possible to argue that asking for a judgement about the comprehensibility of sentences (Experiment 1A) only assesses processing of repairs indirectly, it is difficult to see how such an argument could be made for the case where listeners had to repeat the correct form of a sentence containing an altered word (Experiment 1B). It seems, therefore, that a pause before and/or stress on an altered word influence processing of repairs by listeners. Also, the fact that both pauses and stresses influence performance leaves open the possibility that listeners, like speakers, use these factors as an indication of the position where the repair starts and the start of the alteration, respectively. However, it is also possible that pauses, like stresses, indicate where the alteration starts. To check whether listeners use pauses to ascertain that a repair has started or not, material is used in the following experiments where pauses do not occur immediately prior to the alteration.

GENERAL PROCEDURE FOR STIMULUS PREPARATION: EXPERIMENTS 2A AND 2B

To ascertain whether pauses signal the start of a repair, material is needed where pauses can be inserted at different points in the repair when none of the positions used coincides with the start of the alteration. This can be achieved by using materials that include retraces and repeats. Pauses can then be inserted before the repeat or retrace. The prediction tested in the experiments below (Experiments 2A and 2B) is that conditions where the pause occurs prior to a retrace (i.e. at the start of the repair) will be judged more comprehensible (Experiment 2A) and responded to faster (Experiment 2B) than pauses introduced before the repeat.

Materials

Dictaphone material was employed, as in Experiments 1A and 1B. A total of 120 sentences was selected. The selection criteria were the same as those in Experiments 1A and 1B.

Preparation of Materials

As the interest here is in the material surrounding a reparandum/alteration, the inserted word in the repairs and controls was neither preceded by a pause, nor did it carry stress. Five altered versions of each sentence were produced. These were illustrated (for a case that includes an altered word):

1. retrace alone, introduced with a pause preceding it:

   /shee :"muuvd /tuu /a :'dif-rant :skuul QQQQ /tuu /a :'dif-rant :klars /in :"bar-nit.

2. repeat alone, introduced with a pause preceding it:

   /shee :"muuvd /tuu /a :'dif-rant :skuul /in :"bar-nit :klars QQQQ /in :"bar-nit.

When the repair contains both a retrace and repeat, pause/s were included on

3. the retrace only:

   /shee :"muuvd /tuu /a :'dif-rant :skuul /in :"bar-nit QQQQ /tuu /a :'dif-rant :klars /in :"bar-nit.

4. only on the repeat:

   /shee :"muuvd /tuu /a :'dif-rant :skuul /in :"bar-nit /tuu /a :'dif-rant :klars QQQQ /in :"bar-nit.

and

5. on both the repeat and retrace:

   /shee :"muuvd /tuu /a :'dif-rant :skuul /in :"bar-nit QQQQ /tuu /a :'dif-rant :klars QQQQ /in :"bar-nit.

The baseform for each sentence was the corresponding version without the pause or pauses.

EXPERIMENT 2A

The analyses reported earlier showed that pauses occur at the beginning of a retrace. If pauses in this position indicate to listeners the position where the repair starts, then these positions should be judged more comprehensible and be repeated more quickly than repairs with pauses at other points.

Method

Subjects. Eight female and four male subjects were used.

Procedure. The sentences were split into two groups of 60—one group including a repeated word, and the other including an altered word. The control parameter outputs were used to drive the hardware synthesizer. The task was described to subjects in the same way as in Experiment 1A. The listeners made judgements about all pairs of prosodically altered/baseform combinations for both the set with a repeated and those with an altered word. On each trial, the sentence was presented in its baseform (i.e. the version without the pause) and in one of the corresponding versions with prosody altered. There were five types of baseform/prosodic alteration condition combination, and these were presented 12 times each. Subjects indicated which they judged the easier to comprehend, as they did in Experiment 1A.

Results and Discussion

The results were analysed in a similar way to Experiment 1A, with the number of preferences expressed for the prosodically altered sentence being calculated. The averages of these across listeners are presented in Table 6. The ANOVA examined the effects of alteration condition as before (alteration versus repetition), but there were now five prosodic alteration types.

There was a significant difference between responses in the alteration and repetition conditions, $F(1, 11) = 33.2$, $p < 0.01$. As in Experiment 1A, there were fewer preferences expressed for the prosodically altered versions of the sentences for the material that included a repeated word compared with that for material with an altered word.

The main effect of prosodic change type was significant, $F(4, 44) = 13.2$, $p < 0.01$, as was the interaction of this factor with alteration/repetition condition, $F(4, 44) = 5.7$, $p < 0.01$. The interaction was examined by a Newman–Keuls test. All types of prosodic change with a repeated word yielded lower scores than all prosodic changes with an altered word (all $ps < 0.05$ or better). This outcome shows that prosodic change was only effective at improving the comprehensibility of repaired material, not the controls with a repeated word.

For comparisons of different types of prosodic change made between sentences with an alteration, the only significant differences involved the conditions that include adding a pause solely on the repeat (Types 2 and 4 in the general procedure section for this experiment). The altered prosody version of these sentences was chosen significantly less often than in each of the other prosodic change types (although note that this was still preferred to the prosodic alterations made in the sentences with a repeated word). The difference between pauses introduced before a repeat alone (Type 2) or along with a retrace (Type 4) was not significant.

TABLE 6
Mean Preferences Across Twelve Listeners for the Conditions in Experiment 2A

			Retrace and Repeat		
	(1) Retrace and Pause	*(2) Repeat and Pause*	*(3) Pause on Retrace*	*(4) Pause on Repeat*	*(5) Pause on Both*
Alteration	10.17	8.33	10.25	8.5	10.5
Repetition	6.17	6.67	6.25	6.0	6.25

Note: All values are out of a maximum of 12.

Speakers prefer sentences with a pause at the start of a repair to sentences that have a pause at another position. This applies whether the sentence has a retrace alone or retrace plus repeat. In the current experiment the position of pauses never coincided with the point where the altered word occurred. Thus, this rules out the possibility that pauses are used to indicate the start of the alteration, as discussed in connection with Experiments 1A and 1B.

EXPERIMENT 2B

As discussed earlier, it may be that differences between judgements about repair comprehensibility for repairs that have differences in prosody is not directly related to how listeners process these repairs. The current experiment uses the speech repair task (Experiment 1B) with the material employed in Experiment 2A.

Method

Subjects. Ten subjects (five of each sex) were employed; they were drawn from the same pool as those used in the earlier experiments.

Procedure. The software synthesizer output was used to produce a digital version of the speech. Signal-correlated noise was added at the same level as in Experiment 1B.

In Experiment 1B, there was only a single baseform. Here, there are five baseforms, corresponding to those numbered in the general introduction for these experiments. These would be needed for both the alteration and repetition condition. If all of the baseforms had been included, this would have resulted in an unmanageably large number of conditions and trials. The repetition conditions that correspond to each of the alteration conditions were used as an appropriate basis for assessing how pauses aid processing of repairs. Thus, the five prosodic types for the alteration condition were compared with the corresponding five types for the repetition condition (10 conditions in total). All 120 sentences were used for the test material, and each subject responded to 12 sentences for each of the 10 conditions. The sentences were counterbalanced across the 10 subjects, so that each sentence was given to each subject in only one of its forms.

The type of change to be made to each sentence (repetition or alteration), and prosodic type for each subject were established. Once this had been decided, the order in which the sentences would occur was randomized, and a test tape was prepared for each subject.

In all other respects, the procedure was the same as in the corresponding condition in Experiment 1B.

Results and Discussion

The data for the initiation times were analysed in similar fashion to that for the corresponding condition in Experiment 1B. The mean initiation times, calculated as in Experiment 1B, are presented in Table 7. These were entered into an ANOVA that included alteration condition (alteration/repetition) and prosodic alteration type.

The ANOVA showed that the main effect of alteration condition, $F(1, 9) = 13.3$, $p < 0.01$, and of prosodic change type, $F(4, 36) = 9.1$, $p < 0.01$, and their interaction, were significant, $F(4, 36) = 5.5$, $p < 0.01$. As in Experiment 1B, the data on the speech repair task are consistent with those from the direct judgement task; the initiation times are faster when the sentence contained a repeated word than when it contained an altered word. Newman–Keuls tests showed that there were no differences between the prosodic types in the repetition condition. The only difference between the prosodic types in the alteration condition was that the types with pauses before the retrace (numbered 1, 3, and 4 in the general introduction) were responded to significantly faster than the remaining types, which do not have pauses prior to the retrace. The differences between prosodic types 1 and 2 and between 3 and 4 are of particular note as, with the counterbalancing performed across subjects, the designated pairs do not differ in length. Therefore, the faster responses in prosodic types that have a pause before the retrace (Types 1 and 2) compared with sentences that have equivalent lengths but a pause before the repeat (Types 3 and 4, respectively) show that the positioning of the pause aids processing of the repair. As the pauses are at the start of the repair but not at the start of the alteration, as in Experiment 1A, the data confirm that a pause is used to signal the start of the repair.

Conclusions

The experiments reported used the analysis of a corpus of repairs drawn from unrestricted speech as a basis for hypotheses about what prosodic factors

TABLE 7
Mean Initiation Times for Repetition of Repaired Speech for Sentences Containing an Alteration or Repetition in Experiment 2B

			Retrace and Repeat		
	(1) Retrace and Pause	*(2) Repeat and Pause*	*(3) Pause on Retrace*	*(4) Pause on Repeat*	*(5) Pause on Both*
Alteration	2.91	3.42	3.21	3.79	3.33
Repetition	2.44	2.55	2.39	2.65	2.74

Note: Mean initiation times in seconds.

listeners might attend to in order to follow a speaker's intent in such circumstances. The analysis showed that pauses occur at the start of repairs, whether or not the repair includes a retrace. In addition, speakers stress the first word of the alteration in comparison with the first word of the reparandum. These findings were interpreted as indicating that speakers use pauses to signal where a repair starts and stress to indicate where the altered material begins. As pauses are a prosodic factor and their location depends on whether or not a retrace occurs, this analysis shows that prosody is related to the structure of a repair.

The two perceptual experiments assess whether listeners use these cues to process the information in repairs. In Experiments 1A and 1B, pauses and stress on the alteration were assessed. From the results of this experiment it appears that a 200-msec pause and loudness and durational changes corresponding to primary stress influence listeners' judgements and processing of repairs. The importance of pauses was emphasized in the analyses as highlighting where repairs start in speech. Similarly, the influence of stress appears to be tied up with the start of the alteration—at the point where the alteration starts there is a tendency for speakers to use a higher stress than on the corresponding word in the reparandum, and the significant interaction with stress in Experiments 1A and 1B indicates that listeners are sensitive to this factor.

In Experiments 1A and 1B, stress and pause position were correlated so the interpretation of whether pauses are used to signal where the repair starts is circumstantial; pauses could be an additional cue indicating where the alteration starts. In Experiments 2A and 2B, the influence of pauses when placed at different positions within repairs was investigated. Here it was found that a pause before the retrace (preceding the alteration) aids the listener in perceiving the message, but that a pause before the repeat (following the alteration) does not. This would indicate that listeners use pauses as an indication about where the repair starts.

Finally, why is pausing helpful in indicating the start of a repair for listeners? Continuity of the prosodic contour is important for speech perception (Buxton, 1983). Consequently, interruption of this contour—by a pause, for example—is one way in which the speaker signals that ongoing processing should be interrupted. Of course, stress could also be used to interrupt the contour. However, the scope for variation in prosodic contours is so great that stress at the start of a repair would not constitute an unusual contour. It would not serve therefore to alert the listener that a repair is being made in the way a pause does. Once the prosodic break has been noted by the listener, comparison of the stress of the prosody of the retrace with that on the first occurrence of this section of speech can aid listeners in establishing what the speaker intended to alter.

REFERENCES

Buxton, H. (1983). Temporal predictability of English speech. In A. Cutler & D.R. Ladd (Eds.), *Prosody: Models and measurements*. Berlin: Springer-Verlag.

Crystal, D. (1969). *Prosodic systems and intonation in English*. London: Cambridge University Press.

Crystal, D. (1985). *A dictionary of linguistics and phonetics*. Oxford: Blackwell.

Delattre, P.C., Liberman, A.M., & Cooper, F.S. (1955). Acoustic loci and transitional cues for consonants. *Journal of the Acoustical Society of America*, *27*, 769–773.

Edward, J.A. (1982). Rules for synthesizing the prosodic feature of speech. *Joint Speech Research Unit Report* (no. 1015).

Holmes, J.N. (1983). Formant synthesizers: cascade or parallel? *Speech Communication*, *2*, 251–273.

Holmes, J.N. (1988). *Speech synthesis and recognition*. Wokingham: Van Nostrand Reinhold.

Holmes, J.N., Mattingly, I.G., & Shearme, J.N. (1964). Speech synthesis by rule. *Language and Speech*, *7*, 127–143.

Levelt, W.J.M. (1983). Monitoring and self-repair in speech. *Cognition*, *14*, 41–104.

Levelt, W.J.M. (1989). *Speaking: From intent to articulation*. Cambridge, MA: M.I.T. Press.

Levelt, W.J.M. & Cutler, A. (1983). Prosodic marking in speech repair. *Journal of Semantics*, *2*, 205–217.

Schroeder, M.R. (1968). Reference signal for signal quality studies. *Journal of the Acoustical Society of America*, *44*, 1735–1736.

Sternberg, S., Monsell, S., Knoll, R.L., & Wright, C.E. (1978). The latency and duration of rapid movement sequences: Comparisons of speech and typing. In G.E. Stelmach (Ed.), *Information control in motor control and learning*. New York: Academic Press.

Svartvik, J. & Quirk, R. (1980). *A corpus of English conversation*. Lund: Gleerup.

Revised manuscript received 31 December 1990

Publications Received

Bruce, V. & Green, P.R. (1990). *Visual perception: Physiology, psychology and ecology* (2nd ed.). Hove: Lawrence Erlbaum Associates. Pp. 431. ISBN 0–86377–146–7. Hardback £24.95; paperback £11.95.

Cromer, R.F. (1991). *Language and thought in normal and handicapped children.* Oxford: Blackwell. Pp. 341. ISBN 0–631–14526–5. Hardback £35.00; paperback £10.95.

Graham, N.V.S. (1989). *Visual pattern analyzers.* Oxford: Oxford University Press. Pp. 646. ISBN 0–19–505154–8. Paperback £13.50.

Johnson-Laird, P.N. & Byrne, R.M.J. (1991). *Deduction.* Hove: Lawrence Erlbaum Associates. Pp. 243. ISBN 0–86377–148–3. £14.95.

Joshi, R.M. (Ed.). (1991). *Written language disorders.* Dordrecht: Kluwer Academic Publishers. Pp. 196. ISBN 0–7923–0902–2. £56.50.

Krumhansl, C.L. (1990). *Cognitive foundations of musical pitch.* Oxford: Oxford University Press. Pp. 307. ISBN 0–19–505475–X. £45.00.

Monk, A. (1991). *Exploring statistics with MiniTab: A workbook for the behavioural sciences.* Chichester: John Wiley & Sons. Pp. 247. ISBN 0–471–92391–5. £11.95.

Narmour, E. (1991). *The analysis and cognition of basic melodic structures: The implication-realization model.* Chicago: University of Chicago Press. Pp 485. ISBN 0–226–56845–8. £47.95.

Rosenbaum, D.A. (1990). *Human motor control.* San Diego: Academic Press. Pp. 411. ISBN 0–12–597300–4. $35.90.

Sawyer, D.J. & Fox, B.J. (Eds.). (1991). *Phonological awareness in reading: The evolution of current perspectives.* Heidelberg: Springer-Verlag. Pp 262. ISBN 3–5140–97308–7. DM 92.00.

Siegal, M. (1991). *Knowing children: Experiments in conversation and cognition.* Hove: Lawrence Erlbaum Associates. Pp. 154. ISBN 0–86377–158–0. Hardback £19.95; paperback £8.95.

Stoll, B.A. (Ed.). (1991). *Approaches to breast cancer prevention.* Dordrecht: Kluwer Academic Publishers. Pp 244. ISBN 0–7923–0995–2. £115.00.

Strack, F., Argyle, M., & Schwarz, N. (Eds.). (1991). *Subjective wellbeing: An interdisciplinary perspective.* Oxford: Pergamon Press. Pp. 291. ISBN 0–08–037264–3. £24.95.

Tufte, E.R. (1990). *Envisioning information.* Cheshire, CT: Graphics Press. Pp 126. ISBN 0–961–3921–1–8. $48.00.

Wade, N.J. & Swanston, M. (1991). *An introduction to visual perception.* London: Routledge. Pp. 212. ISBN 0–415–01043–8. £9.99.

Yamada, J.E. (1990). *Laura: A case for the modularity of language.* Cambridge, MA: MIT Press. Pp. 169. ISBN 0–262–24030–0. £24.75.

Subject Index